Equine Clinical Pathology

Equine Clinical Pathology

Edited by

Raquel M. Walton

VMD, PhD, Diplomate ACVP (Clinical Pathology)
Senior Clinical Pathologist
Idexx Laboratories, Inc.
Animal Medical Center
New York, New York, USA

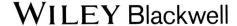

This edition first published 2014 © 2014 by John Wiley & Sons, Inc.

Editorial offices: 1606 Golden Aspen Drive, Suites 103 and 104, Ames,
Iowa 50010, USA
The Atrium, Southern Gate, Chichester, West Sussex, PO19 8SQ, UK
9600 Garsington Road, Oxford, OX4 2DQ, UK

For details of our global editorial offices, for customer services and for information about how to apply for permission to reuse the copyright material in this book please see our website at www.wiley.com/wiley-blackwell.

Library of Congress Cataloging-in-Publication Data

Equine clinical pathology / edited by Raquel M. Walton.
  p. ; cm.
  Includes bibliographical references and index.
  ISBN 978-0-8138-1719-4 (hardback : alk. paper) – ISBN 978-1-118-49197-3 – ISBN 978-1-118-49198-0 – ISBN 978-1-118-49199-7 – ISBN 978-1-118-71870-4
  I. Walton, Raquel M.
  [DNLM: 1. Horse Diseases–pathology.   2. Pathology, Clinical–methods. SF 951]
  SF951
  636.1′089607–dc23

                                                            2013010436

A catalogue record for this book is available from the British Library.

Wiley also publishes its books in a variety of electronic formats. Some content that appears in print may not be available in electronic books.

Cover design by Nicole Teut

Set in 9/12.5pt Interstate Light by Aptara® Inc., New Delhi, India
Printed and bound in Malaysia by Vivar Printing Sdn Bhd

1   2014

Contents

Contributors

Jill Beech, *VMD*
Emeritus Professor of Medicine and Reproduction
Georgia E. and Philip B. Hofmann New Bolton Center
University of Pennsylvania School of Veterinary Medicine
Kennett Square, Pennsylvania, USA

Allison Billings, *VMD, Diplomate ACVP*
(Clinical Pathology)
Contract Clinical Pathologist
Idexx Laboratories, Inc.
Memphis, Tennessee, USA

Andrea A. Bohn, *DVM, PhD, Diplomate ACVP (Clinical Pathology)*
Associate Professor
Department of Microbiology, Immunology, and Pathology
Colorado State University
Fort Collins, Colorado, USA

Karen V. Jackson, *BVSc, MRCVS, Diplomate ACVP (Clinical Pathology)*
Clinical Pathologist
Idexx Laboratories, Inc.
Sydney, Australia

Dennis J. Meyer, *DVM, Diplomate ACVP (Clinical Pathology)*
ACVIM (Internal Medicine)
Executive Director
Navigator Services
Charles River Laboratories
Reno, Nevada, USA

Martina Piviani, *DVM, MSc, MRCVS, Diplomate ACVP (Clinical Pathology)*
Clinical Pathologist
CTDS, Ltd.
Leeds, United Kingdom

Andrea Siegel, *DVM*
Clinical Pathologist
Idexx Laboratories, Inc.
Animal Medical Center
New York, New York, USA

Koranda Wallace, VMD
Instructor in Clinical Pathology
University of Pennsylvania School of Veterinary Medicine
Philadelphia, Pennsylvania, USA

Raquel M. Walton, VMD, PhD, Diplomate ACVP (Clinical Pathology)
Senior Clinical Pathologist
Idexx Laboratories, Inc.
Animal Medical Center
New York, New York, USA

Preface

Veterinary clinical pathology is the study of disease in the living animal and encompasses hematology, clinical chemistry, cytopathology, endocrinology, urinalysis, coagulation, immunohematology, laboratory management, and general pathophysiology. The interpretation of clinical pathologic data often leads to a disease diagnosis, from which treatment and prognosis are derived. Thus, as a discipline, clinical pathology is integral to the practice of veterinary medicine and is essential to the training of veterinary students, technicians, clinicians, and specialists.

While there are general pathophysiologic principles that carry across most genera, species-dependent deviations exist. Disease pathogenesis is a consequence of individual physiology, and species differences produce unique disease characteristics. Significant differences between equids and other common domestic species exist, and yet a comprehensive equine clinical pathology textbook has been lacking. The authors of this book present equine disease from a clinicopathological perspective, which is systems-based rather than problem-based. We hope that *Equine Clinical Pathology* will fill an important need and serve as a valuable resource for all those engaged in the care of equids, from students to specialists.

Equine Clinical Pathology

Chapter 1

General Laboratory Medicine

Raquel M. Walton

Acronyms and abbreviations that appear in this chapter:

Hb	hemoglobin
MCH	mean cell Hb
MCHC	mean cell Hb concentration
MCV	mean cell volume
PCV	packed cell volume
POC	point of care
POCT	point-of-care testing
RBC	red blood cells
TP	total protein
TP_{Ref}	refractometer total protein
TS	total solids

General laboratory medicine

Laboratory medicine, more commonly referred to as clinical pathology (or bioanalytical pathology), is a distinct specialty that overlaps other medicine specialties such as internal medicine and oncology in the area of diagnostics. In contrast to internists, clinical pathologists practice a systems-based rather than problem-based approach when interpreting hematologic and biochemical results. However, in addition to recognizing disease-associated changes, two other phenomena contribute to test interpretation: how test results are generated and how "normal" is defined. Artifacts due to sample preparation, sample condition, or disease processes need to be identified and distinguished from true disease-associated changes. Similarly, test interpretation is always

Equine Clinical Pathology, First Edition. Edited by Raquel M. Walton.
© 2014 John Wiley & Sons, Inc. Published 2014 by John Wiley & Sons, Inc.

performed in context–the context of "health." The accuracy of the test methodology and the reference intervals generated from the methodology are essential to the ability to diagnose disease.

This chapter provides information on hematologic and biochemical test methodologies and validation, and discusses the basic knowledge needed for generating and/or using reference intervals. The remainder of the book addresses test interpretation using a systems-based approach.

Basic hematologic techniques

Packed cell volume and plasma evaluation: Disease and artifacts

Measurement of the packed cell volume (PCV) can provide more information than simply the percentage of red blood cells in whole blood. In addition to the packed erythrocytes at the bottom of a microhematocrit tube, there is the white buffy coat layer and a plasma layer. The size of the buffy coat is related to the white blood cell (and platelet) count; a thick buffy coat would indicate a high leukocyte (and/or platelet) count, whereas a scant buffy coat suggests leukopenia. The character of the plasma can also yield valuable information pertaining to a disease process, as well as contribute to spurious results. The plasma can appear hemolyzed, icteric, or lipemic (Figure 1.1).

Hemolysis in samples from horses usually indicates an in vivo phenomenon due to toxins or immune-mediated disease (see Chapter 3). However, hemolysis can also occur during blood collection if excessive force or a needle gauge that is too small is used in phlebotomy. Whether in vivo or in vitro, hemolysis produces a color change that can make refractometer readings difficult or interfere with spectrophotometric tests.

Icterus indicates hyperbilirubinemia that usually exceeds 1.5 mg/dL (see Chapter 4). However, in herbivorous animals, yellow-colored plasma is not a reliable indicator of hyperbilirubinemia due to the presence of diet-associated carotene pigments, which impart a yellow color to plasma. Icterus has not been demonstrated to interfere with refractometer readings.[4] Depending on the chemistry analyzer, icterus can cause interference with some serum chemistry tests.

Lipemia is visible to the eye as increased turbidity in plasma or serum at triglyceride concentrations >300 mg/dL. Whether physiologic (post-prandial) or pathologic (see Chapter 8), lipemia can cause spuriously high refractometer readings and will interfere with many chemistry tests.

Protein measurement by refractometer

Protein can be rapidly and accurately measured by handheld refractometers. Because refractometers measure protein via a total solids-based technique, the total dissolved solids in the sample affect light refraction. In addition to protein, total solids include electrolytes, glucose, urea, and lipids. The term "total solids" has caused much confusion in the reporting of refractometric protein results. Total protein (TP) and total solids (TS) are not synonymous. Currently the vast majority of all refractometers incorporate a conversion

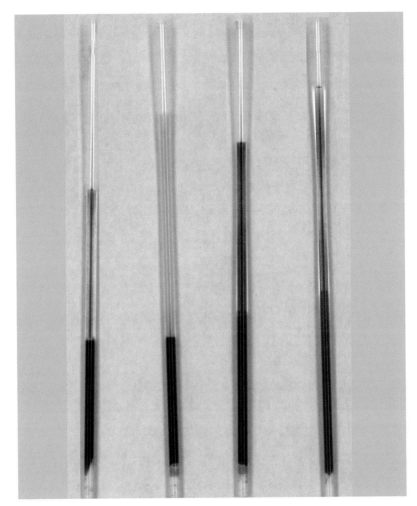

Figure 1.1 Evaluation of plasma. From left to right: normal plasma color and consistency; lipemic and slightly hemolyzed plasma; hemolyzed plasma; icteric plasma.

factor in their design so that the scales report TP and not TS. Contributing to the confusion is the fact that at least one refractometer is named the TS meter (AO Corporation) when it is in fact calibrated to report TP. While the altered refraction of plasma is mostly due to protein content, increases in lipid, glucose, or urea content interfere with refractometric protein measurements. However, marked increases in urea or glucose (273 mg/dL and 649 mg/dL, respectively) are needed to increase protein measurement by 0.4–0.5 g/dL. Increases in plasma cholesterol of 39 mg/dL are shown to increase the refractometer TP (TP_{Ref}) by 0.14 g/dL.[2]

Another potential cause of erroneous refractometer readings is the addition of EDTA from K_3EDTA anticoagulant tubes.[1] At the standard concentration of

EDTA (5 μmol/ml), K_3EDTA by itself has minimal effect on the fluid's refraction ($\leq$0.1 g/dL increase). At higher concentrations of EDTA (10 and 20 μmol/ml), EDTA can increase TP_{Ref} by 0.9–1.0 g/dL. Underfilling of EDTA tubes has the effect of increasing the EDTA concentration and will cause spurious increases in the TP_{Ref}. Some commercial tubes with K_3EDTA anticoagulant may also contain additives to prevent crystallization of the EDTA. Tubes that contain the additive may increase TP_{Ref} readings by up to 0.9 g/dL, even when properly filled. While sodium heparin anticoagulant has no effect on TP_{Ref}, heparin has deleterious effects on cellular morphology and is not recommended for samples that will be evaluated cytologically.

Point-of-care testing

Point-of-care testing (POCT) is defined as testing done at or near the patient with the expectation that results will be available quickly to facilitate immediate diagnosis and/or clinical intervention.[7] While POCT provides quick, relatively inexpensive results with small volumes of blood, it also comes with its own set of risks. Instrument calibrations and quality control measures may be omitted out of ignorance or the need for fast results. Furthermore, in veterinary medicine, analyzers may be used with species for which the instrument has not been validated. It should also be noted that diagnostic instruments for veterinary use are not subject to governmental regulations as they are for human use, which means that devices may not have been independently evaluated or tested.[8] Finally, poorly maintained instruments that are carried from one area to another may be a source of nosocomial infection or may transmit antibiotic-resistant bacterial strains.[7]

As part of the process of ensuring accuracy in an analytical method, calibrators and controls are used. A *calibrator* is a material of known or assigned characteristics that is used to correlate instrument readings with the expected results from the calibrator (or standard). A *control* is a preparation of human or animal origin intended for use in assuring the quality control of the measurement procedure, not for calibration. Controls usually represent abnormal and normal concentrations of the measured analyte. Currently, there are some POC analyzers, marketed as "maintenance-free," that do not come with controls and some that do not have calibrators. These instruments should be used with caution as there is no way to verify assay accuracy.

Hematology analyzers

Impedance technology

Many point-of-care (POC) hematology analyzers are based on impedance methodology. Examples include the HM series (Abaxis, Union City, CA), the HemaVet 950 (Drew Scientific, Oxford, CT), the HemaTrue (Heska, Loveland, CO), and the scil Vet abc (Scil, Gurnee, IL). Impedance technology employs an electric current that flows through a conductive liquid. When cells, which are nonconductive, pass through an aperture containing this fluid, there is an

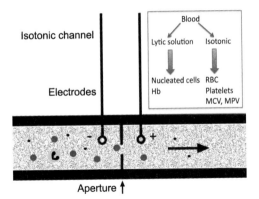

Figure 1.2   Schematic representing standard impedance methodology. Blood is directed into two chambers. In one chamber a lytic solution is used to obtain the WBC count by evaluating bare nuclei and to measure the hemoglobin released from erythrocytes. The second chamber contains isotonic solution and an aperture of limited size through which erythrocytes and platelets are enumerated.

electrical impedance created for each cell that is proportional to the size of the cell. The impedance method facilitates measurement of the mean RBC and platelet volumes, as well as enumeration of white blood cells (WBCs), RBCs, and platelets. The WBCs (and any nucleated RBCs) are counted separately from RBCs and platelets after cell lysis. Hemoglobin (Hb) concentration is also measured after RBC lysis. In the isotonic solution, nucleated cells are pre-vented from being counted along with RBCs and platelets because they are too big to pass through the aperture (see Figure 1.2).

Failure of RBCs to lyse may result in their being counted as WBCs, thereby falsely increasing the WBC count. Similarly, large platelet aggregates may be erroneously counted as WBCs, resulting in spuriously low platelet and high WBC counts. Very large platelets may be miscounted as erythrocytes.

Centrifugal hematology analyzers

Centrifugal analyzers operate by taking quantitative measurements on the cell layers below and within the buffy coat. The quantitative buffy coat (QBC) VetAutoread (Idexx Laboratories, Westbrook, ME) is an example of a centrifu-gal hematology analyzer. Granulocytes, mononuclear cells (monocytes and lymphocytes), erythrocytes, and platelets are separated into layers in an en-larged microhematocrit-like tube using a cylindrical float to further expand the buffy coat layer. Cells separate into layers upon centrifugation according to relative density and fluorescent staining differentiates layers. Centrifugal analyzers can also provide fibrinogen concentrations by rereading the sample after incubating in a precipitator.

Only the spun hematocrit is measured with centrifugal analyzers. Since erythrocyte counts are not determined, the MCV cannot be calculated. The Hb

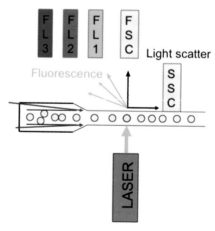

Figure 1.3 Schematic representing the principle of hematologic analysis using laser methodology. Light passing directly through the cells (forward scatter; FSC) and light deflected 90° (side scatter; SSC) is captured by detectors. FSC and SSC correspond to cell size and complexity, respectively. Complexity refers to the character of the cytoplasm (e.g., presence or absence of granules). Fluorescence detectors capture fluorescence from dyes that stain RNA, myeloperoxidase, or reticulum to differentiate leukocytes or to count reticulocytes.

can be estimated assuming a constant relationship between hematocrit and Hb. From Hb and hematocrit, MCHC can be calculated. Estimated WBC counts are obtained from the thickness of layers by assuming an average cell size.

Laser technology

Laser hematology analyzers generate both cell counts and differentials using light scatter. Single cells pass through a laser beam and scatter light at forward and side angles from the cell, which is picked up by photoreceptors (Figure 1.3). Forward, right-angle, and side light scatter represent cell size and complexity.

While this technology affords the opportunity to generate leukocyte differentials, in general there is not good precision with differential leukocyte counts.[3,8] The presence of band neutrophils, toxic change, or reactive lymphocytes can result in poor separation between leukocyte groups, adversely affecting the instrument differential (Figure 1.4). A manual differential from a blood film is still recommended to verify instrument differentials. The most common examples of POC hematology analyzers using light scatter are the ProCyte® and LaserCyte® analyzers (Idexx Laboratories).

Clinical chemistry analyzers

Dry reagent analyzers

The majority of in-clinic chemistry analyzers are based on dry reagent technology, which uses reflectance photometry. Similar to absorbance photometry, a

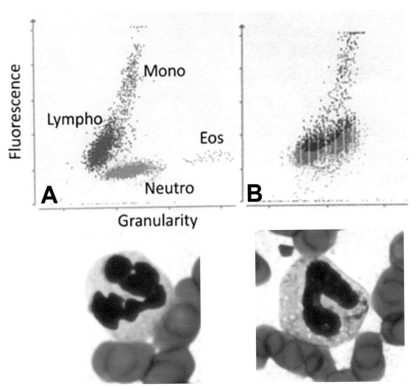

Figure 1.4   Laser-generated leukocyte differentials from the ProCyte.5® Dx point of care hematology analyzer (Idexx Laboratories, Westbrook, ME). The scatterplot is based on side scatter (granularity) and fluorescence from a fluorescent polymethine dye that stains nucleic acids. (A) Scatterplot from a healthy horse. Neutrophils have the least amount of cytoplasmic RNA and are thus located at the base of the y-axis. (B) Scatterplot from a horse with toxic change in neutrophils and a left-shift to band neutrophils. Neutrophils with toxic change and neutrophil bands both have increased RNA content relative to normal mature neutrophils. Note how the increased RNA staining causes the neutrophil plot area to move up on the y-axis, blending into the lymphocyte region.

chemical reaction (occurring within a dry fiber pad or multilayer film) results in a product that absorbs a portion of the light that illuminates it. The remaining reflected light reaches a photodetector that measures its intensity relative to the original illuminating light or a reference surface. There is an inverse relationship between reflected light (transmittance) and absorbance, where T is the percent transmittance. Analyzers will convert transmittance into

$$\text{Absorbance} = 2 - \log \%T \qquad (1.1)$$

absorbance because of the linear relationship between concentration and absorbance. Thus, concentration can be directly calculated from the absorbance.

Dry reagent technology has the advantage of minimal interference from hemolysis, lipemia, and icterus relative to wet chemistry analyzers. While most of the common chemistry analytes can be measured with dry chemistry systems, electrolytes cannot. Common in-clinic analyzers using this methodology include the Spotchem (Heska Corporation), VetTest (Idexx Laboratories), and RefloVet Plus (Scil Animal Care Company, Grayslake, IL).

Reconstituted liquid chemistry analyzers

Liquid chemistry analyzers operate via absorbance photometry. Reconstituted liquid systems use lyophilized rather than liquid reagents in cuvettes attached to rotors so that centrifugation mixes the sample with the reagent. Similar to reflectance photometry, when the sample is added to the reagents, a chemical reaction manifesting as a color change in the liquid occurs. Light of a specific wavelength is then passed through the liquid; the wavelength used is usually the wavelength at which maximum absorbance for the substance being measured occurs. The light transmitted through the fluid post-reaction is measured and converted into absorbance. Liquid chemistry systems are affected by hemolysis, lipemia, and bilirubinemia more than dry reagents systems. If not already known, determining the effect of substances such as these on the measurement of specific analytes should be part of the validation of a methodology.

Examples of this type of chemistry analyzer include VetScan (Abaxis) and Hemagen Analyst (Hemagen Diagnostics, Columbia, MD). Just as with dry reagent systems, most common chemistry analytes, with the exception of electrolytes, can be measured.

Electrochemistry

In order to measure ion concentration, electrochemistry (also known as ion selective electrode methodology) is employed in POC analyzers. Examples include the VitalPath (Heska Corporation), VetLyte and VetStat (Idexx Laboratories), and EasyLyte Plus (Hemagen Diagnostics). Ion selective electrode (ISE) technology relies on development of a membrane potential for the ion being measured. This is achieved by using an electrode with a membrane selective for the ion being measured. The membrane potential that develops when the membrane is in contact with the sample is then proportional to the activity of the ion of interest (Figure 1.5). This is compared to the reference electrode to calculate the ion concentration using the Nernst equation. Unlike flame photometry methods to measure electrolytes, ISE is not affected by lipemia or hyperproteinemia.

Test validation and reference values

Test validation

Laboratory test method validation refers to the multitiered process of evaluating the performance of a new instrument or test methodology, often in relation to an instrument or methodology that is currently in use. In its

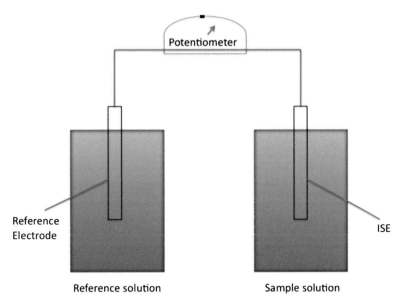

Figure 1.5 Ion selective electrode (ISE) methodology. When a sample is in contact with the membrane selective for the ion to be measured, a membrane potential proportional to the activity of the ion develops. The ion concentration is calculated using the Nernst equation by comparing the sample potential to the potential generated from a reference electrode in a reference solution.

broadest sense, method validation comprises the evaluation of test performance following a change in reagents, instruments, methodology, or–unique to veterinary clinical laboratories–introduction of a new species. The importance of test validation for different species cannot be overstated. As a result of the interspecies structural differences in any given analyte, a methodology that is adequate for one species may be inappropriate for another. Differences in expected reference values may affect whether a test has an appropriate detection limit and analytical range. Species differences exist also in how lipid, hemoglobin, or bilirubin interfere with analyte measurements.[5] Certainly, drug interferences could also be species specific. Thus, in the age of POC instrumentation, it is essential that the instrument be validated for the species in which it is used.

Before evaluating a test for a new species, it is important to know whether the analyte to be measured is clinically relevant. For example, in equids there is little need to validate an alanine aminotransferase (ALT) assay for clinical purposes. The ultimate goal of method validation is to provide objective evidence that the evaluated method will show acceptable reproducibility and accuracy so as to be clinically applicable.

The major steps in test validation consist of estimating the following:

1. Precision
2. Accuracy

3. Sensitivity
4. Specificity
5. Reference intervals

Reproducibility of results is referred to as *precision*. Precision is measured as a coefficient of variation and reflects the amount of variation inherent in the method and is estimated by repeating measurements of the same sample at least 20 times (intra-assay precision). Estimating day-to-day precision (inter-assay precision) requires running aliquots of the same sample over 20 days.

Accuracy or *bias* measures the amount of closeness in agreement between the measured value of an analyte and its "true" value. Accuracy is estimated by comparing the performance of the candidate method with that of a definitive or reference method (gold standard) by performing a recovery experiment or by comparing the candidate method with the established method that is being replaced. Recovery experiments estimate the ability of an analytical method to correctly measure an analyte when a known amount of the analyte is added to authentic biological samples.

Sensitivity is related to precision and refers to a test's ability to detect both small quantities of the analyte and small differences between samples. A "sensitive" methodology has a high level of analytical sensitivity and a low detection limit. The detection limit and analytical sensitivity are related but not synonymous. The detection limit is defined by the International Union of Pure and Applied Chemistry (IUPAC) as the smallest quantity or concentration that can be detected with reasonable certainty. The detection limit depends on the magnitude of the blank measurements and is related to their imprecision.[6] Sensitivity measures the change in signal relative to a defined change in the quantity or concentration of an analyte. This is usually accomplished by measuring a series of dilutions of a known amount of analyte (Figure 1.6).

Analytic *specificity* refers to the ability of a method to detect only the analyte of interest and is related to accuracy. Specificity may be affected by factors such as hemolysis, icterus, or lipemia of serum or plasma, or by drugs and other substances that compete for reagents or affect the physical properties of the sample. Interference studies are performed by adding the interfering material directly and measuring its effects or by comparing measurements from hemolyzed, icteric, or lipemic samples using the candidate method and one that is not affected by these factors.

Reference values are typically generated at the end of the method validation process and should be included with an instrument after the manufacturer has validated the methodology. When considering a POC instrument for purchase, if the manufacturer has truly validated the instrument for horses, species-specific reference values should be available.

Reference values

The use of reference values to diagnose or screen for disease implies that health is a relative concept; clinical examination, evaluation of laboratory data, and diagnostic imaging findings all require comparison to a "normal"

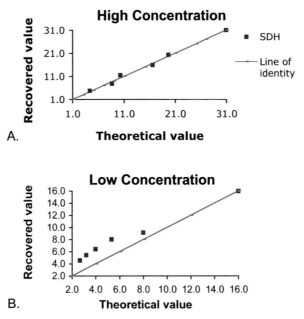

Figure 1.6 Serial dilutions of high and low concentrations of sorbitol dehydrogenase (SDH) to determine assay sensitivity. (A) There is a very good correlation between the expected and recovered values in dilutions made from high-SDH concentrations. (B) In contrast, at low concentrations of SDH, the assay is less sensitive.

standard. "Normality" itself is also relative. What would be considered usual values for a racehorse may vary significantly from values for a cold-blooded working horse. Because health and disease are defined against "normal" or reference standards, the importance of appropriate reference values cannot be overstated. A few general principles regarding the use of reference values should be common knowledge for all veterinary practitioners.

1. When laboratory-specific or instrument-specific reference values are not available, published reference intervals should be used with caution. Published reference values should provide basic information regarding how health was defined for the population, as well as the general characteristics of the population (including number of animals sampled) and the instrumentation from which the values were derived. The practitioner should attempt to match the population and instruments from which the values were generated as closely as possible to the patient to which they are being applied.

2. Reference values obtained from one type of instrument should not be used interchangeably with those for another instrument, especially when different methodologies are involved. Reference values must first be validated before being applied to a second instrument, especially with POCT.

Validation can be achieved using a small sample (n = 20) of "normal" individuals. The values obtained from these healthy individuals can be tested against the RI to be used with another instrument; if two or fewer subjects are outside of the candidate RI, it is considered transferable. If 3 or 4 values fall outside the RI, another 20 patients can be tested and interpreted in the same manner as the original 20 samples. If more than 4 of the original 20 values fall outside the candidate RI, transference is rejected for that analyte and an alternate RI must be used.

References

1. Dubin S and Hunt P. 1978. Effect of anticoagulants and glucose on refractometric estimation of protein in canine and rabbit plasma. *Lab Anim Sci* 28:541-544.
2. George JW. 2001. The usefulness and limitations of hand-held refractometers in veterinary laboratory medicine: an historical and technical review. *Vet Clin Pathol* 30:201-210.
3. Giordano A, Rossi G, Pieralisi C, et al. 2008. Evaluation of equine hemograms using the ADVIA 120 as compared with an impedance counter and manual differential count. *Vet Clin Pathol* 37:21-30.
4. Hayes GM, Mathews K, Floras A et al. 2011. Refractometric total plasma protein measurement as a cage-side indicator of hypoalbuminemia and hypoproteinemia in hospitalized dogs. *J Vet Emerg Crit Care* 21:356-362.
5. Jacobs RM, Lumsden JH and Grift E. 1992. Effects of bilirubinemia, hemolysis, and lipemia on clinical chemistry analytes in bovine, canine, equine, and feline sera. *Can Vet J* 33:605-608.
6. Koch D and Peters T. 2001. Evaluation of methods—with an introduction to statistical techniques. In *Tietz Fundamentals of Clinical Chemistry*, C Burtis and E Ashwood (eds), 5th ed., pp 234-250. Philadelphia: WB Saunders Co.
7. Plebani M. 2009. Does POCT reduce the risk of error in laboratory testing? *Clin Chim Acta* 404:59-64.
8. Weiser MG, Vap LM and Thrall MA. 2007. Perspectives and advances in in-clinic laboratory diagnostic capabilities: hematology and clinical chemistry. *Vet Clin North Am Small Anim Pract* 37:221-236.

Chapter 2
Equine Hematology

Raquel M. Walton

Complete blood count interpretation

The complete blood count (CBC) provides information beyond the concentrations of blood cells. Insight into disease processes and their severity and even diagnoses can be gleaned from a thorough evaluation of the CBC, especially in conjunction with a peripheral blood film.

Blood submitted for a CBC should be mixed well and analyzed as soon as possible after collection. In equine medicine, delays in sample analysis of up to 24 hours commonly occur as a result of restricted access to diagnostic laboratories. Characteristic changes in blood parameters associated with delayed analysis of equine blood samples using a common hematology analyzer (Advia 120; Bayer Corporation, Tarrytown, NY) include increased numbers of normocytic hypochromic red blood cells (RBCs), increased numbers of macrocytic hypochromic RBCs, and misclassification of granulocytes as mononuclear cells using the basophil reagent method. These changes are mitigated by storage at 24 °C rather than at 4 °C.[5] In general, equine blood differential leukocyte counts obtained from the Advia 120 hematology analyzer show less precision compared with classic impedance methods, and these instrument-derived counts should be verified with manual differentials.[13]

Erythrocyte indices

The erythrogram typically comprises the following elements: RBC count ($\times 10^6/\mu L$), hematocrit (Hct) or packed cell volume (PCV) (%), hemoglobin (Hb) concentration (pg/dL), mean cell volume (MCV)(fL), mean corpuscular Hb (MCH)(pg), and mean corpuscular Hb concentration (MCHC)(g/dL).

Equine Clinical Pathology, First Edition. Edited by Raquel M. Walton.
© 2014 John Wiley & Sons, Inc. Published 2014 by John Wiley & Sons, Inc.

Calculated indices are as follows:

$$\textbf{Hematocrit}\ (\%) = \frac{MCV \times RBC}{10} \qquad (2.1)$$

$$\textbf{MCH}\ (pg) = \frac{Hb \times 10}{RBC} \qquad (2.2)$$

$$\textbf{MCHC}\ (g/dL) = \frac{MCH}{MCV}\ \text{ or }\ \frac{Hb}{PCV} \qquad (2.3)$$

The indices that are measured by the hematology analyzer include **RBC count**, **Hb**, **MCV**, and **PCV**. Knowledge of which indices are calculated and which are measured helps to determine possible artifacts in the erythrogram. For example, a discrepancy between the Hct and PCV (>2% difference) points to a spurious MCV or RBC measurement. When there is agglutination, the Hct may be spuriously low as a result of the measured RBC count being lower than the true RBC count because of the presence of RBC aggregates that are not detected by the hematology analyzer. However, agglutination also may spuriously increase the MCV measurement when RBC doublets are measured as individual RBCs. If the artifactually increased MCV is in proportion to the artifactually decreased RBC count, the Hct may not be significantly different from the PCV. Lithium heparin anticoagulant may also cause spuriously high Hct values as a result of RBC swelling.[45] If cell swelling does occur, the increased MCV would similarly affect the centrifuged Hct, so there may not be a mismatch between the calculated Hct and PCV.

As a control for the accuracy of the Hct, a PCV should always be run for comparison with the Hct. In the absence of a spun Hct (i.e., PCV) the universal relationship between the mammalian Hb concentration and Hct can be used to determine the accuracy of the Hct: for mammals other than camelids, the Hb should be one third of the Hct. For example, if the Hb concentration is 11 pg/dL, the Hct should be around 33%.

Changes in indices in response to anemia

Erythropoietin is released in response to hypoxemia caused by decreased erythrocyte circulating mass secondary to loss or hemolysis. The response to erythropoietin from most mammalian species is to release marrow reticulocytes into circulation, which can primarily affect MCV, MCH, and MCHC. The classic change in RBC parameters is macrocytic and hypochromic in most species. In contrast, the typical regenerative response to anemia in horses is macrocytic and normochromic. Horses are unique among domestic mammalian species with respect to the release of reticulocytes following mild to moderate anemia. Although reticulocytes are produced within the marrow and increases in marrow reticulocytes are associated with regenerative erythroid responses, too few reticulocytes are released into circulation to be useful as an indicator of regeneration. Historically, the best indicator of a regenerative response in horses before increasing Hct is evaluation of bone marrow. However, erythrocyte indices can show characteristic changes indicative of a regenerative response, especially in severe hemorrhagic or hemolytic anemias.

A regenerative response to anemia secondary to blood loss in horses is reported to take about 4 days from the onset of RBC loss with a maximal response seen at 9 days.[27] Recovery to normal values after a hemolytic event takes about 1 to 2 months, whereas recovery from hemorrhagic anemia is about 2 to 3 months.[25,26]

Mean cell volume

Macrocytosis, characterized by the release of macrocytes that are roughly twice normal size, is part of the maximal erythrocyte regenerative response. This macrocytosis is not strictly related to reticulocytosis because regenerative macrocytosis in horses and other species does not correlate with reticulocytosis.[6] Macrocytosis is one of the first and most consistent parameters to show change following anemia in horses and is a more sensitive indicator of regeneration than Hct. However, horses with effective regenerative responses do not always have macrocytosis as defined by increases above reference values, especially with mild blood loss or hemolytic anemias. In these cases, serial evaluation of individual MCVs was more sensitive in detecting macrocytosis than comparison with a population-based reference interal.[34] Widening in the red cell distribution width (RDW) (discussed later) can also identify macrocytic subpopulations before the MCV increases above reference values.

In horses, macrocytosis that follows anemia is associated with a decrease in the number of normocytes, which suggests that macrocytes remain large and do not contribute to the normocyte population.[44] Macrocytes persist after Hct and RBC counts have returned to preanemia levels; thus, macrocytosis in the presence of other normal erythrocyte values in horses may be an indicator of a recent past regenerative response.[34,44]

In dogs and cats, microcytosis is typically associated with absolute or functional iron deficiency or portosystemic shunting. The most common cause of microcytosis in horses is physiologic and age-associated, necessitating separate reference values for MCV in horses less than 9 months of age. In horses, microcytosis associated with absolute iron deficiency has not been reported. Documented iron deficiency anemia in a foal was characterized as normocytic and normochromic.[11] Functional iron deficiency attributable to iron storage (i.e., anemia of chronic disease) may result in microcytosis and does appear to occur in horses. Reported cases of larval cyathostominosis associated with microcytosis attributed the finding to systemic inflammation and/or protein exudation associated with intestinal parasitism.[32] Nonregenerative anemia due to anemia of chronic disease may also be normocytic and normochromic, just as nonregenerative anemia due to chronic renal failure.

Red cell distribution width and the distribution histogram

Most hematology analyzers report the RDW with the erythrocyte indices. The RDW value is a coefficient of variation of the erythrocyte volume. Increases in RDW are associated with blood loss, hemolytic anemias, and erythropoietin

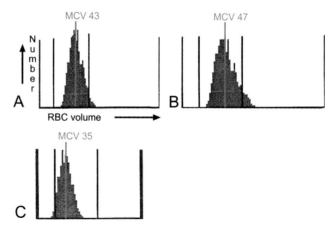

Figure 2.1   Red blood cell (RBC) histograms from the Advia 120 hematology analyzer. (A) Histogram from a hematologically normal horse. The red line shows the mean cell volume (MCV) in femtoliters; the black lines represent the instrument's preset range of equine RBC volume. (B) Histogram from a horse with macrocytic anemia. Note the widening of the histogram to include a right shoulder. The MCV is still within the reference limits established for this instrument (38 to 55 fL), but there is an emerging population of macrocytes suggesting a regenerative response. (C) Histogram from a horse with microcytic anemia. The whole population of RBCs is microcytic, resulting in a shift of the entire histogram to the left. This horse had anemia of chronic disease.

administration.[6,34] Similar to the MCV, increases in RDW secondary to macrocytosis are detectable in serial comparisons of individuals but may not exceed population-based reference intervals. Because the RDW can increase as a result of the emergence of smaller or larger erythrocyte populations, the distribution histogram itself can better identify the cause of increases in RDW. The impedance method generates a histogram depicting the distribution of erythrocyte volumes (Figure 2.1). The RBC histogram is valuable in detecting the emergence of macrocytic and microcytic erythrocyte subpopulations. These subpopulations are best identified by comparing serial histograms from a patient at weekly intervals. In horses, the histogram is especially useful because macrocytic subpopulations representing a regenerative response to anemia can be detected before the MCV rises above the reference interval.[44] As discussed previously, not all horses with regenerative responses show changes in MCV above the reference interval, but macrocytic subpopulations are detectable on the histogram.

Mean corpuscular hemoglobin and mean corpuscular hemoglobin concentration

The MCH and MCHC represent the quantity of Hb and the concentration of Hb, respectively, per average erythrocyte. Any increase in MCH and/or MCHC indicates artifact because it is not physiologically possible for these indices to increase outside of the upper reference limit. Increases in MCH and MCHC are associated with spurious Hb or RBC measurements. RBC agglutination may cause increases in MCH or MCHC secondary to a spuriously low RBC count. However, as discussed previously, decreases in RBC count as a result of ag-glutination may be countered by spuriously increased MCV measurements, resulting in minimal impact on the MCH and MCHC. Another common cause of increased MCH or MCHC or both is the presence of lipemia, which results in spurious increases in the Hb measurement. Heinz bodies also falsely in-crease MCH and MCHC when determined by laser hematology analyzers and spuriously increase the Hb measurement with spectrophotometric methods. In vitro hemolysis also increases the MCH and MCHC because the number of intact RBCs is disproportionately low for the amount of Hb measured.

Decreases in MCH or MCHC or both are typically associated with regenera-tive responses in species that release reticulocytes in large numbers. However, in horses the regenerative response is normochromic. In other species iron deficiency causes microcytic, hypochromic anemia, but iron deficiency anemia is reported to be normochromic in horses.[11,46]

Age and breed effects on RBC parameters

Relative to adults, erythrocyte number, Hb, and Hct are increased at birth, decline sharply within 12 to 24 hours, and show a gradual decline over the subsequent 2 weeks to levels at the lower end of adult reference intervals. The MCV is elevated at birth and subsequently decreases to reach a nadir at 3 to 5 months of age; values are microcytic relative to adult reference intervals until 9 months to 1 year of age.[16,18] The microcytosis is thought to be due to a relative iron deficiency from limited storage of body iron or low concentration of iron in the dam's milk.[11]

Breed effects on erythrocyte indices are reflected in higher Hct, Hb, and RBC counts in "hot-blooded" breeds (Arabians and thoroughbreds) compared with the "cold-blooded" draft horse and pony breeds. In addition, thoroughbreds have a smaller reported MCV compared with draft horses.[16] The use of breed-appropriate and age-specific reference values is very important.

Splenic effects

The equine spleen can store 50% of the RBC mass and rapidly transfer large numbers of erythrocytes into the systemic circulation after epinephrine-induced splenic contraction.[33] Epinephrine-induced splenic contraction is associated with excitement or strenuous exercise. Depending on the base-line PCV, splenic contraction may result in erythrocytosis or a normal PCV. The time taken for the PCV to return to baseline after contraction may range from 40 to 60 minutes to several hours depending on the magnitude of the stimulus. Erythrocytosis in horses may also occur secondary to dehydration and hemoconcentration. Erythrocytosis secondary to hemoconcentration pro-duces concomitant increases in both the PCV and the plasma protein concen-tration, whereas erythrocytosis from splenic contraction is not accompanied by alterations in plasma protein concentration.[24]

In contrast, splenic RBC sequestration and congestion following barbiturate or halothane anesthesia may cause the PCV to decrease below baseline val-ues.[21] The spleen's large storage capacity may have a significant impact on the circulating RBC mass. Anemia potentially could be masked after splenic contraction or simulated secondary to anesthetic-induced splenic congestion and RBC sequestration.

Reticulocytes

Until the advent of automated reticulocyte enumeration methods that evaluate more than 40 times the number of erythrocytes evaluated by manual methods, reticulocytosis was not thought to occur in equine blood. Using laser methodology (Advia 120), small numbers of circulating reticulocytes (0.5 to $85 \times 10^3/\mu L$) can be detected in healthy states.[13] However, because of these very low circulating numbers, the precision of reticulocyte counts in healthy horses is poor. Using automated methods, regenerative responses in reticulocytes can be detected in select situations, such as in hemolytic anemia and with high-dose erythropoietin administration.[6,49]

Leukogram

The leukogram includes the numeric and morphologic data pertaining to white blood cells. Similar to erythrocyte indices, the leukogram can provide information regarding the presence of a pathologic or pathophysiologic process but rarely leads to a specific diagnosis. Distinct leukogram profiles are associated with inflammation, corticosteroids, and epinephrine.

Leukogram patterns

Inflammation

Acute inflammation results in the release of mature neutrophils and bands from the marrow storage and maturation pools; thus, neutrophilia with a left shift is characteristic of an active need for neutrophils. The marrow responds to inflammatory cytokines released into the blood by replenishing the storage and maturation pools from the stem cell and proliferation pools, resulting in a chronic or compensated inflammatory leukogram characterized by a mature neutrophilia (Figure 2.2). A simplified depiction of the growth factors responsible for stimulation of neutrophil production and release is presented in Figure 2.2. The total 7- to 9-day neutrophil transit time in the healthy state decreases with inflammation.

The equine neutrophil storage pool is intermediate in size compared with the canine and bovine pools, which have the largest and smallest pools, respectively. When the storage pool is diminished during an inflammatory response, younger neutrophils (e.g. bands, metamyelocytes) are then released from the maturation pool. This left shift is considered the hallmark of acute inflammation. Horses may have little to no neutrophilia or left shift during inflammation. With severe inflammation, the storage and maturation pools may become depleted resulting in neutropenia. Neutropenia with the presence of immature neutrophils is termed a 'degenerative left shift' and suggests that the neutrophil production and release are not adequate to the demand. Persistence of a degenerative left shift is a poor prognostic sign. In contrast, a regenerative left shift is characterized by neutrophilia with the presence of

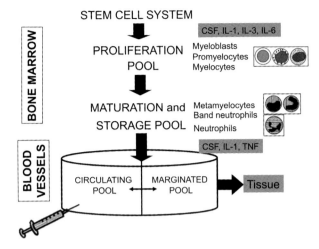

Figure 2.2 Schematic diagram of bone marrow and blood neutrophil pools. Inflammatory mediators released into the blood stimulate the marrow to produce neutrophils via an increase in growth factors and cytokines, mainly colony-stimulating factors (CSF) and interleukins (IL). G-CSF, GM-CSF, IL-1, IL-3, and IL-6 are the most prominent in neutropoiesis. Inflammatory mediators and cytokines such as tumor necrosis factors (TNF), IL-1, and CSF increase neutrophil release from marrow sinuses and migration from blood into tissue. The most mature neutrophil forms preferentially leave the marrow; these forms also preferentially migrate into tissue.

immature neutrophils and indicates the neutrophil response to the inflammatory stimulus is appropriate. Inflammatory neutrophilias in horses exceed 20,000/μL only occasionally, and it is uncommon to see neutrophilias greater than 30,000/μL.

Monocytosis may be a feature of both acute and compensated (chronic) inflammation and generally reflects a need for macrophages. Inflammatory processes that elicit histiocytic responses are associated with monocytosis.

Production of eosinophils from the bone marrow takes 2 to 6 days. The etiologies of eosinophilia in horses are similar to the etiologies in other species and include parasitism, hypersensitivity reactions, and a paraneoplastic phenomenon.[8] Multisystemic eosinophilic epitheliotropic disease, although associated with eosinophilic abdominal effusions and eosinophilic marrow hyperplasia, has not been reported to be associated with peripheral eosinophilias.[23,41]

Antigenic stimulation may produce lymphocytosis; however, lymphocytosis in horses is more commonly attributable to epinephrine-associated responses. The presence of reactive lymphocytes supports an interpretation of antigenic stimulation even in the absence of lymphocytosis.

Corticosteroid response

Endogenous and exogenous glucocorticoids produce a characteristic leukogram pattern consisting of a mature neutrophilia and lymphopenia. In contrast to dogs and cats, horses do not have monocytosis as part of the glucocorticoid response. The neutrophilia is the result of the release of marginated neutrophils into circulation. The ratio of marginated to circulating neutrophils in horses is 1:1; the maximum increase in neutrophil concentration as a result of demargination does not exceed twofold. Lymphopenia is considered the hallmark of the glucocorticoid response and is attributed to margination and emigration of lymphocytes to tissues and lymph nodes; chronic glucocorticoid effects include lymphoid hypoplasia, which contributes to the lymphopenia.

Epinephrine response

Catecholamine-associated leukocytosis occurs more often in young horses and in stallions. A physiologic or excitement leukogram, promoted by the effects of catecholamines, is characterized by lymphocytosis and a mature neutrophilia. Excitement, fear, or vigorous exercise may result in release of catecholamines, which promote an increase in circulating lymphocytes via demargination, especially from the spleen. The concomitant mature neutrophilia is also due to demargination.

Platelets

In horses, platelet number and size are shown to be directly proportional rather than inversely proportional as in some species. Normal platelet counts in horses are the lowest of the common domestic species.[3]

Thrombocytopenia

The causes of thrombocytopenia are increased platelet use, decreased production, increased destruction, and sequestration. Of these etiologies, equine thrombocytopenia is most commonly attributable to consumptive processes related to inflammation and endotoxemia.[39] Prothrombotic stimuli, especially potent platelet activators such as thrombin and platelet activating factor, are produced subsequent to endotoxemia and with severe inflammation. Systemic activation of the coagulation system associated with severe inflammation and/or endotoxemia may result in thrombocytopenia from platelet activation and consumption.[50] Thrombocytopenia may be present in horses with colic with or without disseminated intravascular coagulation (DIC).[7] Thrombocytopenia is a common sequela of snake envenomation, likely through consumption and sequestration secondary to inflammation caused by venom components.[10, 14]

A less frequent cause of equine thrombocytopenia is immune-mediated thrombocytopenia (IMT). Etiologies associated with IMT include infectious, neoplastic, and idiopathic conditions. In equine infectious anemia (EIA), infectious immune complexes consisting of EIA virus particles and antibodies deposit on platelets, targeting them for destruction. In addition, EIA-induced IMT shows a lack of compensatory megakaryocytopoiesis, which contributes to the development of thrombocytopenia.[4, 28] The mechanism of thrombocytopenia in *Anaplasma phagocytophilum* infection also may be immune-mediated.[15] IMT has also been reported in horses with lymphoma, secondary to drugs (e.g., trimethoprim, penicillin), and as an idiopathic disorder.[28, 30, 36, 39] Intermittent thrombocytopenia attributable to decreased production is unusual but has been reported in conjunction with myeloid and megakaryocytic hypoplasia in related standardbreds.[22]

Pseudothrombocytopenia occurs when platelets are not counted in a blood sample. This may occur with traumatic venipuncture resulting in platelet aggregation and clumping or ethylenediamine tetraacetic acid–associated platelet clumping.[20] If the latter is suspected, reevaluation of the blood using lithium heparin anticoagulant is recommended.

Thrombocytosis

Thrombocytosis in most species is most commonly attributable to physiologic or reactive processes. Physiologic thrombocytosis occurs secondary to epinephrine-induced splenic contraction. Reactive thrombocytosis is reported secondary to inflammation, infection, or neoplasia. In one study population, thrombocytosis was reported in 1% of horses over a 5-year period.[40] Thrombocytosis was highly associated with inflammatory or infectious disease. Thrombocytosis was also more likely to occur in younger horses and stallions.

Blood film evaluation

A blood film can be dissected into three parts: the body, the monolayer, and the feathered edge (Figure 2.3).

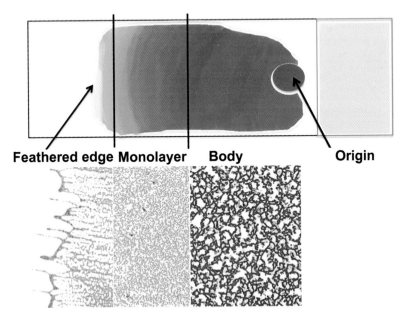

Feathered edge Monolayer   Body   Origin

Figure 2.3   Anatomy of a blood smear. The feathered edge and monolayer should be scanned first at low power (4× to 10×), and then the monolayer should be evaluated at high magnification (50× to 100×). Leukocytes and erythrocytes cannot be evaluated adequately in the smear body because of the thickness of the preparation in this area.

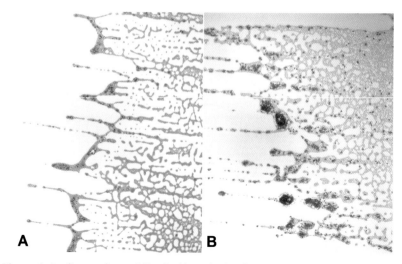

Figure 2.4 Comparison of the feathered edge from two different blood smears. (A) Normal blood smear feathered edge. (B) The presence of large platelet clumps can interfere with both the automated platelet count and the manual platelet estimation.

The general approach to a blood film can be summed up as follows:

1. Low-power scan (4× to 10×) of the feathered edge for platelet clumps, large cells, or microorganisms (Figure 2.4).
2. Low-power scan (10×) of the monolayer to estimate RBC and white blood cell density (Figure 2.5).
3. High-power (40× to 100×) scan of the monolayer to evaluate cellular morphology and perform leukocyte differential and platelet estimation.

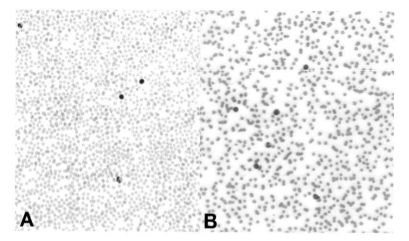

Figure 2.5 Evaluation of red blood cell density at low magnification (10×). (A) Monolayer of a normal blood smear. (B) Monolayer from an anemic blood smear. Note the difference in the concentration of erythrocytes in the monolayers.

The 40× objective was designed for use with samples with coverslips and will not focus properly unless the slide has a coverslip. A coverslip may be temporarily placed on the slide for viewing purposes or permanently fixed to the slide with mounting medium.

Erythrocyte morphology

More than the erythrocytes of any other domestic species, equine erythrocytes have a strong tendency for rouleau formation that is characterized by "coin-stacking." The prominent rouleaux are likely a result of the unique RBC glycocalyx glycoprotein composition of equids.[2] Rouleau formation must be distinguished from agglutination, which also occurs in horses and has been associated with immune-mediated hemolytic anemia, unfractionated heparin therapy, and red maple leaf toxicosis.[9,31,35,49] Agglutination on a blood film is characterized by the formation of grape-like RBC clusters, in contrast to the "coin-stacking" associated with rouleau formation (Figure 2.6). Distinction between agglutination and rouleau formation can be difficult on a blood film but is readily made using a saline dilution test. When RBCs are diluted in saline (1:10 dilution), rouleaux disperse but not agglutinated RBCs.

The umbrella term for variability in erythrocyte morphology is "poikilocytosis," from the Greek term *poikilos*, meaning varied. The types of poikilocytosis encountered in equine hematology are similar to poikilocytosis in other species. Abnormal erythrocyte morphologies reported for horses include eccentrocytes, spherocytes, and ecchinocytes.[12,19,31,35,49] Morphologic abnormalities, such as keratocytes, acanthocytes, ovalocytes, and schistocytes, are less common and have been reported in association with iron deficiency anemia in a foal.[11]

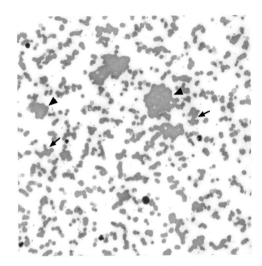

Figure 2.6   Equine blood film showing agglutination (arrowheads) and prominent rouleaux (arrows). There is some overlap in morphology between grape-like agglutination and "coin-stacking" rouleau formation.

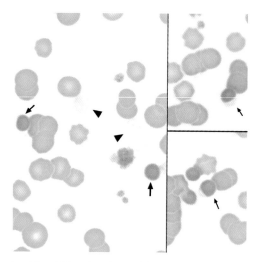

Figure 2.7 Equine blood film showing evidence of erythrocyte oxidative damage. Note the eccentrocytes (right panels; small arrows) and pyknocytes (left panel; large arrows). Ghost cells, indicating intravascular hemolysis, are also present (left panel; arrowheads).

Eccentrocytes

Eccentrocytes are dense, spherocyte-like RBCs with a semilunar cytoplasmic clear area with irregular edges (Figure 2.7). They occur as a result of oxidative injury to erythrocyte membranes causing fusion of opposing areas of the cytoplasmic face of the erythrocyte membrane. Pyknocytes, which need to be distinguished from spherocytes, develop from eccentrocytes following the loss of much of the fused membrane (see Figure 2.7).[17] Eccentrocytes likely represent a more severe form of oxidative damage than Heinz bodies.[35] Hemolytic anemia with eccentrocytosis has been associated with red maple leaf toxicity, glucose-6-phosphate dehydrogenase deficiency, and erythrocyte flavin adenine dinucleotide deficiency.[19, 35, 42]

Heinz Bodies

Heinz bodies are the result of oxidative denaturation and precipitation of the globin portion of Hb into large aggregates, which are more readily seen using a vital stain such as brilliant cresyl blue (Figure 2.8).[17] Hemolytic anemia with Heinz bodies has been reported with copper-associated hepatotoxicity, red maple leaf toxicosis, onion ingestion, phenothiazine, and EIA viral infection.[1, 29, 35] Heinz bodies should not be confused with Howell-Jolly bodies, which represent nuclear remnants remaining in the cytoplasm after mitosis. These can be seen in small numbers in healthy horses (see Figure 2.13).

Spherocytes

In species with small erythrocytes and a lack of central pallor, identification of spherocytes is difficult but not impossible. Spherocytes are dense RBCs

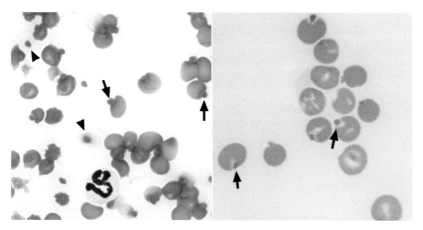

Figure 2.8   Heinz body hemolytic anemia. (Left panel) Heinz bodies are evident as dense round bodies that stain the same color as hemoglobin with Wright-Giemsa stain (arrows). Note the presence of ghost cells with Heinz bodies (arrowheads). (Right panel) A vital stain such as brilliant cresyl blue stains Heinz bodies blue (arrows).

that appear smaller than average RBCs, although volume is not decreased (Figure 2.9). Spherocytes are morphologically similar to pyknocytes, but accurately distinguishing between the two is clinically important. Spherocytosis is the result of macrophage phagocytosis of bits of RBC membrane opsonized with immunoglobulin or complement. The presence of spherocytes usually indicates immune-mediated hemolytic anemia (IMHA). In contrast, pyknocytes are derived from eccentrocytes following the loss of much of the fused

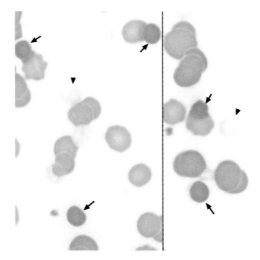

Figure 2.9   Spherocytes can be identified as dense, darkly staining erythrocytes (arrows) that appear smaller than normal erythrocytes. Note the presence of ghost cells (arrowheads).

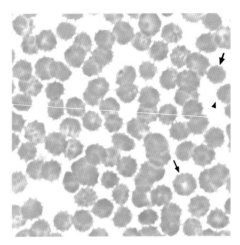

Figure 2.10 Echinocytes can range from erythrocytes with a symmetrically undulating membrane (small arrow) to erythrocytes with symmetric spiculated projections (arrowhead). A spheroechinocyte is a small, dense, darkly staining erythrocyte with sharp projections (large arrow).

membrane and represent oxidative damage to RBCs. Hemolytic anemia with spherocytosis has been reported in EIA viral infection and IMHA.[31,37]

Echinocytes

Echinocytes are characterized by multiple undulations or spicules uniformly distributed around the erythrocyte circumference (Figure 2.10). This morphology can be an artifact associated with slow drying of blood smears or represent a true morphology associated with in vitro or in vivo conditions. Echinocytosis in horses has been strongly associated with hyponatremia, as a result of either disease or diuretic administration.[12,48] Echinocytosis is a common sequela immediately following snakebite envenomation in dogs; however, this does not seem to be the case in horses, likely because of venom dilution with the horse's relatively large circulating blood volume.[43] Aged blood may also have echinocytosis as a result of in vitro adenosine triphosphate depletion and accumulation of lysolecithin in the RBC membrane. An interpretation of in vivo echinocytosis should be made only when fresh blood is evaluated and the smear has been properly prepared.

Spheroechinocytes have been reported in association with *Clostridium perfringens* IMHA.[49] It is thought that these spiculated spherocytes may represent true spherocytes that have been modified by the echinocytic effects of the *C. perfringens* type A alpha toxin.

Schistocytes

Schistocytes are erythrocyte membrane fragments resulting from shearing by mechanical or physical forces. They may be comma-shaped, triangular, or round to irregular bits of membrane (Figure 2.11). Fibrin strands from

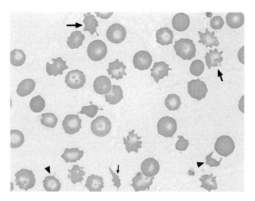

Figure 2.11 Schistocytes (small arrow), keratocytes (arrowheads), and acanthocytes (large arrows) in peripheral blood. These are uncommon in equine blood but have been reported in association with iron deficiency in a foal.

microthrombi, such as occurs with DIC or with vasculitis, can shear off RBC fragments. Schistocytes are not as consistently noted with horses in DIC as with dogs. Schistocytes can also be associated with iron deficiency, likely secondary to oxidative membrane damage or increased susceptibility to trauma in iron-deficient erythrocytes, and have been reported with iron deficiency in a foal.[11]

Keratocytes

Keratocytes are also grouped as products of membrane fragmentation injury. They are erythrocytes that contain a blister-like vesicle or vacuole at the cell periphery that ruptures to form a cell with a crescent-shaped defect and one to two horn-like projections (see Figure 2.11). Similar to schistocytes, they are associated with iron deficiency and microangiopathic disease (e.g., DIC or vasculitis). It is unusual to see keratocytes in horses, although they have been reported in association with iron deficiency in a foal.

Acanthocytes

Acanthocytes are cells with irregular, asymmetrically spaced projections, often with a paddle-like end (see Figure 2.11). The etiopathogenesis of acanthocytes is unknown in domestic animals but in humans is due to lipid membrane changes, such as occur with liver disease. Acanthocytes are associated with hemangiosarcoma in dogs and hepatic lipidosis in cats. These cells are rarely seen or reported in horses.[11]

Platelet evaluation

Of the common domestic species, horses have the lowest platelet counts.[3] An adequate platelet estimation using oil immersion magnification (100× objective) is an average of 7 to 20 platelets per field.[47] Equine platelets are smaller than dog and cat platelets, with a mean platelet volume around 5.0 fL.[3]

Giant forms, approaching the size of erythrocytes, are indicative of increased platelet consumption or destruction.

Leukocytes

Neutrophils

Neutrophils are the predominant leukocyte in blood in healthy horses. Neutrophils circulate about 5 to 10 hours before entering tissues and do not return to circulation. Mature equine neutrophils have a segmented nucleus with three to five segmentations and cytoplasm that is pale pink to nonstaining (Figure 2.12). Fine magenta granules may be evident with Wright-Giemsa staining. Band neutrophils have a nucleus with a uniform diameter that is U-shaped or S-shaped, whereas metamyelocytes have a reniform nucleus (Figure 2.13).

Toxic change

Toxic change is the result of altered bone marrow neutropoiesis and is associated with severe inflammation. Neutrophils and neutrophil precursors have increased amounts of organelles that are normally minimal to absent at later maturation stages, imparting characteristic morphologic changes. Despite these morphologic changes, the cells have normal function. Toxic change is characterized by any or all of the following (Figure 2.14): cytoplasmic basophilia, diffuse or focal (Döhle bodies); foamy cytoplasm; giant size; and less

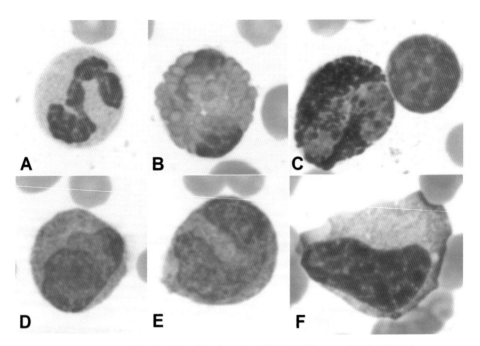

Figure 2.12 Equine blood leukocytes (Wright-Giemsa stain). (A) Mature neutrophil; (B) eosinophil; (C) basophil and small lymphocyte (on right); (D–F) monocytes.

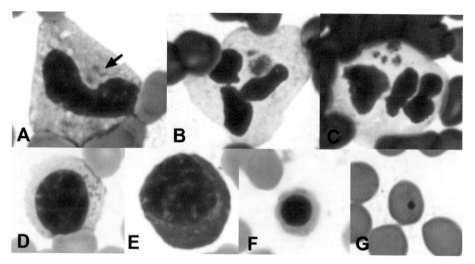

Figure 2.13   (A) Neutrophil band with linear to globular basophilic Döhle bodies (arrow); (B and C) *Anaplasma phagocytophilum* morulae in neutrophils (Diff-Quik stain); (D) granulated lymphocyte; (E) reactive lymphocyte; (F) metarubricyte; (G) Howell-Jolly body in an erythrocyte.

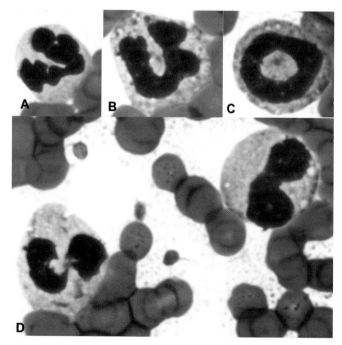

Figure 2.14   Toxic changes in neutrophils (Diff-Quik stain). (A) Normal neutrophil; (B) neutrophil with toxic changes characterized by large size, presence of Döhle bodies, increased cytoplasmic basophilia, and less condensed chromatin; (C) "donut" neutrophil, also considered a toxic morphology; (D) toxic neutrophils with linear Döhle bodies (left) and generalized cytoplasmic basophilia with vacuolization (right).

mature nuclei (more open chromatin pattern with segmented nuclei). Döhle bodies should not be mistaken for *A. phagocytophilum*, which are dark purple to black granular inclusions rather than blue (see Figure 2.13).

Lymphocytes

Lymphocytes are the second most plentiful blood leukocyte in the healthy state. The ratio of circulating neutrophils to lymphocytes is about 1.5:1. Most circulating lymphocytes are T cells (about 60%). B cells constitute about 35% of lymphocytes, and natural killer (NK) cells account for the remaining 5%.[38]

Lymphocytes in blood are morphologically mature. Mature lymphocytes are the smallest of the blood leukocytes (7 to 9 μm diameter) and have a round nucleus, condensed chromatin, and scant basophilic rim of cytoplasm (see Figure 2.12). In comparison, nucleated RBCs (metarubricytes) have a nucleus with much more condensed chromatin and either gray or hemoglobinized cytoplasm (see Figure 2.13). The presence of circulating large lymphocytes (12 to 14 μm diameter) with less condensed, granular chromatin is abnormal and suggests a lymphoproliferative process (Figure 2.15).

Reactive lymphocytes are slightly larger than mature lymphocytes with a mature, condensed chromatin and an increased amount of cytoplasm that is deeply basophilic. Granulated lymphocytes typically contain fine, magenta cytoplasmic granules (see Figure 2.13). Reactive lymphocytes and granulated lymphocytes are associated with antigenic stimulation. Granulated lymphocytes represent either T cell or NK cell phenotypes.

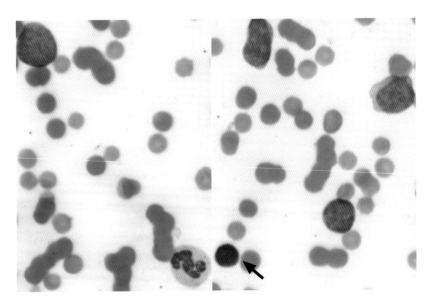

Figure 2.15 Peripheral blood film from a horse with large cell lymphoma (Wright-Giemsa stain). Most lymphocytes are intermediate to large (10 to 16 μm diameter) with immature, granular chromatin. A normal small, mature lymphocyte is indicated by the arrow (right panel).

Monocytes

Monocytes are the third most common peripheral leukocyte, are the largest in size, and usually account for less than 10% of blood leukocytes. Monocytes have a reniform to lobated nucleus with abundant gray-blue cytoplasm that may or may not contain a few punctate vacuoles. Monocytes have varied morphologies and can resemble toxic neutrophils or large lymphocytes (see Figure 2.12).

Eosinophils

In contrast to neutrophils, the half-life of circulating eosinophils is days rather than hours. Eosinophils have a segmented nucleus and prominent round pink-orange secondary granules filling the cytoplasm (see Figure 2.12). Equine eosinophil granules are the largest of the common domestic species.

Basophils

Basophils are uncommon in the peripheral blood of horses (Figure 2.12). The segmented nucleus, when visible under the dark blue-to-purple cytoplasmic granules, distinguishes the basophil from the mast cell, which has similar granules but an oval-to-round nucleus.

References

1. Ankringa N, Wijnberg ID, Boerma S, et al. 2012. Copper-associated hepatic cirrhosis in a Friesian horse. *Tijdschr Diergeneeskd* 137:310-314.
2. Baumler H, Neu B, Mitlohner R, et al. 2001. Electrophoretic and aggregation behavior of bovine, horse and human red blood cells in plasma and in polymer solutions. *Biorheology* 38:39-51.
3. Boudreaux MK, Ebbe S. 1998. Comparison of platelet number, mean platelet volume and platelet mass in five mammalian species. *Comp Haematol Int* 8:16-20.
4. Clabough DL, Gebhard D, Flaherty MT, et al. 1991. Immune-mediated thrombocytopenia in horses infected with equine infectious anemia virus. *J Virol* 65:6242-6251.
5. Clark P, Mogg TD, Tvedten HW, et al. 2002. Artifactual changes in equine blood following storage, detected using the Advia 120 hematology analyzer. *Vet Clin Pathol* 31:90-94.
6. Cooper C, Sears W, Bienzle D. 2005. Reticulocyte changes after experimental anemia and erythropoietin treatment of horses. *J Appl Physiol* 99:915-921.
7. Dolente BA, Wilkins PA, Boston RC. 2002. Clinicopathologic evidence of disseminated intravascular coagulation in horses with acute colitis. *J Am Vet Med Assoc* 220:1034-1038.
8. Duckett WM, Matthews HK. 1997. Hypereosinophilia in a horse with intestinal lymphosarcoma. *Can Vet J* 38:719-720.
9. Feige K, Schwarzwald CC, Bombeli T. 2003. Comparison of unfractioned and low molecular weight heparin for prophylaxis of coagulopathies in 52 horses with colic: a randomised double-blind clinical trial. *Equine Vet J* 35:506-513.
10. Fielding CL, Pusterla N, Magdesian KG, et al. 2011. Rattlesnake envenomation in horses: 58 cases (1992-2009). *J Am Vet Med Assoc* 238:631-635.

11. Fleming KA, Barton MH, Latimer KS. 2006. Iron deficiency anemia in a neonatal foal. *J Vet Intern Med* 20:1495-1498.
12. Geor RJ, Lund EM, Weiss DJ. 1993. Echinocytosis in horses: 54 cases (1990). *J Am Vet Med Assoc* 202:976-980.
13. Giordano A, Rossi G, Pieralisi C, et al. 2008. Evaluation of equine hemograms using the ADVIA 120 as compared with an impedance counter and manual differential count. *Vet Clin Pathol* 37:21-30.
14. Goddard A, Schoeman JP, Leisewitz AL, et al. 2011. Clinicopathologic abnormalities associated with snake envenomation in domestic animals. *Vet Clin Pathol* 40:282-292.
15. Granick JL, Reneer DV, Carlyon JA, et al. 2008. Anaplasma phagocytophilum infects cells of the megakaryocytic lineage through sialylated ligands but fails to alter platelet production. *J Med Microbiol* 57:416-423.
16. Grondin TM, Dewitt SF. 2010. Normal hematology of the horse and donkey. In *Schalm's Veterinary Hematology*, Weiss DJ and Wardrop KJ (eds), 6th ed. pp. 821-828. Ames: Wiley-Blackwell.
17. Harvey JW. 2006. Pathogenesis, laboratory diagnosis, and clinical implications of erythrocyte enzyme deficiencies in dogs, cats, and horses. *Vet Clin Pathol* 35:144-156.
18. Harvey JW, Asquith RL, McNulty PK, et al. 1984. Haematology of foals up to one year old. *Equine Vet J* 16:347-353.
19. Harvey JW, Stockham SL, Scott MA, et al. 2003. Methemoglobinemia and eccentrocytosis in equine erythrocyte flavin adenine dinucleotide deficiency. *Vet Pathol* 40:632-642.
20. Hinchcliff KW, Kociba GJ, Mitten LA. 1993. Diagnosis of EDTA-dependent pseudothrombocytopenia in a horse. *J Am Vet Med Assoc* 203:1715-1716.
21. Jain NC. 1986. The horse: normal hematology with comments on response to disease. In *Schalm's Veterinary Hematology*, Jain NC (ed), 4th ed. pp. 140-177. Philadelphia: Lea & Febiger.
22. Kohn CW, Swardson C, Provost P, et al. 1995. Myeloid and megakaryocytic hypoplasia in related standardbreds. *J Vet Intern Med* 9:315-323.
23. La Perle KM, Piercy RJ, Long JF, et al. 1998. Multisystemic, eosinophilic, epitheliotropic disease with intestinal lymphosarcoma in a horse. *Vet Pathol* 35:144-146.
24. Lording PM. 2008. Erythrocytes. *Vet Clin North Am Equine Pract* 24:225-237.
25. Lumsden JH, Valli VE, McSherry BJ, et al. 1975. The kinetics of hematopoiesis in the light horse. III. The hematological response to hemolytic anemia. *Can J Comp Med* 39:332-339.
26. Lumsden JH, Valli VE, McSherry BJ, et al. 1975. The kinetics of hematopoiesis in the light horse. II. The hematological response to hemorrhagic anemia. *Can J Comp Med* 39:324-331.
27. Malikides N, Kessell A, Hodgson JL, et al. 1999. Bone marrow response to large volume blood collection in the horse. *Res Vet Sci* 67:285-293.
28. McGovern KF, Lascola KM, Davis E, et al. 2011. T-cell lymphoma with immune-mediated anemia and thrombocytopenia in a horse. *J Vet Intern Med* 25:1181-1185.
29. McGuire TC, Henson JB, Keown GH. 1970. Equine infectious anaemia: the role of Heinz bodies in the pathogenesis of anaemia. *Res Vet Sci* 11:354-357.
30. McGurrin MK, Arroyo LG, Bienzle D. 2004. Flow cytometric detection of platelet-bound antibody in three horses with immune-mediated thrombocytopenia. *J Am Vet Med Assoc* 224:83-87.

31. Messer NT, Arnold K. 1991. Immune-mediated hemolytic anemia in a horse. *J Am Vet Med Assoc* 198:1415-1416.

32. Peregrine AS, McEwen B, Bienzle D, et al. 2006. Larval cyathostominosis in horses in Ontario: an emerging disease? *Can Vet J* 47:80-82.

33. Persson S. 1967. On blood volume and working capacity in horses. Studies of methodology and physiological and pathological variations. *Acta Vet Scand Suppl* 19:19-189.

34. Radin MJ, Eubank MC, Weiser MG. 1986. Electronic measurement of erythrocyte volume and volume heterogeneity in horses during erythrocyte regeneration associated with experimental anemias. *Vet Pathol* 23:656-660.

35. Reagan WJ, Carter C, Turek J. 1994. Eccentrocytosis in equine red maple leaf toxicosis. *Vet Clin Pathol* 23:123-127.

36. Reef VB, Dyson SS, Beech J. 1984. Lymphosarcoma and associated immune-mediated hemolytic anemia and thrombocytopenia in horses. *J Am Vet Med Assoc* 184:313-317.

37. Riegel CM, Stockham SL. 2010. Anemia associated with bacteria and viral infections. In *Schalm's Veterinary Hematology*, Weiss DJ and Wardrop KJ (eds), 6th ed. pp. 211-215. Ames: Wiley-Blackwell.

38. Satue K, Hernandez A, Lorente C, et al. 2009. Immunophenotypical characterization in Andalusian horse: variations with age and gender. *Vet Immunol Immunopathol* 133:219-227.

39. Sellon DC, Levine J, Millikin E, et al. 1996. Thrombocytopenia in horses: 35 cases (1989-1994). *J Vet Intern Med* 10:127-132.

40. Sellon DC, Levine JF, Palmer K, et al. 1997. Thrombocytosis in 24 horses (1989-1994). *J Vet Intern Med* 11:24-29.

41. Southwood LL, Kawcak CE, Trotter GW, et al. 2000. Idiopathic focal eosinophilic enteritis associated with small intestinal obstruction in 6 horses. *Vet Surg* 29:415-419.

42. Stockham SL, Harvey JW, Kinden DA. 1994. Equine glucose-6-phosphate dehydrogenase deficiency. *Vet Pathol* 31:518-527.

43. Walton RM, Brown DE, Hamar DW, et al. 1997. Mechanisms of echinocytosis induced by Crotalus atrox venom. *Vet Pathol* 34:442-449.

44. Weiser G, Kohn C, Vachon A. 1983. Erythrocyte volume distribution analysis and hematologic changes in two horses with immune-mediated hemolytic anemia. *Vet Pathol* 20:424-433.

45. Weiser MG, Vap LM, Thrall MA. 2007. Perspectives and advances in in-clinic laboratory diagnostic capabilities: hematology and clinical chemistry. *Vet Clin North Am Small Anim Pract* 37:221-236.

46. Weiss DJ. 2010. Iron and copper deficiencies and disorders of iron metabolism. In *Schalm's Veterinary Hematology*, Weiss DJ and Wardrop KJ (eds), 6th ed. pp. 167-171. Ames: Wiley-Blackwell.

47. Weiss DJ. 1984. Uniform evaluation and semiquantitative reporting of hematologic data in veterinary laboratories. *Vet Clin Pathol* 13:27-31.

48. Weiss DJ, Geor R, Smith CM, et al. 1992. Furosemide-induced electrolyte depletion associated with echinocytosis in horses. *Am J Vet Res* 53:1769-1772.

49. Weiss DJ, Moritz A. 2003. Equine immune-mediated hemolytic anemia associated with Clostridium perfringens infection. *Vet Clin Pathol* 32:22-26.

50. Weyrich AS, Lindemann S, Zimmerman GA. 2003. The evolving role of platelets in inflammation. *J Thromb Haemost* 1:1897-1905.

Chapter 3

Immunohematology and Hemostasis

Karen V. Jackson

Acronyms and abbreviations that appear in this chapter:

ACD	acid citrate dextrose
ACT	activated clotting time
ADP	adenosine diphosphate
aPC	activated protein C
aPTT	activated partial thromboplastin time
ATIII	antithrombin III
ATP	adenosine triphosphate
BMBT	buccal mucosal bleeding time
CBC	complete blood count
DIC	disseminated intravascular coagulation
DS	2% dextrose in 0.9% saline
EDTA	ethylenediamine tetra-acetic acid
EIA/EIAV	equine infectious anemia/equine infectious anemia virus
EPCR	endothelial cell protein C receptor
FDPs	fibrin(ogen) degradation products
FII	factor II or prothrombin
FIIa	activated factor II or thrombin
FIX/FIXa	factor IX/activated factor IX
FV/FVa	factor V/activated factor V
FVIII/FVIIIa	factor VIII/activated factor VIII
FX/FXa	factor X/activated factor X

Equine Clinical Pathology, First Edition. Edited by Raquel M. Walton.
© 2014 John Wiley & Sons, Inc. Published 2014 by John Wiley & Sons, Inc.

FXI/FXIa	factor XI/activated factor XI
FXII/FXIIa	factor XII/activated factor XII
GPIb	glycoprotein Ib
GPIIb-IIIa	glycoprotein IIb-IIIa
HMWK	high-molecular-weight kininogen
IgA	immunoglobulin class A
IgG	immunoglobulin class G
IgM	immunoglobulin class M
IMHA	immune-mediated hemolytic anemia
JFA	jaundiced foal agglutination
MAC	membrane-attack complex
NI	neonatal isoerythrolysis
NO	nitric oxide
PAF	platelet activating factor
PAI-1	plasminogen activator inhibitor-1
PBS	phosphate buffered saline
PDGF	platelet-derived growth factor
PF4	platelet factor 4
PGI_2	prostacyclin
PK	prekallikrein
PL	phospholipid
pRBC	packed red blood cells
PT	prothrombin time
RBC	red blood cell
TAFI/TAFIa	thrombin-activatable fibrinolysis inhibitor/activated thrombin-activatable fibrinolysis inhibitor
TAT	thrombin-antithrombin complex
TBT	template bleeding time
TF	tissue factor
TFPI	tissue factor pathway inhibitor
tPA	tissue plasminogen activator
UA	urinalysis
vWF	von Willebrand Factor

Immunohematology testing

Blood types are surface red blood cell (RBC) antigens that are genetically coded and therefore inherited. Bench-top blood typing uses specialized anti-sera to identify these RBC antigens. In the horse, the clinical significance of blood typing historically lay in parentage testing. However, now parentage testing via blood type is genetic in basis and bench-top blood typing is more often used in the transfusion setting for blood donor and recipient typing and in the investigation of neonatal isoerythrolysis (NI) cases.

Antibody screening and the jaundiced foal agglutination test are most often used combined with blood typing for investigation or prediction of NI. Antibody screening alone can also be used in the transfusion setting for blood donor screening and to identify patients who have developed anti-erythrocyte antibodies through transfusion or pregnancy.

Crossmatching is used to detect potential transfusion incompatibilities between donor sera and RBCs and recipient sera and RBCs to ensure optimal RBC survival post-transfusion. It is often used directly prior to transfusion for selection of a compatible donor for packed RBC (pRBC) and plasma transfusions.

Blood typing

Blood types and clinical relevance

Horses have eight RBC groups or systems: A, C, D, K, P, Q, U, and T. The first seven are recognized by the International Society of Animal Blood Grouping Research, and the remaining T blood group is mainly of research interest.[64] Recently, new nomenclature has been proposed for standardization, with the two letters "EA" for erythrocyte antigen preceding the traditional groups above. Within these groups there are more than 30 factors, which are designated by a lowercase letter that follows the uppercase group/system. A summary of the horse blood groups and factors is presented in Table 3.1. As the equine

Table 3.1 Internationally recognized horse blood groups, factors, and alleles

Blood groups	Factors	Alleles[a]
EAA	a b c d e f g	A^a, A^{adf}, A^{adg}, A^{abdf}, A^{abdg}, A^b, A^{bc}, A^{bce}, A^c, A^{ce}, A^e, A^-
EAC	a	C^a, C^-
EAD	a b c d e f g h i j k l m n o p q r	D^{adl}, D^{adlnr}, D^{adlr}, D^{bcmq}, D^{cefgmq}, $D^{cegimnq}$, D^{cfgkm}, D^{cfmqr}, D^{cgm}, D^{cgmp}, D^{cgmq}, D^{cgmqr}, D^{cgmr}, D^{deklr}, D^{deloq}, D^{delq}, D^{dflkr}, D^{dghmp}, D^{dghmq}, D^{dghmqr}, D^{dkl}, D^{dlnq}, D^{dlnqr}, D^{dlqr}, D^q, D^-
EAK	a	K^a, K^-
EAP	a b c d	P^a, P^{ac}, P^{acd}, P^{ad}, P^b, P^{bd}, P^d, P^-
EAQ	a b c	Q^{abc}, Q^{ac}, Q^a, Q^b, Q^c, Q^-
EAU	a	U^a, U^-

[a]The absence of a factor is denoted as a dash (−).

blood group systems are complex with many factors, identification of a blood donor with an identical blood group profile is difficult, if not impossible. For this reason, while blood typing and/or antibody screening is recommended to select blood donors with a high likelihood of being compatible to other horses, crossmatching is always recommended prior to transfusion.

Although there are many blood groups and factors in horses, and these can be overwhelming when viewed together, the majority of clinically significant transfusion reactions and/or NI cases relate to factor incompatibilities associated with blood groups *EAA* and *EAQ*. Incompatibilities occur when RBC antigens on the surface of one horse's RBCs encounter plasma antibodies from another horse against these same antigens. In practice, blood donors are blood typed to best predict compatible patient-donor pairings for crossmatching and mares are blood typed to determine whether they are at risk for having a foal with NI; mares that lack A^a and/or Q^a have increased chances of having a foal with NI.

Methodology

Blood typing in horses is a time-intensive process requiring 2.5–3 hours to complete. It is also specialized and only performed by select laboratories because the reagents are not commercially available. A sampling of laboratories

Table 3.2   Equine blood typing laboratories

University of California, Davis
  Hematology Laboratory
  Room 1012, Veterinary Teaching Hospital
  One Garrod Drive
  University of California, Davis
  Davis, CA, 95616
  +1-530-752-1303
  www.vetmed.ucdavis.edu/vmth/large_animal/equine/featured_services
    .cfm
University of Kentucky
  Animal Genetic Typing and Research Laboratory
  108 Gluck Equine Research Center
  University of Kentucky
  Lexington, KT, 40546
  +1-859-218-1212
  http://www.ca.uky.edu/gluck/AGTRL.asp
Rood and Riddle Veterinary Laboratory
  2150 Georgetown Rd,
  Lexington, KY, 40511
  +1-859-233-0331
  http://www.roodandriddle.com/laboratory.html
Hagyard Equine Medical Institute
  4520 Iron Works Pike
  Lexington, KY, 40511
  +1-859-259-3685
  http://www.hagyard.com/Hagyard-Laboratory.html

that perform equine blood typing is provided in Table 3.2. Either an ethylene-diamine tetra-acetic acid (EDTA) (purple-top tube) or acid citrate dextrose (ACD) (yellow-top tube) whole blood sample is recommended for submission to the laboratory. Briefly, the procedure involves incubating aliquots of 2% washed RBC saline suspension with aliquots of each specific antiserum at 37°C. A positive reaction, visualized as either hemolysis or agglutination depending on the known reaction of each antiserum, indicates the presence of a blood factor. A negative reaction, visualized as a lack of hemolysis or agglutination, indicates the absence of a blood factor. This has to be performed for each blood factor individually. The hemolytic reactions require addition of complement before incubation. The complement is derived from rabbit serum that has been adsorbed at 4°C with equine RBCs to remove nonspecific hemolysins.

A rapid agglutination method for equine blood typing has been developed for equine RBC blood antigens A^a and C^a, which requires only 15–30 minutes and is performed at room temperature.[43] This may be practical for pre-transfusion testing but particularly because this method does not assess for blood group *EAQ*, it cannot replace crossmatching or complete blood typing and antibody screening for donor-patient compatibility testing pre-transfusion.

Crossmatching

Clinical relevance

Crossmatching is used to detect incompatible antibodies in plasma/serum of the donor and patient that will react with RBC blood types of the patient and donor, respectively. Even in patients that have been blood typed, crossmatching should be performed prior to transfusion to minimize the likelihood of a transfusion reaction secondary to antibody incompatibilities. Crossmatching does not specify to which RBC blood types the incompatibility occurs, and does not predict all transfusion reactions such as those caused by anti-platelet or anti-leukocyte antibodies, pRBC bacterial contamination, urticarial reactions, or hypocalcemia secondary to excessive citrate administration.

All horses can develop antibodies to RBC antigens they do not have themselves if they are sensitized via blood transfusion or pregnancy. These antibodies are called **acquired** alloantibodies. They develop if a horse is exposed to RBC antigens it does not recognize as self. Approximately 10% of Thoroughbred horses and 20% of Standardbred horses have naturally occurring RBC alloantibodies that target RBC antigens that they do not have themselves.[2] Whether these acquired or naturally occurring alloantibodies cause transfusion reactions or NI depends on their action and their strength. Antibodies can be either agglutinins or hemolysins, or both. Anti-A^a and anti-C^a alloantibodies are both agglutinins and hemolysins whereas anti-Q^a alloantibodies are solely hemolysins. This is important to understand mainly for interpreting blood typing and crossmatching results.

The majority of alloantibodies present in horses are either anti-A^a or anti-C^a with fewer anti-Q^a alloantibodies.[2] Anti-A^a and anti-Q^a alloantibodies are likely to cause clinically significant transfusion reactions and/or NI whereas anti-C^a alloantibodies cause blood typing and crossmatch reactions that may not cause a significant transfusion reaction and have not been reported to cause NI. Other alloantibodies that have been reported to rarely cause NI include anti-A[b], Q[b], Q[c], Q[rs], D[a], D[b], D[c], D[g], K[a], P[a], and U[a].[7,11,28,74] Based on this information, blood typing for A[a], C[a], and Q[a] blood types and antibody screening for anti-A, anti-C, and anti-Q antibodies should be the minimum performed on blood donors and when managing NI cases or at-risk pregnancies. Crossmatching should be used prior to transfusion.

Methodology

As horses have naturally occurring and acquired alloantibodies that are both hemolysins and agglutinins, crossmatching should be performed with both a saline-agglutinating technique and a technique that can detect hemolysis. The hemolysis technique requires the addition of complement usually from rabbit serum that has been adsorbed at 4°C with equine RBCs to remove nonspecific hemolysins. Although the saline-agglutinating technique is often performed by many veterinary practices and is a good screening test prior to transfusion, a hemolytic technique should also be performed as clinically significant transfusion reactions often occur secondary to the presence of hemolytic anti-Q antibodies that will not be detected with an agglutinating crossmatch alone.

Patient and donor(s) anticoagulated blood (either EDTA or ACD samples) and serum are required for crossmatching. It has recently been shown that the patient and donor blood samples need to be fresh rather than stored for accurate crossmatching and the best chance of finding a compatible donor.[20] If blood typing cannot be performed prior to donor selection, consider untransfused geldings of the same breed as the recipient as the best donor options. As blood types are hereditary, being of the same breed helps minimize blood type incompatibilities, while the choice of an untransfused gelding avoids the possibility of alloantibodies acquired through transfusion or pregnancy. Donkeys should not be used as donors for horses because they have a donkey-specific RBC antigen that will cause sensitization.[33]

The crossmatch procedures are outlined in Table 3.3. Briefly, in the agglutination crossmatch, aliquots of saline washed RBCs and serum from both the recipient and donor are mixed for the major and minor crossmatches and incubated at 37°C for 15 minutes. For the hemolysin crossmatch, an aliquot of rabbit complement is also added and the incubation is at 37°C for 90 minutes. Autocontrols are also performed for both the agglutination and hemolysin crossmatches. The tubes are then centrifuged and assessed for agglutination (macroscopically and microscopically) and hemolysis. The agglutination can be graded (0-4 + for macroscopic [see Table 3.4] and positive or negative for microscopic), whereas hemolysis is either positive or negative.[31, 43]

Antibody screening and jaundiced foal agglutination test

Antibody screening and the jaundiced foal agglutination (JFA) test are modified crossmatch procedures. Antibody screening uses patient serum added to washed RBCs of known blood types to determine if the patient serum causes

Table 3.3   Crossmatching procedure

1. Obtain anticoagulated blood (EDTA or ACD, i.e., purple-top or yellow-top) and serum (coagulated blood, i.e. red-top) from the recipient and donor(s)
2. Centrifuge and separate the samples into multiple tubes[a]:
   a. Patient RBCs
   b. Patient serum
   c. Donor(s) RBCs
   d. Donor(s) serum
3. Wash patient and donor(s) RBCs separately by adding saline, phosphate-buffered saline (PBS), or 2% dextrose in 0.9% saline solution (DS) to a small amount of pRBCs from each. Mix, then centrifuge and pour off supernatant. Repeat at least three times.
4. After the last wash, resuspend the pRBCs in saline, PBS, or DS to a 2-4% RBC suspension. This can be subjectively judged on color (i.e., "Kool-Aid" or "weak tomato juice" in color) or calculated (i.e., 0.05 ml pRBCs in 2.4 mL saline gives a 2% suspension).
5. Have a source of complement that has been adsorbed at 4°C on equine RBCs to remove nonspecific hemolysins.
6. Make the following mixtures in appropriately labeled tubes (label abbreviations given in parentheses):

Agglutination crossmatch	Hemolysin crossmatch
a. Major agglutination (MaA) crossmatch: 2 drops patient serum, 2 drops donor 2-4% RBC	a. Major hemolysin (MaH) crossmatch: 2 drops patient serum, 2 drops donor 2-4% RBC, 2 drops complement
b. Minor agglutination (MiA) crossmatch: 2 drops donor serum, 2 drops patient 2-4% RBC	b. Minor hemolysin (MiH) crossmatch: 2 drops donor serum, 2 drops patient 2-4% RBC, 2 drops complement
c. Autocontrol 1 (CTL1A): 2 drops patient serum, 2 drops patient 2-4% RBC	c. Autocontrol 3 (CTL1H): 2 drops patient serum, 2 drops patient 2-4% RBC, 2 drops complement
d. Autocontrol 2 (CTL2A): 2 drops donor serum, 2 drops donor 2-4% RBC	d. Autocontrol 4 (CTL2H): 2 drops donor serum, 2 drops donor 2-4% RBC, 2 drops complement

7. Incubate at 37°C for **15 min**	7. Incubate at 37°C for **90 min**
8. Centrifuge for 15-20s (3400 rpm/1000 × g)	8. Centrifuge for 15-20s (3400 rpm/1000 × g)
9. Read and record results:	9. Read and record results:
a. First examine tubes for hemolysis and record if present	a. Positive or negative for hemolysis
b. Then gently rotate and shake the tube to cause RBCs to swirl off the RBC "button" at the bottom of the tube.	
c. Evaluate the suspension for the presence of aggregates/agglutinates:	
i. Macroscopically: Grade 0-4 + (see Table 3.4) depending on the strength of the agglutination	
ii. Microscopically: Place a drop of the mixture on a slide with a coverslip and examine unstained. If rouleaux is present, recentrifuge the original sample and try again with the pRBC and saline. This is either negative or positive.	

**If autocontrols are positive for either hemolysis or agglutination, that portion of the crossmatch is invalidated
[a]Tubes are 12 × 75 mm glass test tubes

Table 3.4 Macroscopic agglutination

0	No visible agglutination
Weak	Few small aggregates of RBCs
1+	Many small aggregates of RBCs
2+	Large aggregates with some smaller aggregates of RBCs
3+	Several large aggregates of RBCs
4+	Single solid aggregate of RBCs

agglutination or hemolysis of the known blood type RBCs (Table 3.4). The mixtures positive for agglutination and/or hemolysis indicate the antibodies that are present within the patient's serum. Horses without antibodies to *EAA*, *EAC*, and *EAQ* are good plasma donors, and if they are negative for these antibodies within the final four weeks of pregnancy, they are unlikely to have a foal with NI.

The JFA test is a modified agglutination crossmatch procedure mixing colostrum from the mare in various saline dilutions with RBCs from the foal. Anticoagulated blood from the foal and colostrum from the mare are required for this test. Colostrum contains the mare's antibodies that are transferred to the foal for immunity, which may include an alloantibody against the foal's RBCs. If there is a blood type mismatch between the mare and the foal, and the mare either has naturally occurring alloantibodies or has acquired alloantibodies (from a previous pregnancy or transfusion), the result is NI. This test is considered clinically significant if there is agglutination at or greater than a dilution of 1:16 in horse foals and 1:64 in mule foals.[1,60] NI is discussed further in the next section.

Immune-mediated hemolytic anemia

Immune-mediated hemolytic anemia (IMHA) is the premature destruction of RBCs due to the presence of antibodies directed against RBC antigens. This can be either a primary (autoimmune) or secondary process. In contrast to dogs and cats, equine IMHA is not considered common and when it occurs it is most often a secondary disease process associated with RBC parasites, infection, neoplasia, or drugs. Excluding NI cases, approximately 45 cases of IMHA have been reported in the horse and of these the most common causes were clostridial infection (20-29% of reported cases), penicillin administration (13% of reported cases), and lymphoma (13% of reported cases).[4,5,10,21,24,27,30,34,35,39,45,48,50-52,59,61,63,70-73] Regardless of whether the cause is primary or secondary, the mechanism of RBC destruction is the same and occurs through antibody binding to the surface of the RBCs causing either intravascular or extravascular hemolysis. Extravascular hemolysis is most common and occurs when the RBC-bound antibody binds to the Fc receptors on tissue macrophages predominantly in the spleen, but also liver and other organs, causing premature removal and breakdown of the RBCs within macrophages. Intravascular hemolysis is less common and a more severe clinical entity that requires complement binding to the antibody-bound RBC surface with subsequent activation of the complement cascade and formation of the membrane-attack complex (MAC) on the RBC surface, which results in lysis within the vascular space. Extravascular hemolysis is clinically associated with icterus, hyperbilirubinemia, and bilirubinuria due to the excessive hemoglobin breakdown. Intravascular hemolysis is clinically similar except there is also hemoglobinemia and hemoglobinuria as free hemoglobin is released into the vascular space and cleared directly by the kidneys. Most often the antibody type responsible for IMHA in the horse is immunoglobulin class G (IgG), with rare cases involving immunoglobulin class M (IgM). Currently there have been no reported cases of immunoglobulin class A (IgA) IMHA reported, but this may be due to the difficulty in identifying IgA in horses.[73]

Primary and secondary IMHA cannot be clinically or diagnostically distinguished. If secondary causes of IMHA are excluded, a primary etiology is assumed. Common clinical signs associated with IMHA are due to anemia and RBC breakdown and include fever, depression, pallor, icterus, hemoglobinuria (if intravascular), tachycardia, and weakness. IMHA is diagnosed if multiple of the following criteria are present: (1) an anemia (often regenerative); (2) autoagglutination after RBC washing (persistent autoagglutination); (3) a positive Coombs' test; (4) RBC morphologic changes reported with equine IMHA (e.g., spheroechinocytes, agglutination); and (5) elimination of other causes of regenerative anemia.[72]

Laboratory testing in cases of suspect IMHA should start with a complete blood count (CBC), biochemical panel, and urinalysis (UA). If the CBC is supportive of an immune-mediated process (i.e., anemia with concurrent hyperbilirubinemia without evidence of oxidative damage and with agglutination or spheroechinocytes), then consider Coombs' testing. Although IMHA is most often regenerative, this is difficult to determine on a single CBC in horses, as reticulocytes are only very rarely noted in the peripheral blood of horses, even in severe anemia. Regeneration is therefore confirmed either through bone marrow aspiration or rising PCV with stable plasma/total protein.

Coombs' testing (otherwise called direct antiglobulin testing) is used to confirm the presence of anti-RBC antibodies. The test involves incubation of washed patient RBCs with antiserum specific to equine IgG, IgM, and/or complement. If IgG, IgM, or complement is present on the washed RBCs, there will be agglutination of the RBCs and a positive result. This same method of incubating washed RBCs with specific antiserum can also be evaluated using flow cytometry instead of positive agglutination to detect bound antibody; however, it is currently uncertain if flow cytometry is a more sensitive or specific method than the traditional Coombs' test. Flow cytometry was shown to accurately document decreasing antibody concentrations in a foal with NI, so it may also have a use in disease monitoring.[73] Although a positive result often indicates an immune-mediated process, negative results via conventional Coombs' testing do not preclude an immune-mediated etiology. Negative Coombs' tests are relatively common even in cases in which all other causes of anemia are ruled out or another method is used to confirm IMHA such as flow cytometry or the detection of anti-penicillin antibodies.[35,54,65] Unfortunately a defined sensitivity for Coombs' testing is not known in equine IMHA given the low number of overall cases. Coombs' testing is still recommended, however, as a positive result indicates that an immune-mediated process is the most likely cause.

Other testing to consider is based on assessment for secondary causes of IMHA and would include targeted investigation of body systems for infection or neoplasia, depending on clinical signs and presentation, and serology and/or PCR testing for infectious diseases with known associations with IMHA (e.g., equine infectious anemia [EIA], leptospirosis, *Streptococcus equi*, *Clostridium* spp.).

Neonatal isoerythrolysis

Neonatal isoerythrolysis is the most common cause for icterus and hemolytic anemia in the neonatal foal. Studies have shown that RBC incompatibilities between mare and foal are common (up to 14%), and that antibody development by the mare is also common and breed specific, with 10% of Thoroughbred and 20% of Standardbred mares having detectable antibodies in serum; however, despite this, for unknown reasons the occurrence of NI is much lower.[2,3] There were only 1% and 2% of incompatibilities between mare and foal in Thoroughbreds and Standardbreds, respectively, that were associated with NI.[2] The rate of NI in mules (donkey sire with horse dam) is as high as 8–10%, as donkey's have a unique RBC antigen to which the mare becomes sensitized from prior pregnancies.[33]

Pathogenesis

Neonatal isoerythrolysis is caused by alloantibodies produced in the mare that are directed against RBC antigens that are only present on the foal's RBCs. These alloantibodies are produced during pregnancy or delivery if there is leakage of blood across the placenta (e.g., placentitis or difficult delivery) or produced secondary to a previous mismatched blood transfusion. Alloantibodies can persist for years and are often strongest in late-term pregnancy, so if antibody screening is to be performed to predict NI, it is recommended in the final four weeks of pregnancy. These alloantibodies are usually IgG and do not cross the placenta, but are transmitted to the foal in colostrum. Passive transfer of immunity occurs as immunoglobulins are transferred from the mare's colostrum to the foal's plasma via uptake of whole immunoglobulin through the gastrointestinal mucosa. Immunoglobulin uptake can occur only in the first 24 hours of life and provides the foal with immunity to environmental pathogens until its own immune system is fully functional. Unfortunately if the mare has developed antibodies to foal-specific RBC antigens during this or previous pregnancies, or a blood transfusion, then these will also be transmitted in the colostrum, resulting in hemolysis and/or hemagglutination. Anti-A[a] alloantibodies are agglutinins and hemolysins, whereas anti-Q^a alloantibodies are solely hemolysins. There are 8 known blood groups and within these groups are 35 known RBC antigens (see Table 3.1) to which alloantibodies could be developed, yet the RBC antigens and serum antibody incompatibilities that commonly cause NI are mostly related to blood groups *EAA* and *EAQ*. Anti-A^a and anti-Q^a alloantibodies are most commonly implicated in NI. Anti-A^b, Q^b, Q^c, Q^{rs}, D^a, D^b, D^c, D^g, K^a, P^a, and U^a alloantibodies are also implicated, albeit rarely.[7,11,28,74]

Clinical features

Because alloantibodies are transferred in colostrum, the foals are normal at birth, with clinical signs appearing only after alloantibody absorption. Hemolysis and associated clinical signs can develop as early as 5 hours and as late as 12 days postpartum, but more commonly are seen within 12 to 48 hours after birth.[7,28] Clinical presentation is associated with the severity of anemia and rapidity of hemolysis and varies from lethargy and icterus to weakness, tachypnea, tachycardia, hemoglobinuria, and hypovolemic shock that can result in death through multiorgan failure and disseminated intravascular coagulation (DIC). Liver failure +/- kernicterus is the major cause of death in NI patients with complications of sepsis noted as the other common cause.[7,46] The development of liver failure +/− kernicterus was found to be statistically associated with the volume of blood products administered (>4 L resulted in a 19.5 times higher likelihood of liver failure) and the maximum total bilirubin concentration (>27 mg/dL resulted in a 17 times higher likelihood of kernicterus) during hospitalization.[46]

Diagnosis

As other causes of IMHA are considered very uncommon in the neonate, any neonate (less than two weeks old) presenting with a hemolytic anemia should be considered to have NI until proven otherwise. The CBC should be considered essential as a first step in diagnosis. Anemia +/− hyperbilirubinemia/hemoglobinemia with normal total/plasma protein is considered supportive of a diagnosis of NI. Definitive tests include: crossmatching (between the mare serum and foal RBCs – submit serum from the mare and anticoagulated blood from the foal); jaundiced foal agglutination test (submit anticoagulated blood from the foal with colostrum from the mare); direct Coombs' test of the foal (submit anticoagulated blood from the foal); and antibody screening of the mare with concurrent blood typing of the mare and foal or stallion if prefoaling (submit anticoagulated blood from mare and foal with serum from the mare). The alloantibodies associated with NI are often stronger hemolysins than agglutinins, so if a crossmatch or antibody screening is performed, it should include incubation with complement to assess for hemolysins. The jaundiced foal agglutination (JFA) test can be used stallside and has been shown to correlate well with the hemolysis-based crossmatch if performed by trained personnel.[1] As this takes place stallside, it can be used before the foal ingests colostrum to predict if the foal would develop NI, as well as being used as a confirmatory test in diagnosing NI as the cause for a foal presenting hyperbilirubinemic and anemic.

Prevention

Prevention is best achieved by identifying mares that are at risk of producing NI-inducing alloantibodies and breeding them accordingly; however, if this is not possible or the mare is already pregnant, then prevention of NI involves determining if the foal is at risk and protecting the foal from exposure to alloantibody. Blood typing of the mare prior to mating can help choose appropriate stallions. If the mare is Q^a or A^a negative, it should only be bred to stallions that are also negative for these blood group factors.

Blood typing during pregnancy can be used to identify mares that are at risk and that would benefit from antibody screening during the last three to four weeks of pregnancy. While antibody screening will determine whether the mare has alloantibodies to RBC antigens she does not carry, determination of whether this will cause NI will require crossmatching and/or blood typing of the foal or stallion with the mare. Antibody screening $+/-$ blood typing of the stallion is recommended prefoaling in mares with a history of NI.

If the foal and mare have incompatible RBC antigens and alloantibodies, it is recommended that the foal be muzzled to prevent colostrum ingestion for the first 36–48 hours postpartum. The mare should be stripped to ensure milk production for when the foal is allowed to return to nursing. The foal needs to receive colostrum from another source to ensure passive transfer of immunity. If a transfusion is required in a clinical NI case, washed pRBCs from the mare are considered the transfusion of choice. Blood from the stallion should never be used for transfusion purposes because it is the sire's RBC antigens (which the foal has inherited) that are causing the mismatch.

Infection-associated (Clostridial, EIA, *R. equi*, *S. equi*)

Pathogenesis

The mechanisms of IMHA associated with clostridial, *Rhodococcus equi*, and *Streptococcus equi* infections are unknown. Proposed mechanisms in clostridial-associated IMHA include RBC membrane damage by clostridial toxins exposing new antigens to which the body develops autoantibodies, and/or membrane damage resulting in morphologic alterations such as spheroechinocytosis and mechanical lysis.[52,72]

The mechanism of anemia in equine infectious anemia (EIA) is threefold. While intravascular immune-mediated hemolysis can rarely be seen in acute disease, more commonly there is an extravascular IMHA in acute and chronic disease paired with an impaired bone marrow response. The IMHA is associated with complement binding to the surface of RBCs causing activation of the intravascular complement cascade (intravascular hemolysis) and phagocytosis by tissue macrophages (extravascular hemolysis). The complement binding in EIA is thought to be secondary to either a hemagglutinin—one of the surface proteins of EIAV—or circulating virus-antibody immune complexes attaching to the RBCs and attracting and activating complement.[58]

Clinical features

Patients with IMHA associated with clostridial, *Rhodococcus equi*, and *Streptococcus equi* infections will have features of both IMHA and the respective infectious disease. IMHA manifests clinically as anemia, icterus, normal/high plasma protein, and Coombs' positivity +/− spheroechinocytes. In horses, clostridial disease most often manifests as a clostridial myositis.[44,72] *Rhodococcus equi*-associated IMHA is rare, and patients with IMHA also present with pulmonary abscesses, neutrophilic inflammation in respiratory wash samples, and fever.[24,53] *Streptococcus equi*-associated IMHA is also rare; in these cases, IMHA is noted with concurrent retropharyngeal lymph node abscessation and positive *S. equi* culture and/or PCR. Occasionally *S. equi* cases can also develop purpura hemorrhagica, thought to be secondary to precipitation of IgA immune complexes with a protein associated with *S. equi* in the blood vessel walls.[21]

One of the major features of EIA is anemia, most often seen in the chronic disease form as an extravascular IMHA. The clinical presentation of EIA can be categorized into three forms: acute, chronic, and inapparent carrier status. The acute disease form is often not noticed clinically as there is usually only a transient, three- to five-day fever and thrombocytopenia associated with the original viremia. Whether the patient develops the chronic form or becomes an inapparent carrier relates to the host-virus immune interaction. The chronic form is seen when the patient experiences multiple febrile episodes associated with recurrent viremia. Classic symptoms of the chronic form include recurrent fevers, ventral edema and edema of the hind limbs, depression, and weight loss concurrent with marked thrombocytopenia (occasionally causing petechiation and ecchymoses) and anemia +/− hyperbilirubinemia. Because the anemia is complement mediated, the patient is Coombs' positive during the recurrent febrile episodes.

Diagnosis

For IMHA associated with clostridial, *Rhodococcus equi*, and *Streptococcus equi* infections, the presence of IMHA combined with confirmed bacterial infection (culture and sensitivity testing, PCR analysis, or toxin quantification [clostridial]) is diagnostic. Often the response to therapy for the bacterial infection is also used to support the diagnosis of infection-associated IMHA.

Diagnosis of IMHA associated with EIAV infection requires a combination of antibody positivity, appropriate clinical signs, and the hallmarks of IMHA. Because the virus is never cleared and there is a good immune response to the virus, affected animals are assured to be antibody positive if tested >45 days after exposure via the AGID test (Coggins test). If the patient is negative via AGID and thought to be an acute case (exposed <45 days ago), consider other testing methods such as ELISA or PCR. Note that these are more sensitive tests but prone to false positives, so an AGID should always be used as confirmation >45 days after original exposure.[58]

Drug-associated

Drug-associated IMHA in the horse is most commonly reported secondary to penicillin, but has also been reported with trimethoprim-sulphamethoxazole administration.[5,34,54,61,65,73] In the case of penicillin, it is known that the penicillin coats the surface of RBCs and that in a small number of patients an antibody develops either to the penicillin itself or to an antigen that represents a combination of the penicillin and RBC membrane. Ultimately, as the penicillin is bound to the RBC, the presence of an antibody, usually IgG, to either penicillin or a combination of penicillin and RBC membrane causes immune-mediated hemolysis, most often through extravascular hemolysis.[5,61] It is hypothesized that the mechanism of antibody development is the same in the case of trimethoprim-sulphamethoxazole-induced IMHA.[65]

Clinically drug-associated IMHA is indistinguishable from other causes of IMHA except for the temporal association with drug administration. The diagnosis of drug-induced IMHA involves the presence of classic IMHA components (anemia with a normal total/plasma protein, icterus, Coombs' positivity, and persistent agglutination) with a history of drug administration in the previous 5-10 days without other identifiable causes of IMHA. Often this diagnosis is supported by the cessation of hemolysis upon removal of the drug and further supported by recurrence of the hemolysis with drug readministration.[65] In cases where penicillin is suspected as the cause, a specialized Coombs' test using both untreated and penicillin-coated RBCs from the patient and from healthy horses can assess for the ability of the patient's serum to cause agglutination of these altered RBCs.

Neoplasia-associated

Neoplasia-associated IMHA is most often reported secondary to lymphoma but has also been reported associated with other neoplasms (e.g., melanoma).[29,30,35,40,48,52] Anemia is considered one of the most common presenting hematologic abnormalities in equine patients, with lymphoma with anemia present in 30-60% of reported cases.[29,40] The anemia can be due to anemia of chronic/inflammatory disease, blood loss, immune-mediated hemolysis, and myelophthisis. Depending on the study, 10-30% of anemias reported with lymphoma are due to IMHA.[29,40] The antibodies directed against RBCs are hypothesized to be produced either due to inappropriate activation or inactivation of T-cells, autoantibodies produced by the neoplastic cells themselves, and/or the presence of a common genetic rearrangement in the patient associated with both lymphoma and immune-system dysregulation allowing immune-mediated disease.[35] Clinically the presentation of IMHA associated with neoplasia is indistinguishable from other IMHAs except there may be evidence of neoplasia. As with all secondary IMHA, ruling out other causes (e.g., infection or drugs) is required.

Coagulation testing

Physiology of hemostasis

Hemostasis is the arrest of bleeding or stoppage of blood flow through a vessel required for the control of bleeding associated with daily trauma or surgery. It also refers to the intricate processes involved in maintaining blood flow in healthy vessels and the reestablishment of vessel patency once the damage that caused the original bleeding has been resolved. Hemostasis results from a delicate balance between procoagulant components (vasoconstriction, exposed tissue factor, activated platelets, coagulation proteins), anticoagulant components (normal vessel endothelium, vasodilation, anticoagulant proteins), and fibrinolytic components (fibrinolytic proteins). The importance of both cellular and protein components of hemostasis has been emphasized in the more recently proposed cell-based model of hemostasis. An understanding of the classic description of hemostasis is useful in the interpretation of coagulation testing, so both classical and cell-based hemostatic models are discussed in this chapter.

Blood vessels

Vascular endothelial cells are the primary components of the vessel wall involved in maintenance of normal blood flow through antiplatelet, anticoagulation, and fibrinolytic activities in healthy vessels. Because they are also essential in inducing and maintaining coagulation when there is vessel damage, they are considered dynamic and pivotal in hemostasis.

During homeostasis, endothelial cells produce prostacyclin (PGI_2), adenosine, and nitric oxide (NO) that inhibit platelet-platelet and platelet-endothelial binding while also ensuring vasodilation. Proteoglycans such as heparin, heparan sulfate, and dermatan sulfate are expressed on the endothelial surface to inhibit clotting factors and platelet aggregation. Endothelial cells also express thrombomodulin on the luminal surface that binds thrombin, thereby inhibiting platelet activation, coagulation cascade initiation, and coagulation cascade amplification. Thrombomodulin also activates protein C to downregulate the amplification effects of any activated factor V (FVa) and VIII (FVIIIa). Tissue pathway factor inhibitor (TFPI) is synthesized by endothelial cells and prevents co-localization of tissue factor (TF) and factor VII. Tissue plasminogen activator (tPA) from endothelial cells activates plasmin, which starts the fibrinolytic cascade, ensuring that any fibrin produced is quickly broken down and does not form a clot.

During vessel damage, the initial reaction of the vessel is transient vasoconstriction to restrict blood flow, which both reduces blood loss and aids in fibrin formation. Vasoconstriction is mediated by an autonomic neurogenic reflex, vasoactive mediators, and potentially reduced production of the normal vasodilators. As the endothelium is metabolically active, environmental changes associated with damage cause the homeostatic anticoagulant effect of the endothelium to alter and become procoagulant so that fibrin clot formation occurs. The alterations include: increased expression of TF on the luminal surface causing activation of the extrinsic cascade/initiation; loss of thrombomodulin and heparan sulfate expression allowing platelet and coagulation protein adherence; release of von Willebrand Factor (vWF) from within the endothelium aiding in platelet adherence to exposed subendothelial collagen; release of plasminogen activator inhibitor-1 (PAI-1) that negates the plasmin activation by tPA stopping fibrinolysis and allowing the fibrin formation to build up; release of thromboxane A2 and platelet-activating factor (PAF), encouraging platelet aggregation and activation; and increase in expression of P-selectin and other adhesion molecules to aid in platelet tethering. Note that the endothelium can alter from anticoagulative to procoagulative due to stimuli other than direct damage (e.g., systemic inflammation, certain viral infections, gram negative bacterial infections, some rickettsial agents, vasculitis) with the same effects. When this is inappropriate or excessive, the procoagulant effect can result in localized or even disseminated intravascular coagulation (DIC).

Primary hemostasis

Primary hemostasis provides primary hemostatic plugs to repair small vascular defects. Platelet interaction with activated endothelium or subendothelial collagen is the basis of primary hemostasis. The activated platelets are also then involved in secondary hemostasis as binding sites for coagulation factors (discussed later). Platelets are anuclear, cytoplasmic fragments from megakaryocytes within the bone marrow and contain dense granules, α-granules, and lysosomal granules, which store most of the proteins and ions required for platelet function in hemostasis. The largest population of granules is the α-granules, which contain proteins that are either synthesized by the megakaryocyte or endocytosed during circulation. The proteins that are predominantly involved in platelet aggregation, adhesion, and vascular repair include fibrinogen, Factor V (FV), fibronectin, thrombospondin, platelet-derived growth factor (PDGF), and platelet factor 4 (PF4). Dense granules contain predominantly ions and amines rather than proteins and those involved in platelet aggregation, adhesion, and vascular repair include calcium, magnesium, adenosine diphosphate (ADP), adenosine triphosphate (ATP), serotonin, and histamine. Lysosomal granules contain hydrolases similar to neutrophils that are responsible for degradation of unwanted cell debris after fibrin formation.[6]

Platelet involvement in primary hemostasis is split into three major categories: adhesion, aggregation, and granule release. Platelets are the first responders to vessel damage through adhesion to either P-selectin on activated endothelium or more often to vWF, which forms a bridge between the subendothelial collagen and platelet glycoprotein Ib (GPIb). When platelets adhere, they can flatten to form a monolayer that effectively halts blood loss. If the damage is minor, adhesion alone may be adequate for hemostasis; however, if the damage is more extensive, platelet aggregation and granule release occur, with subsequent activation of secondary hemostasis.

Platelet aggregation is stimulated by ADP, thrombin, and collagen, although unlike other species, ADP-induced aggregation is reversible in horses.[57] The stimulation causes a conformational membrane change that allows glycoprotein IIb-IIIa (GPIIb-IIIa) expression, which then binds fibrinogen, resulting in cross-linking or aggregation of the platelets, firming the platelet plug. With platelet aggregation the granules release their contents, which amplifies platelet aggregation and activation and, combined with the activated platelet membrane, allows for secondary hemostasis where the platelet plug has formed.

Secondary hemostasis

Secondary hemostasis is a series of enzyme activations and reactions that ultimately cause soluble fibrinogen to form a stable, insoluble fibrin clot. Until recently this was described in the traditional cascade model with intrinsic, extrinsic, and common pathways. The classic cascade model is useful when interpreting and understanding coagulation testing; however, the more recent cell-based model of hemostasis shows that these cascades are very interconnected *in vivo* and should not be thought of as separate.[22]

The coagulation cascade model (Figure 3.1A) is centered around the soluble factors and describes a series of interconnected enzyme and cofactor activations resulting in fibrin formation that is now best used to understand *in vitro* coagulation testing rather than *in vivo* hemostasis. The intrinsic pathway starts with the activation of factor XII (FXII) through contact with a negatively charged surface (e.g., activated phospholipid membrane, collagen, glass tube, or kaolin). Contact proteins including high-molecular-weight kininogen (HMWK) and prekallikrein (PK) interact with FXII to accelerate its activation. Activated FXII causes activation of FXI, which in the presence of free calcium and an activated phospholipid (PL) membrane (often platelet) causes activation of factor IX (FIX). Activated FVIII, a cofactor, in the presence of free calcium and an activated PL membrane (often platelet) binds FIXa and activates factor X (FX), which heralds the start of the common pathway. The extrinsic pathway is simpler and starts with activation of factor VII by tissue factor (TF), which is either exposed due to tissue damage or is upregulated on the surface of activated leukocytes, platelets, and endothelium. The TF-FVIIa complex then activates FX in the presence of free calcium and an activated PL membrane (often platelet), starting the common pathway.

The common pathway begins with FXa, which in the presence of activated factor V (FVa), a cofactor, calcium and an activated PL membrane (often platelet), activates prothrombin (factor II) to thrombin (FIIa). Thrombin is central to hemostasis as it has both procoagulant and anticoagulant effects, the

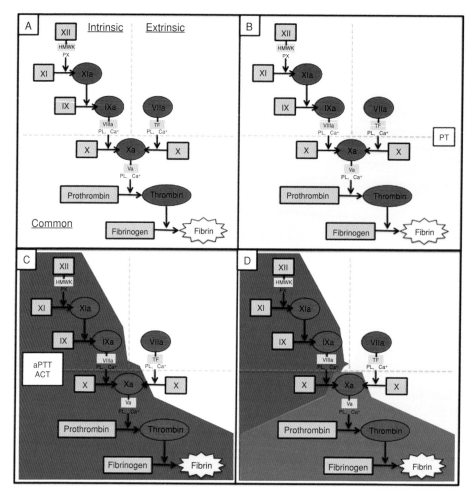

Figure 3.1 (A) The coagulation cascade model: intrinsic, extrinsic, and common pathways. (B) Shaded area represents the pathway tested with the PT assay. (C) Shaded area represents the pathway tested with the aPTT and ACT assays. (D) If only PT or aPTT is prolonged, the common pathway (green shaded area) is not affected, leaving only the factors in the upper shaded areas as potential deficiencies. If PT prolonged and aPTT not prolonged, an FVII deficiency is implicated; if aPTT prolonged but PT is not prolonged, then FXII, FXI, FIX, or FVIII are deficient. Roman numerals indicate factors. HMWK, high-molecular-weight kininogen; PK, prekallikrein; PL, phospholipid; Ca^{++}, calcium; TF, tissue factor.

most important of which is the conclusion of the common cascade: conversion of fibrinogen to fibrin. Factor XIIIa then stabilizes the fibrin clot through cross-linking of the fibrin strands.

The cell-based model (Figure 3.2), which is better used to understand *in vivo* hemostasis, occurs in three overlapping phases: initiation, amplification, and propagation.[22] The same factors are involved but the importance of the

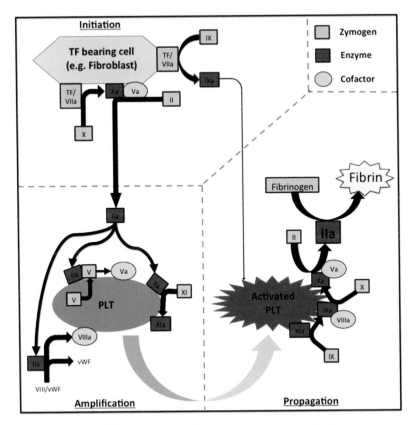

Figure 3.2   The cell-based model of hemostasis showing initiation, amplification, and propagation phases. Roman numerals indicate factors. TF, tissue factor; PLT, platelet; vWF, von Willebrand factor.

activated PL membrane localization, the overlapping activation of the intrinsic, extrinsic, and common pathways from the cascade model, and the concept of a point of no return within the coagulation model are highlighted.

Initiation occurs due to TF, which is either present on damaged or exposed tissue (e.g., fibroblasts) or upregulated on activated endothelium, leukocytes, and other cells, often associated with systemic inflammation. FVII is circulating in plasma and when it binds to tissue-bound TF, it is activated. If the procoagulant stimulus is strong enough, this complex, TF-FVIIa-PL, in the presence of calcium, activates FX and FIX. Activated FX that is tissue-bound with FVa, a cofactor, causes the generation of small amounts of thrombin. The free FXa generated in plasma is rapidly cleared to avoid systemic coagulation and to localize coagulation to where it is needed. This small amount of thrombin generated allows the movement of coagulation to the platelet surface and subsequent **amplification** of coagulation through platelet activation, activation of cofactors, and the localization of the activated cofactors on the platelet surface at the site of tissue damage. Platelet activation occurs through thrombin, which moves platelet proteins and ions to the surface and causes the platelet membrane to flip, exposing the negatively charged phosphatidylserine. After platelet granule release, factor V is one protein that is now available on the platelet surface in a partially activated form (directly from platelet alpha granules). It is fully activated in the presence of thrombin and Xa. The vWF that has bound the platelet to the site is also bound to VIII, which the thrombin now cleaves, releasing VIII to the platelet surface for activation and vWF to encourage more platelet adhesion. Thrombin also activates XI using the platelet surface as an activated PL membrane cofactor.

The third phase, **propagation**, occurs on the activated platelet membrane and involves the localization of the coagulation complexes. FIXa with FVIIIa forms the tenase complex, which then activates FX, which then binds FVa to form the prothrombinase complex, and large amounts of thrombin are generated (thrombin burst). FIXa can either be activated on the platelet surface (through XIa from the amplification phase) or directly diffuse to the platelet surface from the initiation phase because there is no soluble inactivator for FIXa. The larger amounts of thrombin generated in the thrombin burst are required for fibrin polymerization, whereas the small amounts generated during the initiation phase can only activate platelets and start activating the coagulation factors. This is a feature of physiologic hemostasis that ensures fibrin polymerization only occurs where it is needed (i.e., where there is an activated PL membrane and all the appropriate hemostatic factors). Table 3.5 summarizes the coagulation factors, their abbreviations, and their role within each hemostasis model.

Fibrinolysis

At the same time the coagulation system is activated, so is the fibrinolytic system. This is another built-in balance ensuring that thrombus formation occurs exactly where it is needed and only for the time it is needed. Quick restoration of blood flow through clot dissolution occurs once the damage is repaired. Plasminogen, an inactive zymogen produced mostly in the liver and present in circulating blood, binds to fibrin. Plasminogen activators—tissue plasminogen activator (tPA) and urokinase plasminogen activator (uPA)—are released from damaged or activated endothelial or circulating cells and activate plasmin, which then degrades fibrinogen and fibrin to soluble fibrin(ogen) degradation products (FDPs). Note thrombin is a cofactor for plasmin activation, which is yet another way to localize the fibrinolysis to the areas of active coagulation. Kallikrein and XIIa can also activate plasmin. Plasmin also degrades the amplifiers of coagulation (FVa and FVIIIa) as well as PK, HMWK, and vWF, thus downregulating coagulation while also playing a major role in fibrinolysis.

FDPs are the plasmin-generated fragments of fibrinogen and the fibrin monomer (fragment X, fragment Y, fragment D, and fragment E). When plasmin degrades cross-linked fibrin polymers, D-dimers are generated. Both are cleared through the liver. Increased FDPs and D-dimers are therefore used as indicators of increased coagulation and fibrinolysis with D-dimers being thought of as more specific for clinically significant coagulation such as DIC

Table 3.5 Coagulation factors, abbreviations, and roles within each hemostasis model

Factor	Name	Cascade model	Cell-based model	Function
I	Fibrinogen	Common	Propagation	Substrate for thrombin–converted to fibrin
II	Prothrombin	Common	Initiation Amplification Propagation	Proenzyme: IIa (thrombin) cleaves fibrinogen to fibrin, activates V, VIII, XI, XIII, protein C, platelets, plasmin
(III)	Tissue factor (TF), tissue thromboplastin factor	Extrinsic	Initiation	Cofactor: TF binds and activates VII; the TF/VIIa complex activates IX and X
(IV)	Free ionized Ca	Extrinsic Intrinsic Common	Initiation Amplification Propagation	Cofactor for IIa, VIIa, IXa, Xa, and XIIIa
V	Proaccelerin	Common	Initiation Amplification Propagation	Pro-cofactor for Xa; cofactor after activation to Va
VII	Proconvertin, stable factor	Extrinsic	Initiation	Proenzyme: VIIa activates IX and X
VIII	Antihemophilic factor	Intrinsic	Amplification Propagation	Pro-cofactor for IXa; cofactor after activation to VIIIa
IX	Christmas factor	Intrinsic	Initiation Amplification Propagation	Proenzyme: IXa activates X
X	Stuart factor, Stuart-Prower factor	Common	Initiation Amplification Propagation	Proenzyme: Xa activates II
XI	Plasma thromboplastic antecedent	Intrinsic	Amplification Propagation	Proenzyme: XIa activates IX
XII	Hageman factor	Intrinsic	Unnecessary for coagulation	Proenzyme: XIIa activates XI, PK, HMWK, and plasminogen
XIII	Fibrin-stabilizing factors, fibrinase	Common	Propagation	Proenzyme: XIIIa cross-links fibrin and protects it from plasmin degradation
HMWK	Fitzgerald factor	Intrinsic	Unnecessary for coagulation	Cofactor for activation of XII and XI
PL	Phospholipid membrane	Intrinsic Common	Initiation Amplification Propagation	Negatively charged plt mmb lipoproteins important for in vivo activation of X and II and localization of hemostasis to sites of injury
PK	Fletcher factor	Intrinsic	Unnecessary for coagulation	Proenzyme: kallikrein activates XII and PK, generates bradykinin from HMWK, and leads to plasmin generation

and thrombotic disease. However, they can also elevate with hemorrhage, surgery, and inflammatory disease. Horses have higher FDP and D-dimer concentrations when healthy than companion animals and humans.[62]

Inhibitors of coagulation and fibrinolysis

Physiologic inhibitors of coagulation help prevent excessive coagulation. They include a group of proteins that complex with and enzymatically inactivate many enzymatic coagulation factors as well as cause the degradation and removal of activated cofactors. The main inhibitors of coagulation are antithrombin III (ATIII), heparin, protein C, and tissue factor pathway inhibitor (TFPI).

Antithrombin III is the major inhibitor of coagulation enzymes. Its most important anticoagulant function lies in its ability to inhibit thrombin. It inactivates thrombin through binding and forming a stable, measurable, inactivated complex (thrombin-antithrombin complex or TAT), which is cleared by the reticuloendothelial system primarily in the liver and spleen. ATIII's thrombin binding capacity is markedly enhanced, up to 1,000-fold, by its cofactors heparin and heparan sulfate, which are present endogenously in mast cells (heparin) and on endothelial cells (heparan sulfate). As well as binding thrombin, ATIII is also able to bind and inactivate IXa, Xa, XIa, and XIIa. The horse has higher concentrations of ATIII than humans and other companion species.[26]

In addition to enhancing ATIII's ability to bind thrombin, heparin releases membrane-bound TFPI from endothelial cells. TFPI is also produced by monocytes, macrophages, and hepatocytes with most body TFPI within the endothelial cells of the microvasculature and a small amount present bound to circulating lipoproteins. TFPI inhibits coagulation by forming a stable quaternary complex (TF-VIIa-Xa-TFPI), which prevents further IXa and Xa generation by TF-VIIa, thereby dramatically reducing initiation of coagulation. The complex is cleared by receptor-mediated endocytosis.

Protein C is a vitamin K-dependent proenzyme that, when activated, has both anticoagulant and profibrinolytic action. Activation of protein C occurs through thrombomodulin-thrombin complexes. Thrombomodulin is a thrombin receptor present on most endothelial cell membranes. The endothelial cell protein C receptor (EPCR) on the endothelial membrane accelerates thrombin mediated activation of protein C and concentrates the activated protein C (aPC) near the surface of the vessel wall. More EPCR is expressed in large vessels than small vessels, centering aPC's action in large vessels. When aPC is released into circulation, it becomes associated with membrane-bound protein S, another vitamin K-dependent cofactor produced by endothelial cells, hepatocytes, and megakaryocytes, which in combination with aPC and inactive FV inactivates factors Va and VIIIa, the cofactors associated with amplification and propagation.

Activated protein C's profibrinolytic action is through inhibition of plasminogen activator inhibitor (PAI-1), which normally blocks the conversion of plasminogen to plasmin by tPA or uPA. PAI-1 is synthesized and secreted by endothelial cells in its active form. Once plasmin is formed, its major inhibitor is α-2-antiplasmin, which acts by binding and clearing plasmin from the circulation. These two methods prevent premature fibrinolysis and clot dissolution. Thrombin-thrombomodulin complexes as well as activating protein C cause activation of thrombin-activatable fibrinolysis inhibitor (TAFI), which is another fibrinolytic inhibitor. TAFI can also be activated by thrombin itself (although more slowly), plasmin, and trypsin. TAFIa cleaves plasminogen-binding sites from fibrin and as such inhibits fibrinolysis. Table 3.6 summarizes the major inhibitors of coagulation and fibrinolysis and their actions.

Table 3.6   Major inhibitors of coagulation and fibrinolysis and their functions

Factor	Function
ATIII	Major anticoagulant associated with thrombin inhibition. Binds, inactivates, and removes most coagulation enzymes from circulation. Specifically binds IIa, IXa, Xa, XIa, XIIa, kallikrein, plasmin, urokinase. Action markedly enhanced by heparin or heparan sulfate.
aPC	Major anticoagulant and profibrinolytic that is vitamin K dependent. Activated by thrombin bound to thrombomodulin (often large vessels). Anticoagulant through inactivation Va and VIIIa. Profibrinolytic through inhibition of PAI-1.
TFPI	Major anticoagulant through inhibition of TF-VIIa and Xa by forming a quaternary complex (TF-VIIa-Xa-TFPI). Heparin can increase TFPI in circulation by releasing the membrane bound TFPI from endothelial cells.
Heparin	Anticoagulant. Cofactor in ATIII action—increases the binding affinity of ATIII for thrombin by up to 1000×. Increased TFPI concentrations in circulation.
α_2-antiplasmin	Major inhibitor of fibrinolysis. Binds, inhibits, and clears plasmin from circulation.
α_2-macroglobulin	Minor inhibitor of fibrinolysis. Binds, inhibits, and clears plasmin from circulation.
PAI-1	Inhibitor of fibrinolysis through decreasing production of plasmin. Produced by endothelial cells. Inactivates tPA and uPA.
TAFI	Inhibitor of fibrinolysis. Zymogen activated by thrombin and thrombomodulin; TAFIa cleaves plasminogen binding sites from fibrin thus inhibiting fibrinolysis.

ATIII, antithrombin III; aPC, activated protein C; TFPI, tissue factor pathway inhibitor; PAI-1, plasminogen activator inhibitor; tPA, plasminogen activator, tissue type; uPA, plasminogen activator, urokinase type; TAFI, thrombin activatable fibrinolysis inhibitor

Coagulation testing and disorders causing abnormalities

Coagulation testing is used clinically when a patient is bleeding without obvious trauma, bleeding excessively from a surgical/traumatic wound, suspected of being in a hypercoagulable or hypocoagulable state associated with inflammation or DIC, or has an underlying disease that can predispose to bleeding. The tests requested depend on the clinical signs and which component(s) of hemostasis are thought to be affected. Most coagulation testing is designed to assess for disorders associated with excessive bleeding (hypocoagulable states); however, more recently developed tests are also helping investigate procoagulant states of inflammation and/or DIC and protein losing enteropathy.

Disorders of primary hemostasis often present with mucosal/small vessel bleeding characterized by petechiation, ecchymoses, epistaxis, melena, hematuria, or bleeding from the gums. Disorders of secondary hemostasis are characterized by large vessel or cavitary bleeding causing hematomas, hemarthrosis, hemothorax, hemoperitoneum, or excessive bleeding post-surgery. Disorders of fibrinolysis are more difficult to detect on physical examination; however, they can be expected in patients with systemic inflammatory conditions that may lead to DIC.

Primary hemostasis

If the patient presents with mucosal or small-vessel bleeding, testing for primary hemostatic disorders should be considered first. Testing should commence with a CBC to evaluate for thrombocytopenia as this is the most common cause for a primary hemostatic defect. Thrombocytopenia must be marked (<50,000/uL) to cause bleeding, and as platelet clumping is common in horses, a blood smear should always be evaluated in concert with the instrument CBC results to confirm that the automated platelet count is accurate. Causes of marked thrombocytopenia include vasculitis, certain infectious causes (EIAV, *Anaplasma phagocytophilum*), immune-mediated thrombocytopenia, neoplasia, and rarely idiosyncratic drug reactions.[8] If platelet numbers are not markedly decreased or are within or above reference interval with mucosal bleeding, platelet function tests should be considered. The most clinically available test of platelet function is the template bleeding time (TBT), which can be performed on the buccal mucosa (BMBT) or a shaved region of skin on the medial forelimb. The BMBT uses a commercial device with a spring-loaded blade to cause multiple small cuts of defined length and depth (typically 5 mm long and 1mm deep). Venostasis is required prior to instituting the cuts. The length of time until the cuts stop bleeding is the template or buccal mucosal bleeding time. This will be prolonged if there is thrombocytopenia, thrombopathia, or vWF deficiency, and might be prolonged with vasculitis. Unfortunately, the variation between horses and within the same horse at different times has been shown to be too wide to determine a sufficiently narrow reference interval for clinical use. Only if the test is repeatedly markedly prolonged (>860 seconds) can a diagnosis of primary hemostatic defect be made.[55] Other platelet function assays are available primarily at referral institutions and include the PFA-100, platelet aggregation studies, and flow cytometry assessing platelet activation and membrane protein and glycoprotein expression.[56,57] vWF deficiency is very uncommon in the horse, compared to the dog and humans, and has only been reported as individual case reports. vWF deficiency should be considered as a differential if there is mucosal bleeding or prolonged post-surgical bleeding and a normal platelet count and other functional assays.[8,49]

Secondary hemostasis

If the patient presents with large vessel or cavitary bleeding without surgery or significant trauma, or there is excessive bleeding post-surgery or trauma, then consider testing for secondary hemostatic defects. Most of the tests used for secondary hemostatic disorders are functional tests of the coagulation proteins and involve the addition of free calcium $+/-$ activators to platelet-poor citrated plasma with an incubation step and then measurement of the time to fibrin clot formation. These measurements can be manual (time to visible fibrin formation), mechanical (steel ball with a magnetic sensor that notes when the ball is not moving freely within the sample), or optical. Optical methods involve turbidimetry (light transmittance through the fluid) or nephelometry (detection of light scatter through a fluid). The automated assays have increased the precision and decreased operator error.

Sample collection and processing techniques are critical to retain protein function and so derive clinically useful information from the results of the coagulation testing. First, blood sampling should be minimally traumatic, with the samples representing a "clean stick." This reduces the activation of platelets, coagulation, and/or fibrinolytic systems prior to placement within the tube. Secondly most coagulation assays involve citrate as the anticoagulant with the ratio of citrate to whole blood important for accurate results. Citrate causes anticoagulation by reversibly binding calcium, which allows for the subsequent re-addition of calcium in the laboratory to reverse the anticoagulation. The ratio of citrate to blood is critical at 1:9 with either 3.2% of 3.8% citrate tubes depending on the laboratory. If the tubes are over- or underfilled, the ratio will not be accurate and this can cause falsely shortened or prolonged coagulation testing results, respectively. After confirming the absence of any clots in the sample, the citrated blood should be centrifuged for 10-15 minutes at $1,500 \times g$. General recommendations are to centrifuge and remove the plasma within one hour and test within four hours; however, recently in humans and dogs, it has been shown whole blood transport times of up to 48 hours at ambient temperature had no significant effects on prothrombin time (PT) and activated partial thromboplastin time (aPTT) in humans, and no significant effects on PT and only mildly shortened aPTT measurements in dogs, allowing for the possibility of accurate measurements even without rapid sample processing. However, this has not yet been evaluated in the horse, so prompt separation is still advised at this stage.[32,75]

Once the blood sample has been collected, commonly used screening tests include PT, aPTT, and activated clotting time (ACT). The PT and aPTT tests are performed predominantly on citrated plasma; however, some machines, often point of care, are also able to perform this on citrated whole blood. The aPTT and ACT measure the function of the intrinsic and common pathways (Figure 3.1C), so deficiencies in FXI, FIX, FVIII, FX, FV, prothrombin, and fibrinogen will cause prolongations. Note that both aPTT and ACT will also be prolonged with PK, HMWK, and FXII deficiencies. However, even if the patient is deficient in these factors, this should not cause a bleeding tendency and is likely an incidental finding. The ACT is performed as a bedside test on non-anticoagulated whole blood. The whole blood is added to a tube containing an intrinsic pathway activator, often diatomaceous earth, but other materials including kaolin and celite have also been used. The tube is maintained at 37°C and the time to first clot formation is measured as the ACT. It is expected to be between 2 and 3 minutes in healthy horses.[8] The ACT can be performed patient side, which is its major benefit. However, it is less sensitive than the aPTT for detection of deficiencies and so is often not useful unless used as a quick screening test to guide potential further investigation. The aPTT test is performed by mixing excess procoagulant PLs in the form of partial thromboplastin and a surface activator such as kaolin, silicates, or ellagic acid with platelet-poor citrated plasma and then measuring the time to clot formation when incubated at 37°C. The PT measures the function of the extrinsic and common pathways (Figure 3.1B), so deficiencies in FVII, FX, FV, prothrombin, and fibrinogen will cause prolongations. Platelet-poor plasma is mixed with thromboplastin (containing PL and excess TF) and calcium, and the time to clot formation at 37°C incubation is reported as the PT result.

Both PT and aPTT results should be interpreted in light of the reference interval either provided with the results from the reference laboratory or with the point-of-care instrument being used because different activators and methodologies result in markedly different reference intervals. It is important to note that both PT and aPTT are relatively insensitive for the detection of factor deficiencies. A 50–75% deficiency in an individual factor is necessary before a prolongation is noted.

The PT and aPTT should be interpreted together to help narrow the cause for any prolongation (Figure 3.1D). If only one of the two is prolonged, the common pathway factors (FX, FV, prothrombin, and fibrinogen) can be ruled out as the cause for the prolongation. Prolongations in PT indicate that FVII is deficient, whereas aPTT prolongations are due to deficiencies of PK, HMWK, FXII, FXI, FIX, and/or FVII. If solely the aPTT or ACT is prolonged with a normal PT, the exact factor deficiency causing the prolongation cannot be determined. In these circumstances, individual factor analysis could be considered to further characterize the prolongation; however, this is usually only performed only at referral institutions. Inherited individual factor deficiencies are very uncommon in the horse and should not be thought of as the likely cause for any prolongations. Reported inherited defects include deficits in PK, FVIII,

FIX, and FXI, which would cause prolongations in aPTT and/or ACT without a prolongation in PT.

Acquired secondary hemostatic defects are much more likely as the cause of any prolongations. Causes to consider for acquired secondary hemostatic defects include inappropriate heparin administration, severe liver disease/hepatic insufficiency, vitamin K deficiency (e.g., secondary to biliary obstruction, chronic oral antibiotic administration, severe infiltrative bowel disease, rodenticide toxicity, and sweet clover mold ingestion), DIC, or severe systemic inflammation. Most often, the coagulation panel abnormalities associated with acquired secondary hemostatic disease will cause prolongations in both PT and aPTT/ACT as many factors are affected. With vitamin K deficiency, only the vitamin K–dependent factors (II, VII, IX, and X) are affected, resulting in a prolongation of both PT and aPTT while leaving fibrinogen concentration and function unaffected.

Fibrinogen measurement as part of a coagulation profile is an attempt to document hypofibrinogenemia, which is seen with DIC due to consumption and hepatic insufficiency due to decreased production. Most often in horses, fibrinogen is being measured as a sign of inflammatory disease because fibrinogen is a positive acute-phase protein. Severe inflammatory disease is a common cause of DIC in horses, so true hypofibrinogenemia (<150 mg/dL) is often masked with an inflammatory rise in fibrinogen. Horses with subclinical DIC from colitis have been documented to have lower-than-expected fibrinogen concentrations, and a precipitous drop in fibrinogen concentrations (>100 mg/dL) in this same patient population was associated with poor prognosis suggesting that serial measurement of fibrinogen could be useful in the evaluation of DIC.[16] Fibrinogen can be measured by heat precipitation, the von Clauss method, or detection of fibrinogen antigen (see Chapter 7). Heat precipitation is not accurate enough for hemostasis testing as precision is too low at low measurement values.

Anticoagulant testing can also be performed, although this is done less commonly because anticoagulants measurement is usually only performed at specialized coagulation laboratories due to the requirement for species-specific standards and controls.[66-69] The clinical utility of anticoagulant testing lies in the detection of the subclinical or hypercoagulable state of DIC. The most commonly measured anticoagulants would be ATIII and aPC, with TAT measurement also reported. Decreases in ATIII have been associated with DIC, protein loss (often renal and GI), or with failure of production (i.e., hepatic insufficiency). ATIII has been shown to be a sensitive test for the diagnosis of DIC while also being prognostic for outcome.[19,23,25,41] Decreases in aPC are also associated with DIC and a hypercoagulable state but as with fibrinogen aPC is a positive acute-phase protein, so true decreases are often masked when there is concurrent inflammation.[67]

Fibrinolysis

Fibrin(ogen) degradation products and D-dimers are formed after plasmin-mediated degradation of fibrinogen, fibrin monomers, fibrin polymers, and cross-linked fibrin polymers. Thus, their presence indicates excessive clot formation. Excessive clot formation in the horse is most often associated with the procoagulant state associated with inflammation and leading into DIC; however, it can also be seen with hemorrhage and post-surgically. FDPs have been evaluated in horses, but the sensitivity for detection of DIC is low.[12,16,41,62] D-dimers are formed solely from cross-linked fibrin polymer degradation and are therefore thought to be more specific for clinically significant thrombosis or DIC in humans and other companion species.[9,42] When D-dimers were evaluated in horses with severe inflammatory conditions and ischemic disease, they have been shown to be significantly elevated, supporting their clinical significance in the horse as well.[13]

Global hemostasis testing

As previously discussed, the coagulation cascade model, although helpful for understanding coagulation testing, is recognized as not highlighting the importance of the cellular components of coagulation and for falsely separating the intrinsic, extrinsic, and common coagulation pathways, which is not the case *in vivo*. The cell-based model of hemostasis attempts to correct these misconceptions. Along similar lines, there has been a movement to evaluate global hemostasis rather than individual coagulation assays with the advent of viscoelastic hemostatic testing. Available viscoelastic testing devices include thromboelastography (TEG), rotational thromboelastometry (ROTEM), automated thromboelastometer (TEM-A), and Sonoclot analyzers. These analyzers evaluate all phases of clot formation and retraction with all cellular components present and therefore are a better assessment of global hemostasis. Theoretically, they are able to detect hypercoagulable as well as the more commonly assessed hypocoagulable states, which—if this proves true in the horse—will help identify early DIC patients. Briefly, a small ($\sim$350 uL) whole blood aliquot (either anticoagulated or non-anticoagulated if the machine is patient-side) is placed in a cup with a central metal pin or wire. Activators are added, with calcium if required, and the cup is oscillated in a small rotation left to right. As the blood clots, the metal pin is held away from the center of the cup and a tracing is formed whose dimensions are defined by the rate and strength of clot formation and retraction. The main differences between the machines are whether the cup or the pin/wire are rotating or whether the pin/wire moves up and down within the sample. Measurements from the tracing are used to evaluate not only for hypocoagulable states but also platelet plug formation, hypercoagulable states, and—if the test is run to completion until clot dissolution—for disorders associated with fibrinolysis. Discussing TEG abnormalities with disease states in detail is beyond the scope of this chapter; however, this has recently been well reviewed by Mendez-Angulo and colleagues, and readers are referred to this work for more information.[36] TEG in the horse has shown good precision when run in duplicate; however, marked interindividual variation has been noted as well as significant overlap between healthy and sick horses, indicating that the main use of viscoelastic studies will likely be in serial monitoring of cases to determine changes from baseline/admission and response to therapy.[17,18,37,38] Of all the TEG variables, maximum amplitude (MA) has been shown to have the lowest variability, perhaps suggesting this will be the most reliable variable to compare between horses.[37]

Laboratory diagnosis of DIC

Disseminated intravascular coagulation (DIC) is an acquired coagulopathy characterized by overactivation of the coagulation system. When DIC overwhelms the natural inhibitory systems, there is exaggerated intravascular fibrin formation with widespread fibrin deposition and microvascular thrombus formation in different tissues with mild consumption of platelets, coagulation factors, and inhibitors of coagulation. The microvascular thrombus formation can lead to ischemic tissue lesions and multiorgan dysfunction/failure. With time and in a small subset of equine patients, if the fibrin formation is not halted by the inhibitory systems, significant consumption of platelets, coagulation factor depletion, and consumption of coagulation inhibitors occurs, leading to a consumptive coagulopathy (clinical or fulminant DIC), which presents clinically with signs of spontaneous hemorrhage. It is uncommon for most cases of equine DIC to present with spontaneous hemorrhage; most patients present in subclinical DIC with some coagulation panel abnormalities but no overt signs of bleeding. Also, clinical evidence of hypercoagulability is not common in the horse except for jugular thrombophlebitis.[14,15]

DIC always develops secondary to an underlying disease that induces systemic activation of coagulation combined with depression of the anticoagulant system. A common example is sepsis with gram-negative bacteria, often from GI disease, in which endotoxemia is thought to trigger DIC by the induction of TF expression on circulating monocytes and endothelial cells within the vascular space.

The diagnosis of DIC is based on the presence of a disease that can cause increased coagulation combined with clinical and laboratory abnormalities consistent with DIC. Laboratory test results that are considered features of DIC include: thrombocytopenia (usually <100,000/uL), prolonged PT, prolonged aPTT, low fibrinogen (<150 mg/dL), low ATIII activity, and increased FDPs or D-dimers. In clinical reports, DIC is diagnosed if at least three of the six features are present. Reports have shown that with this diagnostic system the presence of DIC is a negative prognostic indicator, with one study reporting an eight times higher likelihood of death in patients with DIC compared to those without.[16,19,23,25] Other laboratory tests that have been reported with DIC to be prognostic for survival include: increased TATs, decreased ATIII, decreased protein C, and increased PAI-1.[25,41,47,66] Given that GI disease is a common inciting cause for DIC, and that DIC is prognostic for survival, a coagulation panel is advised in horses presenting with colic. Prompt therapy of both the underlying disease and the procoagulant state are associated with better survival.

References

1. Axon JE, Palmer JE. 2008. Clinical pathology of the foal. *Vet Clin North Am Equine Pract* 24:357-385.
2. Bailey E. 1982. Prevalence of anti-red blood cell antibodies in the serum and colostrum of mares and its relationship to neonatal isoerythrolysis. *Am J Vet Res* 43:1917-1921.
3. Becht JL, Semrad SD. 1985. Hematology, blood typing, and immunology of the neonatal foal. *Vet Clin North Am Equine Pract* 1:91-116.
4. Beck DJ. 1990. A case of primary autoimmune haemolytic anaemia in a pony. *Equine Vet J* 22:292-294.
5. Blue JT, Dinsmore RP, Anderson KL. 1987. Immune-mediated hemolytic anemia induced by penicillin in horses. *Cornell Vet* 77:263-276.
6. Boudreaux MK. 2008. Characteristics, diagnosis, and treatment of inherited platelet disorders in mammals. *J Am Vet Med Assoc* 233:1251-1259.
7. Boyle AG, Magdesian KG, Ruby RE. 2005. Neonatal isoerythrolysis in horse foals and a mule foal: 18 cases (1988-2003). *J Am Vet Med Assoc* 227:1276-1283.
8. Brooks MB. 2008. Equine coagulopathies. *Vet Clin North Am Equine Pract* 24:335-355.
9. Carrier M, Le Gal G, Bates SM, et al. 2008. D-dimer testing is useful to exclude deep vein thrombosis in elderly outpatients. *J Thromb Haemost* 6:1072-1076.
10. Cottle HJ, Hughes KJ. 2010. Haemolytic anaemia in a pony associated with a perivascular abscess caused by *Clostridium perfringens. Equine Vet Educ* 22:13-19.
11. Cox L. 1984. *A survey of equine red blood cell antibody frequencies and their relevance to neonatal isoerythrolysis.* MS thesis, Genetics Laboratory, University of California at Davis, Davis, California.
12. Dallap-Schaer BL, Epstein K. 2009. Coagulopathy of the critically ill equine patient. *J Vet Emerg Crit Care (San Antonio)* 19:53-65.
13. Delgado MA, Monreal L, Armengou L, et al. 2009. Peritoneal D-dimer concentration for assessing peritoneal fibrinolytic activity in horses with colic. *J Vet Intern Med* 23:882-889.
14. Divers TJ. 2003. Prevention and treatment of thrombosis, phlebitis, and laminitis in horses with gastrointestinal diseases. *Vet Clin North Am Equine Pract* 19:779-790.
15. Dolente BA, Beech J, Lindborg S, et al. 2005. Evaluation of risk factors for development of catheter-associated jugular thrombophlebitis in horses: 50 cases (1993-1998). *J Am Vet Med Assoc* 227:1134-1141.
16. Dolente BA, Wilkins PA, Boston RC. 2002. Clinicopathologic evidence of disseminated intravascular coagulation in horses with acute colitis. *J Am Vet Med Assoc* 220:1034-1038.
17. Epstein KL, Brainard BM, Gomez-Ibanez SE, et al. 2011. Thrombelastography in horses with acute gastrointestinal disease. *J Vet Intern Med* 25:307-314.
18. Epstein KL, Brainard BM, Lopes MAF, et al. 2009. Thrombelastography in 26 healthy horses with and without activation by recombinant human tissue factor. *J Vet Emerg Crit Care (San Antonio)* 19:96-101.
19. Feige K, Kästner SBR, Dempfle CE, et al. 2003. Changes in coagulation and markers of fibrinolysis in horses undergoing colic surgery. *J Vet Med A Physiol Pathol Clin Med* 50:30-36.
20. Harris M, Nolen-Walston R, Ashton W, et al. 2012. Effect of sample storage on blood crossmatching in horses. *J Vet Intern Med* 26:662-667.

21. Heath SE, Geor RJ, Tabel H, et al. 1991. Unusual patterns of serum antibodies to *Streptococcus equi* in two horses with purpura hemorrhagica. *J Vet Intern Med* 5:263-267.

22. Hoffman M, Monroe DM. 2001. A cell-based model of hemostasis. *Thromb Haemost* 85:958-965.

23. Holland M, Kelly AB, Snyder JR, et al. 1986. Antithrombin III activity in horses with large colon torsion. *Am J Vet Res* 47:897-900.

24. Johns IC, Desrochers A, Wotman KL, et al. 2011. Presumed immune-mediated hemolytic anemia in two foals with *Rhodococcus equi* infection. *J Vet Emerg Crit Care (San Antonio)* 21:273-278.

25. Johnstone IB, Crane S. 1986. Haemostatic abnormalities in horses with colic— their prognostic value. *Equine Vet J* 18:271-274.

26. Johnstone IB, Petersen D, Crane S. 1987. Antithrombin III (ATIII) activity in plasmas from normal and diseased horses, and in normal canine, bovine and human plasmas. *Vet Clin Pathol* 16:14-18.

27. Lokhorst HM, Breukink HJ. 1975. Auto-immune hemolytic anemia in two horses. *Tijdschr Diergeneeskd* 100:752-757.

28. MacLeay JM. 2001. Neonatal isoerythrolysis involving the Qc and Db antigens in a foal. *J Am Vet Med Assoc* 219:79-81.

29. Mair TS, Hillyer MH. 1992. Clinical features of lymphosarcoma in the horse: 77 cases. *Equine Vet Educ* 4:108-113.

30. Mair TS, Taylor FG, Hillyer MH. 1990. Autoimmune haemolytic anaemia in eight horses. *Vet Rec* 126:51-53.

31. Marsh WL. 1972. Scoring of hemagglutination reactions. *Transfusion* 12:352-353.

32. Maunder CL, Costa M, Cue SM, et al. 2012. Measurement of prothrombin time and activated partial thromboplastin time in citrated whole blood samples from clinically ill dogs following storage. *J Small Anim Pract* 53:531-535.

33. McClure JJ, Koch C, Traub-Dargatz J. 1994. Characterization of a red blood cell antigen in donkeys and mules associated with neonatal isoerythrolysis. *Anim Genet* 25:119-120.

34. McConnico RS, Roberts MC, Tompkins M. 1992. Penicillin-induced immune-mediated hemolytic anemia in a horse. *J Am Vet Med Assoc* 201:1402-1403.

35. McGovern KF, Lascola KM, Davis E, et al. 2011. T-cell lymphoma with immune-mediated anemia and thrombocytopenia in a horse. *J Vet Intern Med* 25:1181-1185.

36. Mendez-Angulo JL, Mudge MC, Couto CG. 2012. Thromboelastography in equine medicine: technique and use in clinical research. *Equine Vet Educ* 24:629-639.

37. Mendez-Angulo JL, Mudge MC, Vilar-Saavedra P, et al. 2010. Thromboelastography in healthy horses and horses with inflammatory gastrointestinal disorders and suspected coagulopathies. *J Vet Emerg Crit Care (San Antonio)* 20:488-493.

38. Mendez-Angulo JL, Mudge M, Zaldivar-Lopez S, et al. 2011. Thromboelastography in healthy, sick non-septic and septic neonatal foals. *Aust Vet J* 89:500-505.

39. Messer NT, Arnold K. 1991. Immune-mediated hemolytic anemia in a horse. *J Am Vet Med Assoc* 198:1415-1416.

40. Meyer J, Delay J, Bienzle D. 2006. Clinical, laboratory, and histopathologic features of equine lymphoma. *Vet Pathol* 43:914-924.

41. Monreal L, Anglés A, Espada Y, et al. 2000. Hypercoagulation and hypofibrinolysis in horses with colic and DIC. *Equine Vet J Suppl* 32:19-25.

42. Nelson OL, Andreasen C. 2003. The utility of plasma D-dimer to identify throm-boembolic disease in dogs. *J Vet Intern Med* 17:830–834.
43. Owens SD, Snipes J, Magdesian KG, et al. 2008. Evaluation of a rapid aggluti-nation method for detection of equine red cell surface antigens (Ca and Aa) as part of pretransfusion testing. *Vet Clin Pathol* 37:49–56.
44. Peek SF, Semrad SD, Perkins GA. 2003. Clostridial myonecrosis in horses (37 cases, 1985–2000). *Equine Vet J* 35:86–92.
45. Perdrizet JA, Callihan DR, Rebhun WC, et al. 1987. Successful management of malignant edema caused by *Clostridium septicum* in a horse. *Cornell Vet* 77:328–338.
46. Polkes AC, Giguère S, Lester GD, et al. 2008. Factors associated with outcome in foals with neonatal isoerythrolysis (72 cases, 1988–2003). *J Vet Intern Med* 22:1216–1222.
47. Prasse KW, Topper MJ, Moore JN, et al. 1993. Analysis of hemostasis in horses with colic. *J Am Vet Med Assoc* 203:685–693.
48. Raidal SL, Clark P, Raidal SR. 2006. Angiotrophic T-cell lymphoma as a cause of regenerative anemia in a horse. *J Vet Intern Med* 20:1009–1013.
49. Rathgeber RA, Brooks MB, Bain FT, et al. 2001. Clinical vignette. Von Willebrand disease in a Thoroughbred mare and foal. *J Vet Intern Med* 15:63–66.
50. Rebhun WC, Shin SJ, King JM, et al. 1985. Malignant edema in horses. *J Am Vet Med Assoc* 187:732–736.
51. Reef VB. 1983. *Clostridium perfringens* cellulitis and immune-mediated hemolytic anemia in a horse. *J Am Vet Med Assoc* 182:251–254.
52. Reef VB, Dyson SS, Beech J. 1984. Lymphosarcoma and associated immune-mediated hemolytic anemia and thrombocytopenia in horses. *J Am Vet Med Assoc* 184:313–317.
53. Reuss SM, Chaffin MK, Cohen ND. 2009. Extrapulmonary disorders associated with *Rhodococcus equi* infection in foals: 150 cases (1987–2007). *J Am Vet Med Assoc* 235:855–863.
54. Robbins RL, Wallace SS, Brunner CJ, et al. 1993. Immune-mediated haemolytic disease after penicillin therapy in a horse. *Equine Vet J* 25:462–465.
55. Segura D, Monreal L. 2008. Poor reproducibility of template bleeding time in horses. *J Vet Intern Med* 22:238–241.
56. Segura D, Monreal L, Espada Y, et al. 2005. Assessment of a platelet function analyser in horses: reference range and influence of a platelet aggregation inhibitor. *Vet J* 170:108–112.
57. Segura D, Monreal L, Pérez-Pujol S, et al. 2006. Assessment of platelet function in horses: ultrastructure, flow cytometry, and perfusion techniques. *J Vet Intern Med* 20:581–588.
58. Sellon DC, Fuller FJ, McGuire TC. 1994. The immunopathogenesis of equine infectious anemia virus. *Virus Res* 32:111–138.
59. Sockett DC, Traub-Dargatz J, Weiser MG. 1987. Immune-mediated hemolytic anemia and thrombocytopenia in a foal. *J Am Vet Med Assoc* 190:308–310.
60. Sprayberry KA. 2003. Neonatal transfusion medicine: The use of blood, plasma, oxygen-carrying solutions, and adjunctive therapies in foals. *Clinical Tech Equine Pract* 2:31–41.
61. Step DL, Blue JT, Dill SG. 1991. Penicillin-induced hemolytic anemia and acute hepatic failure following treatment of tetanus in a horse. *Cornell Vet* 81:13–18.
62. Stokol T, Erb HN, De Wilde L, et al. 2005. Evaluation of latex agglutination kits for detection of fibrin(ogen) degradation products and D-dimer in healthy horses and horses with severe colic. *Vet Clin Pathol* 34:375–382.

63. Taylor FG, Cooke BJ. 1990. Use of erythrocyte fragility profiles for monitoring immune-mediated haemolysis in horses. *Res Vet Sci* 48:138–140.

64. The International Society for Animal Blood Group Research. 1987. Proceedings of the 20th International Conference on Animal Blood Groups and Biochemical Polymorphisms. Helsinki, Finland, 28 July-1 August 1986. *Anim Genet* 18(s1):1–145.

65. Thomas HL, Livesey MA. 1998. Immune-mediated hemolytic anemia associated with trimethoprim-sulphamethoxazole administration in a horse. *Can Vet J* 39:171–173.

66. Topper MJ, Prasse KW. 1996. Use of enzyme-linked immunosorbent assay to measure thrombin-antithrombin III complexes in horses with colic. *Am J Vet Res* 57:456–462.

67. Topper MJ, Prasse KW. 1998. Analysis of coagulation proteins as acute-phase reactants in horses with colic. *Am J Vet Res* 59:542–545.

68. Topper MJ, Prasse KW. 1998. Chromogenic assays for equine coagulation factors VII, VIII:C, IX, and X, and C1-esterase inhibitor. *Am J Vet Res* 59:538–541.

69. Topper MJ, Prasse KW, Morris MJ, et al. 1996. Enzyme-linked immunosorbent assay for thrombin-antithrombin III complexes in horses. *Am J Vet Res* 57:427–431.

70. Underwood C, Southwood LL. 2008. Haemolytic anaemia as a complication following colic surgery in a 10-year-old Arabian stallion. *Equine Vet Educ* 20:422–426.

71. Weiser G, O'Grady M. 1983. Erythrocyte volume distribution analysis and hematologic changes in dogs with iron deficiency anemia. *Vet Pathol* 20:230–241.

72. Weiss DJ, Moritz A. 2003. Equine immune-mediated hemolytic anemia associated with *Clostridium perfringens* infection. *Vet Clin Pathol* 32:22–26.

73. Wilkerson MJ, Davis E, Shuman W, et al. 2000. Isotype-specific antibodies in horses and dogs with immune-mediated hemolytic anemia. *J Vet Intern Med* 14:190–196.

74. Zaruby JF, Hearn P, Colling D. 1992. Neonatal isoerythrolysis in a foal, involving anti-Pa alloantibody. *Equine Vet J* 24:71–73.

75. Zürcher M, Sulzer I, Barizzi G, et al. 2008. Stability of coagulation assays performed in plasma from citrated whole blood transported at ambient temperature. *Thromb Haemost* 99:416–426.

Chapter 4

The Liver

Dennis J. Meyer and Raquel M. Walton

> ### Acronyms and abbreviations that appear in this chapter:
>
> ALP   alkaline phosphatase
>
> AST   aspartate aminotransferase
>
> BA   bile acids
>
> BR   total bilirubin
>
> GGT   gamma-glutamyltransferase
>
> GLD   glutamate dehydrogenase
>
> SDH   sorbitol dehydrogenase

While the diagnostic and prognostic gold standard for hepatic disease is histologic evaluation, biopsy is an invasive procedure. Diagnosis of hepatic disease can be achieved with noninvasive procedures such as evaluation of serum biochemical data in conjunction with clinical findings, history, and ultrasound examination. Clinical signs of hepatic disease in horses can include dullness, anorexia, abdominal pain, encephalopathy, weight loss, jaundice, diarrhea, photosensitization, and coagulopathy.[5] In one study, the diagnostic specificity of clinical signs for the presence of hepatic disease was good (81%), but sensitivity poor (28%), while the most useful noninvasive prognostic test in mature horses with suspected liver disease was the severity of clinical signs.[12,14] Certain biochemical tests have better sensitivity than clinical signs in predicting the presence of liver disease when they are abnormal; however, normal test results do not preclude the presence of liver disease.

Liver enzymes

Liver enzymes are generally categorized as hepatocellular and hepatobiliary for diagnostic purposes. The hepatocellular enzymes are comprised of

Equine Clinical Pathology, First Edition. Edited by Raquel M. Walton.
© 2014 John Wiley & Sons, Inc. Published 2014 by John Wiley & Sons, Inc.

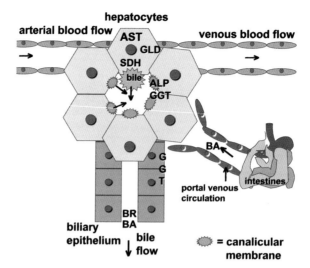

Figure 4.1 The cells and the structures they form along with their constituent enzymes are illustrated. The hepatocellular enzymes, AST, SDH, and GLD, are preformed and located within the hepatocyte. Altered integrity of the hepatocyte membrane, generally due to some type of injury, allows increased "leakage" of these enzymes into the circulation as a reflection of the underlying pathology.

The hepatobiliary enzymes, ALP and GGT, are associated with the bile canaliculi and biliary epithelium. Minimal activity is preformed and a stimulus is required to increase their production. An increase in their synthesis and release into the circulation is generally due to impairment of bile flow (cholestasis). Bile acids and bilirubin are eliminated via bile. An increase in their concentrations in the circulation occurs if the cause of the cholestasis is acute and severe (attendant high activities of SDH, GLD, and AST) or chronic and diffuse (high activities ALP and/or GGT). An increase in bile acids generally precedes an increase in bilirubin.

Modified from Meyer, Denny J, Harvey, John W. 2004. *Veterinary Laboratory Medicine-Interpretation and Diagnosis*, 3rd ed. Elsevier, Inc.

aspartate aminotransferase (AST), sorbitol dehydrogenase (SDH), and glutamate dehydrogenase (GLD). Alanine aminotransferase (ALT), a hepatocellular enzyme that is identified as "liver specific" in humans, dog, and cat, has limited activity in the horse liver and, therefore, no correlative diagnostic utility. Alkaline phosphatase (ALP) and gamma-glutamyltransferase (GGT) constitute the hepatobiliary enzymes. In contrast to the use of alkaline phosphatase in humans, dog, and cat, GGT is considered the preferable hepatobiliary enzyme in the horse. The location of these enzymes is illustrated in Figure 4.1.

Patterns of enzyme changes are associated with different types of liver pathology. An acute, severe, predominantly hepatocellular injury is initially associated with high activity of hepatocellular enzymes with increased values for GGT gradually developing over days and even persisting after the hepatocellular enzymes have returned within the reference interval after complete

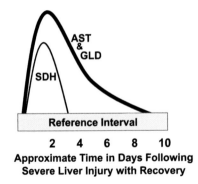

Figure 4.2 The approximate magnitude and duration of SDH, AST, and GLD increases in the circulation following severe hepatic injury with recovery is illustrated. Persistent increases for several weeks in one or more of these enzymes with repeat testing, especially if accompanied by an increase in hepatobiliary enzymes, is suggestive of persistent, progressive (chronic) liver pathology.

Modified from Meyer, Denny J, Harvey, John W. 2004. *Veterinary Laboratory Medicine-Interpretation and Diagnosis*, 3rd ed. Elsevier, Inc.

recovery. Persistent injury is associated with minimal to mild changes in both hepatocellular and hepatobiliary enzymes and requires other diagnostics to define the causation of their persistent increase. A disorder that causes predominantly cholestasis is associated with increases in GGT with low elevations for the hepatocellular enzymes developing over days to weeks. Sufficiently severe liver pathology, acute or chronic and persistent, is likely to alter one or more tests of liver function.

Hepatocellular enzymes

The hepatocellular enzymes are preformed and located in high activity within the hepatocyte. Altered membrane permeability, generally as a result of some type of injury, permits increased leakage into the circulation; the magnitude of increase generally correlates with the number of affected hepatocytes when the pathology is acute and severe. The time to return to reference values following complete recovery is dependent on their respective plasma half-life; that of SDH is shorter than that of AST and GLD (Figure 4.2). Incomplete return to reference values after several weeks of repeated testing suggests persistent pathology, referred to as chronic persistent (active) hepatitis.

Sorbitol dehydrogenase

Sorbitol dehydrogenase (SDH) is considered a liver-specific enzyme, present in high concentrations in the equine liver but in low concentrations in other tissues. The enzyme is free within hepatocyte cytoplasm and is more specific than AST or GDH in detecting hepatocellular damage. The half-life is less than

12 hours, so serum concentrations can return to reference values within days after a single insult. The *in vitro* stability is much less than other diagnostic enzymes, which can limit the utility of the test; it should be performed on serum within 5 hours if stored at room temperature and within 48 hours if frozen.[17] While SDH is very specific for liver disease, its sensitivity is lower than either GDH or AST for detection of hepatic lipidosis, cirrhosis, and necrosis in horses.[38]

Glutamate dehydrogenase

Similar to SDH, glutamate dehydrogenase (GDH) is a liver-specific enzyme present in high concentrations in hepatocytes but in low concentrations in other tissues. It is located primarily in the central lobular region. In contrast to SDH, it is mitochondrial rather than cytosolic, and is therefore typically released only with irreversible cell injury. The half-life of GDH is slightly longer than for SDH but shorter than AST. The *in vitro* stability of enzyme activity is considered greater than SDH. The activity of bovine GDH is reported to be stable for a month at -20°C.[39]

The sensitivity of GDH for diagnosis of hepatic disease in mature horses is reported to be 63%, which exceeds the reported sensitivity of SDH.[12] As a liver-specific enzyme with greater stability than SDH, GDH is a valuable tool for the diagnosis of acute liver injury in horses, but the limited availability of the assay in the United States restricts its use in practice.

Aspartate aminotransferase

Aspartate aminotransferase (AST) is present in high concentrations in hepatocytes and myocytes (see Chapter 9). Creatine kinase (CK) has high activity in skeletal muscle but is not present in the liver. An enzyme profile of marked increases in AST and CK (without increases in SDH and GLD) is indicative of primarily skeletal muscle injury. Erythrocytes also contain AST, so the presence of hemolysis in samples will increase AST activity. The enzyme is present both in the cytosol and mitochondria of hepatocytes, but in higher concentrations in the mitochondria. In theory, higher magnitude increases in AST would be expected with irreversible than reversible hepatocyte (or myocyte) injury, but this has not been proven. *In vitro* stability at room temperature or refrigerated is days rather than hours, in contrast to SDH or GDH.

Marked increases in serum AST and SDH suggest acute or active hepatocellular injury, whereas marked increases in serum AST with mild to moderate increases in SDH suggests chronic hepatic injury or recovery from acute liver injury (Figure 4.2). For horses, the diagnostic sensitivity of AST is 100% for hepatic lipidosis and 72% for hepatic necrosis.[38]

Hepatobiliary enzymes

The hepatobiliary enzymes require a stimulus for increased production with resultant increase in the circulation. Retained bile is generally considered the primary stimulant for increased production by the liver with GGT having relatively greater responsiveness and magnitude of production compared to ALP in the horse. Both GGT and ALP, when increased, have high diagnostic value for the presence of cholestatic liver disease.

Alkaline phosphatase

Alkaline phosphatase (ALP) is present in multiple tissues, but serum ALP activity does not necessarily correlate with tissue concentrations. ALP is present in relatively low concentrations in liver and yet liver ALP is found in serum, whereas in horses, intestinal ALP, present in high tissue concentrations, is not. In hepatocytes the majority of ALP is bound to bile canalicular surface membranes.

In health, serum ALP originates primarily from liver and bone, and is therefore higher in growing horses. In foals, serum ALP may be 100-fold greater than in adults due to bone ALP. In mature horses, roughly 80% of serum ALP is liver ALP and 20% is bone ALP. The ALP isoforms can be distinguished on the basis of differences in heat stability, electrophoretic migration, and wheat germ lectin precipitation. The bone isoform is more susceptible to wheat germ lectin precipitation than the liver, has slower anodal electrophoretic migration, and is more sensitive to heat inhibition. Bone ALP can be directly measured using commercially available antibodies for human bone ALP that have been validated for use in the horse.[19] Often evaluation of ALP in conjunction with another biliary-specific enzyme such as GGT is sufficient in determining the origin and significance of increased serum ALP concentrations.

The most common cause of increased serum ALP concentrations is cholestasis. Cholestasis induces the synthesis of ALP, which concentrates on the basolateral hepatocyte membrane where it is released into blood or lymphatics.[16] The highest concentrations of serum ALP are associated with cholangitis, biliary cirrhosis, or extrahepatic bile duct obstruction.

Gamma-glutamyltransferase

Gamma-glutamyltransferase (GGT; also known as gamma-glutamyltranspeptidase) is a membrane-bound enzyme that is primarily associated with biliary epithelial cells in horses, like other domestic animals. Most serum GGT activity originates from the liver, although it is present in high concentrations in the kidney, intestine, and pancreas. This is attributable to its presence on the luminal surfaces in these organs. Serum half-life of GGT in horses is thought to be around three days, similar to ALP.[16]

Increases in GGT are associated with cholestasis and biliary hyperplasia. Serum GGT concentrations are more sensitive than ALP in the diagnosis of cholestatic diseases; in horses with cholestasis, GGT increased ninefold whereas ALP activity only increased twofold.[15] GGT activity is high in colostrum and increased serum GGT concentrations are present in calves and goats during suckling, but not in foals. There is no significant difference in GGT concentrations pre- and post-suckling in foals; however, GGT concentrations are higher in foals relative to adults.[29]

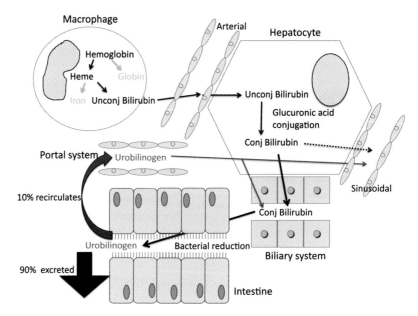

Figure 4.3   Bilirubin metabolism. Unconjugated bilirubin is released into the plasma from macrophages after the breakdown of hemoglobin to heme, which is further degraded into iron and bilirubin. Unconjugated bilirubin is bound by albumin and transported to the liver where it is then conjugated to glucuronic acid. Conjugated bilirubin is excreted into bile via biliary canaliculi and then into the intestinal tract, where it is reduced to urobilinogen or stercobilinogen by the action of bacteria. About 10% of urobilinogen returns to the liver via the portal system and the majority is excreted into bile; a small proportion (1–5%) enters the circulation to be excreted via the kidneys. In cases of biliary obstruction or impaired bilirubin excretion due to hepatocellular dysfunction, conjugated bilirubin will efflux into the plasma (dotted line).

Liver function tests

Excretory function tests

Total bilirubin

Total bilirubin is comprised of two forms, unconjugated and conjugated. The primary source of bilirubin is from the degradation of hemoglobin from aged erythrocytes, termed unconjugated (indirect-reacting) bilirubin. Unconjugated bilirubin is transported to the liver via albumin for receptor-mediated uptake by hepatocytes, internalized and altered to form conjugated (direct-reacting) bilirubin, and actively secreted by the specialized portion of the hepatocyte membrane (canalicular membrane) into bile for delivery to the small intestine (Figure 4.3).

A relatively unique feature of bilirubin removal by the horse is at the site of uptake by the hepatocyte. Lack of food intake is commonly associated with moderate to marked increases in total bilirubin due to increases in the uncon-jugated form. It is likely that free fatty acids and other metabolic constituents that are increased in the fasted state compete for uptake of unconjugated bilirubin; it decreases once appetite returns.

Another cause of increased unconjugated bilirubin is acute, severe hemolysis. Concomitant moderate to marked decreases in circulating red cell mass as measured by the hematocrit are supportive of a hemolytic process. Intrahepatic diseases and extrahepatic obstruction both can cause increases in total bilirubin, with conjugated bilirubin comprising less than half of the total bilirubin.

Bile acids

The circulating concentrations of bile acids are dependent on an intact enterohepatic circulation. Bile acids are efficiently removed from the intestines into the portal circulation, transported to the liver, efficiently extracted from the blood by receptor-mediated uptake by the hepatocyte, processed by the hepatocyte, and actively excreted by the canalicular membrane into bile for delivery to the intestine where the process is repeated (Figure 4.1). Serum bile acid concentrations in foals are significantly higher than in adult horses in the first six weeks of life, and age-specific reference values should be used in interpreting results.[3]

Bile acids increase in the circulation before an increase in total bilirubin due to liver disease. In contrast to total bilirubin, serum bile acid concentrations in the horse are not affected by short-term fasting (less than three days).[15,38] Post-prandial increases are also not observed given the lack of gall bladder in equids. The measurement of bile acids is a diagnostic adjunct when abnormal liver enzyme tests are detected; a concomitant increase in bile acids suggests substantial liver pathology precluding their removal from the sinusoidal blood and supports further diagnostics such as liver biopsy. Congenital abnormalities of the portal circulation, often manifested as encephalopathy, cause bile acids to bypass the liver, resulting in increases in the circulation; total bilirubin will not be increased as a result of the shunt, but in equids it may be increased due to fasting.[7]

Tests dependent on synthetic/metabolic functions

Albumin

Albumin is produced exclusively by hepatocytes. The formation of albumin is relatively well preserved, and decreases are not significant until there is substantial loss of hepatocellular mass due to disease (>60–80% of functional mass). Moreover, the half-life of albumin in horses is longer than in other species (19.4 days). Hypoalbuminemia is an infrequent finding with severe acute or chronic liver disease, occurring in only 13% to 16% of cases in two studies.[25,28] Hypoalbuminemia occurred more frequently in chronic rather than acute liver disease.

When there are no liver test abnormalities to suggest liver disease, other causes should be considered. These primarily include losses of albumin due to diseases involving the intestines and kidney. Mild decreases in albumin production can occur when globulins are increased in association with chronic inflammation, referred to as a negative acute-phase protein response (see Chapter 7).

Ammonia

Ammonia is formed in the intestines and carried to the liver by the portal circulation where it is metabolized in hepatocytes via the Krebs-Henseleit urea cycle with urea nitrogen as one by-product. Loss of hepatocellular mass due to severe disease and congenital portosystemic shunts permits high concentrations to enter the circulation where it can cause cerebral dysfunction (hepatic encephalopathy). A concomitant decrease in blood urea nitrogen (BUN) may be noted, although this is not a consistent finding.[25, 40]

Hepatic encephalopathy is a common clinical feature of hepatic failure in horses. While ammonia has neurotoxic effects, the etiopathogenesis of hepatic encephalopathy is currently unclear and it is not attributable solely to hyperammonemia as signs cannot be experimentally induced by injection of ammonia in similar concentrations to those associated with encephalopathy.[24] Hyperammonemia with encephalopathy in the absence of detectable hepatic disease has been reported in horses (also referred to as intestinal hyperammonemia).[11, 33, 35] In these cases hyperammonemia is thought to be due to gastrointestinal disease resulting in increased ammonia production by gastrointestinal bacteria in conjunction with increased gut permeability.[35] In cases of intestinal hyperammonemia, bile acids concentrations have been within reference limits. The measurement of bile acids is a more dependable liver function test for the differential diagnosis of hepatic encephalopathy; moreover, ammonia is labile in blood samples, which limits its diagnostic utility.

Globulins

Nearly half of horses with severe liver disease showed hyperproteinemia attributable to hyperglobulinemia in one study.[28] Hyperglobulinemia has high diagnostic value for the presence of liver disease with intermediate sensitivity (56%) and good specificity (80%).[14] Hyperglobulinemia is a result of increased synthesis of alpha-, beta-, and/or gamma-globulins.[28]

Beta-gamma bridging, an electrophoretic pattern observed when there is poor demarcation between the beta and gamma globulin peaks, in conjunction with a decreased albumin to globulin ratio, has been reported in many veterinary textbooks to be pathognomonic for chronic active hepatitis or hepatic cirrhosis. Recent data show that beta-gamma bridging in horses does not have a strong predictive value for hepatic disease; of three horses with beta-gamma bridging, two had liver disease and one had pulmonary carcinoma with no liver involvement.[8]

Glucose

Glucose is dependent on the liver as one of several organs for maintenance of normal concentrations in the circulation. However, liver-related decreases in glucose are uncommon and develop only after severe loss of hepatocellular mass due to disease. In a study of primary hepatic disease in adult horses, of the 28 cases for which glucose concentrations were available, none were hypoglycemic.[25] However, in foals with hepatic disease, hypoglycemia is reported, likely as a result of decreased hepatic gluconeogenesis capacity relative to adults.[6,18]

Coagulation factors

Coagulation factors (except Factor XIII) are formed by the liver. Acute, severe, or chronic loss of hepatocellular mass can result in sufficient deficiency of one or more coagulation factors resulting in prolongation of the prothrombin time and/or activated partial thromboplastin time. It is important to note that with liver disease no biopsy procedure should be considered until coagulation testing is conducted.

Other tests

Increases in liver enzyme tests often are the initial indication that liver disease may be present and the cause of clinical signs. Liver function tests can further support the presence of liver disease and define the extent of the liver pathology. Repeated testing is helpful to determine if the liver disease is recovering or persistent. Further assessment of the cause of abnormal liver tests includes ultrasound evaluation and microscopic examination of a cytology aspirate or biopsy.

Biopsy

Hepatic biopsy is considered the gold standard for diagnosis and prognosis of hepatic disease, but is an invasive procedure. Depending on the distribution of lesions, biopsy—especially single biopsy—may not detect liver disease. While ultrasound guidance may increase the chances of sampling a diseased area, histologic lesions can be present in ultrasonographically normal liver.

Histologic evaluation of the liver succeeds most often in establishing presence of disease, but may fail in identifying a specific etiology. A recent study evaluating the prognostic use of hepatic biopsy for equine liver disease showed that the most useful negative prognostic indicators were hepatic fibrosis and biliary hyperplasia.[13] Previous findings support fibrosis as a negative prognostic factor.[21]

Table 4.1   Etiologies of Liver Disease in Horse

Toxic	Parasitic	Infectious	Miscellaneous	Idiopathic	Primary Neoplasms
Pyrrolizidine alkaloid	*Fasciola hepatica*	*Clostridium piliforme*	Cholelithiasis	Theiler's disease	Hepatoblastoma
Panicum grasses	*Heterobilharzia americana*	Cholangiohepatitis *Salmonella* spp.	Lipidosis		Hepatocellular carcinoma
Xanthium (cocklebur)	*Parascaris equorum*	*E. coli* *Pseudomonas* spp.			Cholangiocellular carcinoma
Mycotoxins	Strongyle larvae	*Actinobacillus equuli*			
Alsike clover					
Iron					

Hepatic diseases

Toxins

Toxic hepatopathies are relatively common in equids as a result of grazing behavior. Common toxicoses and their associated lesions are listed in Tables 4.1 and 4.2, respectively. The distribution of lesions is often similar with most hepatotoxins, but unique histologic features are noted with some toxins (e.g., megalocytes with pyrrols and mycotoxins). The type (acute necrosis or chronic

Table 4.2   Lesions Associated with Various Etiologies of Liver Disease

Etiology	Lesions
Pyrrolizidine alkaloid	Megalocytosis, periacinar necrosis, biliary hyperplasia, periportal fibrosis
Panicum grasses	Biliary fibrosis, periacinar necrosis, crystalline material in bile ducts
Alsike clover	Portal fibrosis, biliary hyperplasia
Mycotoxins	Central lobular necrosis, biliary hyperplasia, megalocytosis
Cocklebur (*Xanthium* spp.)	Periacinar necrosis
Iron	Portal necrosis, increased iron stores
Clostridium piliforme	Liver necrosis with neutrophilic infiltrate, intrahepatocellular filamentous bacteria
Salmonella spp., *Pseudomonas* spp., *Actinobacillus equuli*, *E. coli*	Cholangiohepatitis: biliary hyperplasia, periductular inflammation, periportal fibrosis
Parasitic (*Heterobilharzia americana*, *Fasciola hepatica*)	Multifocal granulomas with eosinophilic and lymphocytic inflammation
Theiler's disease	Acute hepatitis: centrolobular necrosis, inflammatory cell infiltrates

disease) and distribution of hepatocellular damage will influence the pattern of enzyme increases.

Pyrrolizidine alkaloids

Pyrrolizidine alkaloids (PA) are found in several species of plants, including *Senecio, Crotalaria, Amsinkia, Heliotropium*, and *Cynoglossum*. The toxic principle is the pyrrols, which are broken down from the alkaloids in the liver and cross-link with DNA. Liver enzymes typically are elevated before clinical signs appear, and the dehydrogenases (SDH, GDH) may be within reference limits by the time the animals present with signs of disease. Serum GGT, ALP, and bile acids are more sensitive indicators of PA toxicity because the disease is typically chronic. In one study, serum GGT is shown to be relatively sensitive (75%) and specific (90%) as a screening test for subclinical PA toxicosis, defined by histologic evidence of PA toxicity in the absence of clinical signs.[10] In this same study, ALP was shown to have lower sensitivity (58%) and higher specificity (100%) as a screening test.

Mycotoxins

There are a number of mycotoxins that are hepatotoxic. Some of the more common ones include aflatoxins and fumonisin. Like pyrrolizidine alkaloids, mycotoxins can cause megalocytosis. In addition to megalocytosis, histologic changes seen with mycotoxins include hepatocellular necrosis, depletion of centrilobular hepatocytes, lobular disarray, and biliary hyperplasia.[37]

Alsike clover, Cocklebur, and Panicum grasses

It is thought that the toxic principles associated with alsike clover (*Trifolium hybridum*) and *Panicum* grasses are mycotoxins or plant metabolites because the hepatotoxicity is sporadic and often weather-related.[5] Deposition of crystalline substances in bile ducts that are plant saponin derivatives has been reported with *Panicum coloratum*. In a recent report of Panicum toxicosis, increases in SDH, AST, GGT, and ALP were documented along with hepatic necrosis.[20] The toxic principle in cocklebur (*Xanthium*) inhibits the exchange of ATP for ADP in the mitochondria and cytosol, respectively, resulting in hepatic necrosis with a periacinar distribution. Serum chemistry changes reflect the acute hepatocellular necrosis.

Iron

Iron toxicosis causes acute hepatotoxicity with massive periacinar necrosis and deposition of iron in Kupffer cells. Toxicosis is typically the result of administration of ferrous fumarate or sulfate containing vitamin supplements and has been reported in foals and adult horses, although foals are much more susceptible to iron toxicosis than adults.[2,27] Iron hepatotoxicity was reported as a result of administration of 16 mg/kg ferrous fumarate to neonatal Shetland ponies, whereas administration of 50 mg/kg of ferrous sulfate for 8 weeks was not sufficient to induce hepatotoxicity in adult ponies.[30] Although in one of the reported cases of adult iron toxicity a dose of approximately 390 mg iron/kg (ferrous fumarate) over a period of 5 days was reported, concomitant selenium/vitamin E deficiency with iron excess may have been a contributing factor in other cases of adult iron toxicosis.[2]

Cases of hemochromatosis in adult horses characterized by hepatic cirrhosis with marked increases in iron storage in hepatocytes, Kupffer cells, and portal macrophages are described.[23,25,31] Whether these cases represent hepatotoxicity secondary to iron overload or a primary hepatopathy with secondary iron overload is uncertain. Iron intake was not excessive in any of the horses for which it was evaluated.

Infections

Clostridium piliforme (Tyzzer's disease)

Infection by *Clostridium piliforme* usually occurs in foals one to six weeks old and causes acute or peracute hepatitis that usually causes death within hours or days. The infection causes multifocal to confluent central coagulation necrosis with inflammatory cells and degenerate hepatocytes at the periphery. A definitive diagnosis is made by identifying filamentous bacteria within hepatocytes at the periphery of the necrotic areas; this may be accomplished via cytology or histology. Use of silver stains such as Warthin-Starry facilitates visualization of the organisms on histologic sections. There is a marked increase in SDH concentration due to the severe necrosis with moderate to marked hyperbilirubinemia and mild to moderate increases in GGT concentration; ALP is not increased.[6]

Cholangiohepatitis

Ascending infection from the intestinal tract with *Salmonella* sp., *E. coli, Pseudomonas* sp., *Actinobacillus equuli*, and (less commonly) *Pasteurella* sp., *Streptococcus* sp., or *Clostridium* sp. is associated with inflammation of the biliary tracts and adjacent liver. Histologically there is biliary hyperplasia, periductular inflammation, and periportal fibrosis. Cholangiocellular enzymes GGT and ALP may be disproportionately high relative to SDH or GDH; however, this depends on the amount of hepatocellular involvement. Hyperglobulinemia can be seen with chronic (>3 weeks) conditions. Cholelithiasis is frequently encountered with cholangiohepatitis, possibly as a result of decreased biliary flow.[32]

Parasites

Parascaris equorum and strongyle larvae migrate through the liver and can cause hemorrhagic tracts with necrosis, inflammatory cells (especially eosinophils), and fibrosis. Histopathologic findings with liver flukes (*Fasciola hepatica*) include multifocal granulomas with eosinophilic and lymphocytic inflammation. Experimental infection with *F. hepatica* resulted in increases in GDH and GGT three to five months post-infection.[36]

The schistosome *Heterobilharzia americana* has recently been recognized as a cause of multifocal fibrosing eosinophilic and lymphocytic granulomas in the liver of horses in the southern United States.[9] These disseminated granulomas present grossly as a starry-sky appearance to the liver. *H. americana*, similar to other schistosomal species, can infect the liver from the intestinal tract via the portal circulation. In many of the reported cases, the granulomas were incidental findings unrelated to a primary disease for which the horse was presented.

Hepatic lipidosis

Hepatic lipidosis in equids is associated with hyperlipemia, a disorder of lipid metabolism that is discussed in depth in Chapter 8. Hyperlipemia frequently occurs secondary to primary disease processes such as enterocolitis/colitis and colic that produce a negative energy balance and affect insulin sensitivity. Ponies and donkeys can present with primary hyperlipemia; stress and obesity are predisposing factors. Both stress and obesity induce decreases in insulin sensitivity, which is considered the primary predisposing factor (see Chapter 8). There appears to be a genetic predisposition to hyperlipemia in the case of Shetland ponies.

Stimulation of hormone-sensitive lipase in adipocytes by glucagon, corticosteroids, ACTH, or epinephrine (hormones associated with illness) catalyzes the hydrolysis of stored triglycerides and releases nonesterified fatty acids (NEFA). When there is increased release of fatty acids from adipocytes, the NEFA not utilized by peripheral tissues are taken up by hepatocytes to be oxidized for energy, converted into ketones, or used to synthesize triglycerides that are either stored or released as very-low-density lipoproteins (VLDL). Equids have a limited ability to form ketones, and thus increases in circulating fatty acids contribute to hepatic triglyceride storage and hypertriglyceridemia via hepatic VLDL synthesis.

Serum hepatitis (Theiler's disease)

In horses, acute central lobular necrosis has been associated with administration of tetanus antitoxin, antiserum for various diseases (influenza, equine encephalomyelitis, strangles), vaccines prepared from equine fetal tissues, and commercial plasma.[1,26] There is a seasonal incidence of serum hepatitis, which in conjunction with its association with the use of equine serum and plasma products suggests a possible infectious etiology. Pregnant lactating mares appear to have an increased risk of developing serum hepatitis.[26] The majority of serum hepatitis cases have been associated with tetanus antitoxin administration 4-10 weeks prior to clinical presentation. Clinical presentation is acute and increases in both hepatocellular and hepatobiliary enzymes are seen, although hepatocellular enzyme increases are typically of greater magnitude.

Hepatocellular neoplasia

Primary liver neoplasms are rare in the horse and comprise hepatoblastoma, hepatocellular carcinoma, and cholangiocarcinoma.[4] Hepatoblastomas are reported in neonates and juveniles up to four years of age. Hepatocellular carcinomas occur in juveniles and mature horses, whereas reports of cholangiocarcinomas are in mature horses. A single case report of a biliary cystadenoma morphologic variant (biliary adenofibroma) has been described as an incidental finding in a mature horse.[34]

References

1. Aleman M, Nieto JE, Carr EA, et al. 2005. Serum hepatitis associated with commercial plasma transfusion in horses. *J Vet Intern Med* 19:120-122.
2. Ambjerg J. 1981. Poisoning in animals due to oral application of iron. *Nord Vet Med* 33:71-76.
3. Barton MH, LeRoy BE. 2007. Serum bile acids concentrations in healthy and clinically ill neonatal foals. *J Vet Intern Med* 21:508-513.
4. Beeler-Marfisi J, Arroyo L, Caswell JL, et al. 2010. Equine primary liver tumors: a case series and review of the literature. *J Vet Diagn Invest* 22:174-183.
5. Bergero D, Nery J. 2008. Hepatic diseases in horses. *J Anim Physiol Anim Nutr* 92:345-355.
6. Borchers A, Magdesian G, Halland S, et al. 2006. Successful treatment and polymerase chain reaction (PCR) confirmation of Tyzzer's disease in a foal and clinical and pathologic characteristics of 6 additional foals (1986-2005). *J Vet Intern Med* 20:1212-1218.
7. Buonanno AM, Carlson GP, Kantrowitz B. 1988. Clinical and diagnostic features of portosystemic shunt in a foal. *J Am Vet Med Assoc* 192:387-389.
8. Camus MS, Krimer PM, LeRoy BE, et al. 2010. Evaluation of the positive predictive value of serum protein electrophoresis beta-gamma bridging for hepatic disease in three domestic animal species. *Vet Pathol* 47:1064-1070.
9. Corapi WV, Birch SM, Carlson KL, et al. 2011. *Heterobilharzia americana* infection as a cause of hepatic parasitic granulomas in a horse. *J Am Vet Med Assoc* 239:1117-1122.
10. Curran JM, Sutherland RJ, Peet RL. 1996. A screening test for subclinical liver disease in horses affected by pyrrolizidine alkaloid toxicosis. *Aust Vet J* 74:236-240.
11. Dunkel B, Chaney KP, Dallap-Schaer BL, et al. 2011. Putative intestinal hyperammonemia in horses: 36 cases. *Equine Vet J* 43:133-140.
12. Durham AE, Newton JR, Smith KC, et al. 2003a. Retrospective analysis of historical, clinical, ultrasonographic, serum biochemical and haematological data in prognostic evaluation of equine liver disease. *Equine Vet J* 35: 542-547.
13. Durham AE, Smith KC, Newton JR, et al. 2003b. Development and application of a scoring system for prognostic evaluation of equine liver biopsies. *Equine Vet J* 35:534-540.
14. Durham AE, Smith KC, Newton JR. 2003c. An evaluation of diagnostic data in comparison to the results of liver biopsy in mature horses. *Equine Vet J* 35:554-559.
15. Hoffman WE, Baker G, Rieser S, et al. 1987. Alterations in selected serum biochemical constituents in equids after induced hepatic disease. *Am J Vet Res* 48:1343-1347.

16. Hoffman WE, Solter PF. 2008. Diagnostic enzymology of domestic animals. In *Clinical Biochemistry of Domestic Animals*, Kaneko JJ, Harvey JW, and Bruss ML (eds), 6th ed., pp 351-378. Burlington: Academic Press.

17. Horney BS, Honor DJ, MacKenzie A, et al. 1993. Stability of sorbitol dehydrogenase activity in bovine and equine sera. *Vet Clin Pathol* 22:5-9.

18. Humber KA, Sweeney RW, Saik JE, et al. 1988. Clinical and clinicopathologic findings in two foals infected with *Bacillus piliformis. J Am Vet Med Assoc* 193:1425-1428.

19. Jackson B, Eastell R, Russell RGG. 1996. Measurement of bone specific alkaline phosphatase in the horse: a comparison of two techniques. *Res Vet Sci* 61:160-164.

20. Johnson AL, Divers TJ, et al. 2006. Fall panicum (*Panicum dichotomiflorum*) hepatotoxicosis in horses and sheep. *J Vet Intern Med* 20:1414-1421.

21. Johnston JK, Divers TJ, Reef VB, et al. 1989. Cholelithiasis in horses: 10 cases (1982-1986). *J Am Vet Med Assoc* 194:405-409.

22. Kaneko JJ, Rudolph WG, Wilson DW, et al. 1992. Bile acid fractionations by high-performance liquid chromatography in equine liver disease. *Vet Res Commun* 16:161-172.

23. Lavoie JP, Teuscher E. 1993. Massive iron overload and liver fibrosis resembling haemochromatosis in a racing pony. *Equine Vet J* 25:552-554.

24. Maddison JE. 1992. Hepatic encephalopathy. *J Vet Intern Med* 6:341-353.

25. McGorum BC, Murphy D, Love S, et al. 1999. Clinicopathological features of equine primary hepatic disease: a review of 50 cases. *Vet Rec* 145:134-139.

26. Messer NT, Johnson PJ. 1994. Idiopathic acute hepatic disease in horses: 12 cases (1982-1992). *J Am Vet Med Assoc* 204:1934-1937.

27. Mullaney TP, Brown CM. 1988. Iron toxicity in neonatal foals. *Equine Vet J* 20:119-124.

28. Parraga ME, Carlson GP, Thurmond M. 1995. Serum protein concentrations in horses with severe liver disease: a retrospective study and review of the literature. *J Vet Intern Med* 9:154-161.

29. Patterson WH, Brown CM. 1986. Increase of serum gamma-glutamyltransferase in neonatal Standardbred foals. *Am J Vet Res* 47:2461-2463.

30. Pearson EG, Andreasen CB. 2001. Effect of oral administration of excessive iron in adult ponies. *J Am Vet Med Assoc* 218:400-404.

31. Pearson EG, Hedstrom OR, Poppenga RH. 1994. Hepatic cirrhosis and hemochromatosis in three horses. *J Am Vet Med Assoc* 204:1053-1056.

32. Peek SF. 2004. Cholangiohepatitis in the mature horse. *Equine Vet Educ* 16:72-75.

33. Peek SF, Divers TJ, Jackson CJ. 1997. Hyperammonemia associated with encephalopathy and abdominal pain without evidence of liver disease in four mature horses. *Equine Vet J* 29:70-74.

34. Salvaggio A, Caracappa S, Gurrera A, et al. 2003. Hepatic biliary adenofibroma: a hitherto unrecognized tumor in equines. Report of a case. *Vet Pathol* 40:114-116.

35. Sharkey LC, DeWitt S, Stockman C. 2006. Neurologic signs and hyperammonemia in a horse with colic. *Vet Clin Pathol* 35:254-258.

36. Soulé C, Boulard C, Levieux D, et al. 1989. Experimental equine fascioliasis: evolution of serologic, enzymatic, and parasitic parameters. *Annales de Recherches Vétérinaires* 20:295-307.

37. Stalker MJ, Hayes MA. 2007. Liver and biliary system. In *Jubb, Kennedy, and Palmer's Pathology of Domestic Animals*. Maxie MG (ed). Vol. 2, 5th ed. pp. 297-388. Philadelphia: Elsevier Saunders.

38. West HJ. 1989. Evaluation of total plasma bile acid concentrations for the diagnosis of hepatobiliary disease in horses. *Res Vet Sci* 46:264-270.
39. West HJ. 1991. Evaluation of total serum bile acids concentrations for the diagnosis of hepatobiliary disease in cattle. *Res Vet Sci* 51:133-140.
40. West HJ. 1996. Clinical and pathological studies in horses with hepatic disease. *Equine Vet J* 28:146-156.

Chapter 5

Laboratory Evaluation of the Equine Renal System

Andrea A. Bohn

Abnormalities in laboratory values can help determine the presence and severity of urinary tract disease. Many different disorders of the equine urinary tract have been described and include pre-renal, intra-renal, and post-renal processes. Routine laboratory data are used to assess glomerular filtration rate as well as other functions of the kidney. The kidney is very important in filtering wastes from the blood as well as maintaining electrolyte, water, and acid-base balances. The kidney also plays an important role in erythropoiesis and vitamin D activation.

Comprehensive evaluation of the equine renal system requires a complete blood count (CBC), serum biochemical panel, and full urinalysis. The CBC can help detect inflammatory conditions and the presence of anemia. Serum biochemical analysis will detect increases in nitrogenous waste products normally excreted by the kidneys, reveal electrolyte and protein abnormalities, and provide information regarding acid-base status. Urinalysis is essential in differentiating causes of azotemia as well as providing clues as to the presence, location, and cause of urinary tract disorders (Table 5.1).

Laboratory assessment of the kidney

In examining laboratory data for evaluation of the urinary tract, the functions of the kidney can essentially be broken down into three main actions (Figure 5.1). The first is the filtering of blood through the glomerulus; total plasma volume is filtered approximately 60-70 times every day.[12] While this is essential for removal of waste substances, essential blood solutes are also filtered during this process. Therefore, the second major action of the kidney is to reabsorb those solutes so that appropriate plasma concentrations are maintained. The third major action of the kidney is the maintenance of blood volume or body water. This is predominantly regulated in the collecting ducts under the influence of vasopressin.

Equine Clinical Pathology, First Edition. Edited by Raquel M. Walton.
© 2014 John Wiley & Sons, Inc. Published 2014 by John Wiley & Sons, Inc.

Table 5.1   Common laboratory finding associated with different renal diseases

	CRF	ARF	Early Disease	Glomerular Disease	Bladder Rupture	Strenuous Exercise	Dehydration
Azotemia	+	+	–	–/+	–/+	–/+	+
Urea/Creat	>1:10	<1:10					
USG	1.008–1.012	1.008–1.012	Variable	Variable	Variable	>1.025	>1.035
Proteinuria	+	+	+/–	+++	–	+	–
Other potential findings	Nonregenerative anemia HyperMg Hyperlipidemia Hypoalbuminemia Metabolic acidosis	Glycosuria High FE HyperMg Enzymuria Urine casts and WBCs Metabolic acidosis	Glycosuria High FE Enzymuria	Red cell casts		Hematuria Hemoglobinuria Myoglobinuria	
Serum Electrolytes							
Na&Cl	N-L	N-L	N	N	L	L-N-H	N-H
K	N-H	L-N-H	N	N	N-H	N	N
Ca	N-H	L-N-H	N	N-L	N	N-L	N
Phosphorus	N-L	H	N	N-H	N	N	N-H
Additional testing			FE Enzymuria USG Water deprivation test	UPC ratio	Ratio of abdominal fluid creat to serum creat	Retest later	

Creat, creatinine; FE, fractional excretion; Mg, magnesium; L, low; N, normal; H, high; UPC, urine protein creatinine ratio; USG, urine-specific gravity.

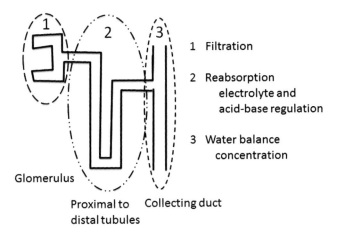

1 Filtration

2 Reabsorption
    electrolyte and
    acid-base regulation

3 Water balance
    concentration

Figure 5.1 Simplified illustration of the three major functions of the kidney that can be assessed by laboratory methods.

Glomerular filtration rate

The ability of the kidneys to filter blood can be evaluated by determining the glomerular filtration rate (GFR). While there are more complicated methods to precisely determine GFR, serum urea and creatinine provide a readily available estimation of GFR. If there is an elevation of these nitrogenous waste products in serum, termed azotemia, it indicates that GFR is decreased. Unfortunately, this is a rather insensitive method of detecting a decrease in renal functional capacity, as three-fourths of function is typically lost before azotemia is seen.

Decreases in GFR can be due to pre-renal, renal, or post-renal factors or a combination of these processes. If the rate of glomerular filtration decreases, serum urea and creatinine concentrations will increase. Urea concentrations can rise faster than creatinine because of the tubules' ability to reabsorb urea, particularly with a pre-renal cause of decreased GFR. Other values that increase with a decrease in GFR are serum phosphorous and total magnesium concentrations.

If the cause for a decrease in GFR is purely pre-renal and there are no extenuating circumstances, a horse should have a urine-specific gravity >1.025 in the face of azotemia. If a horse is not able to concentrate its urine in the face of azotemia (and the animal has not been treated with fluids), the kidney is not functioning properly, and one of the most common causes is renal disease. There are, however, other reasons for the kidneys not to be able to concentrate urine as discussed below. These factors need to be considered before a definitive diagnosis of renal failure is made. With post-renal azotemia, urine-specific gravity can be variable and is often isosthenuric in the post-obstructive phase. The diagnosis of most post-renal urinary tract disorders is usually predominantly based on history and clinical signs.

Both urea and creatinine concentrations can be elevated for reasons other than decreased GFR. Urea is a by-product of protein metabolism, therefore urea concentration can increase with a high protein diet or urea supplementation. Mild increases in urea may be seen with protein catabolism associated with fasting or prolonged exercise.[12] Interestingly, while urea concentration may increase with fasting in horses, it tends to decrease in ponies.[12] Decreases in urea can occur with protein-poor diets or liver failure.

Creatinine is a by-product of muscle metabolism and therefore is correlated with total muscle mass. Heavily muscled animals may have creatinine concentrations that are normally slightly above reported reference intervals. Release of creatinine from muscle during exercise, fasting, muscle wasting, or rhabdomyolysis can influence creatinine concentration. In addition, if the Jaffe's colorimetric method is used to measure creatinine, the concentration of creatinine may be artifactually increased in the presence of non-creatinine chromagens; this may actually be the main reason for the increase in creatinine associated with fasting. Spurious increases in creatinine have also been associated with various metabolic disorders and administration of cephalosporin antibiotics.[10] Hyperbilirubinemia can interfere with the measurement of creatinine, resulting in falsely low values. During the first few days of a foal's life, creatinine concentration can be quite high relative to adult reference values, but should decrease to adult reference values by the age of three to five days if the kidneys are healthy.[3, 12]

The BUN:creatinine ratio is not very useful in determining whether azotemia is pre-renal, renal, or post-renal, but it has been used to help differentiate between acute and chronic renal disease. In many (but not all) cases, the ratio will be <10:1 in acute renal failure and >10:1 in chronic renal failure.[10] If the ratio becomes >15:1 with chronic renal failure, this may be an indication of excess protein in the diet.[13]

Reabsorption and electrolyte regulation

For many of the solutes that are filtered through glomeruli, reabsorption predominantly occurs in the proximal tubules, whereas additional regulation may occur further along the nephron. Because all glucose is normally absorbed in the proximal tubules unless the serum concentration exceeds the renal threshold, the presence of glycosuria without hyperglycemia is an indication of proximal tubule dysfunction. Glycosuria is more commonly seen with acute renal failure than chronic.

Serum electrolyte abnormalities can also be seen with tubular dysfunction, including hyponatremia, hypochloremia, hyper- or hypocalcemia, hypophosphatemia, hyper- or hypokalemia, and increased or decreased bicarbonate levels. Horses normally excrete a large amount of calcium, and serum calcium concentrations are often abnormal with equine renal failure. Hypercalcemia is commonly seen with chronic renal failure, whereas hypocalcemia is more commonly associated with acute renal failure.

A relatively easy way to assess whether there is decreased reabsorption of electrolytes by the kidney is to determine their fractional excretion (FE). The FE of sodium is most commonly determined; the second most common electrolyte used is phosphorous. FE is calculated using the concentrations of the electrolyte and creatinine in both serum and urine and plugging those numbers into the following equation:

$$\frac{\text{Serum creatinine}}{\text{Urine creatinine}} \times \frac{\text{Urine sodium}}{\text{Serum sodium}} \times 100 \qquad (5.1)$$

The fractional excretion of sodium and phosphorous is normally <1%. Values greater than 1% (0.8%) imply tubular dysfunction, unless the animal is receiving a diet very high in sodium or phosphorous, has been administered polyionic intravenous fluids or certain medications (furosemide), recently performed low-intensity exercise, or there is aldosterone or parathormone deficiency.[5]

Water conservation and blood volume regulation

Greater than 99% of what is filtered through the glomerulus is reabsorbed by the renal tubules. Water is largely reabsorbed in the proximal tubules and additional water is reabsorbed as the tubular fluid travels through the descending limb of the loop of Henle. The final concentration of urine is determined by processes within the collecting ducts. Glomerular filtrate, as it enters proximal tubules, has a specific gravity of 1.008–1.014. Therefore, if urine leaving the bladder has a similar specific gravity, it is considered isosthenuric. The specific gravity becomes more concentrated (hypersthenuric) as the tubular fluid travels through the descending limb of the loop of Henle but then becomes less concentrated (hyposthenuric) as electrolytes are actively reabsorbed in the ascending limb, which is relatively impermeable to water. Hyposthenuric urine, therefore, requires energy and functioning tubules. As the tubular fluid travels through collecting ducts, final water regulation occurs under the influence of vasopressin. Vasopressin causes the collecting ducts to become permeable to water so that water can flow from the less concentrated tubular fluid to the highly osmotic medullary interstitium. Hypertonicity of the medulla is necessary for this water movement and is reliant on adequate urea and sodium concentrations in maintaining an osmotic gradient.

If an animal becomes dehydrated, the urine should become concentrated before azotemia occurs. Therefore, if an animal is azotemic with a urine specific gravity <1.025, the kidneys are not able to concentrate appropriately. This is most often due to renal disease, which should be a differential anytime one sees azotemia with lack of urine concentration, but it is possible that the kidneys are not concentrating urine for other reasons. Marked hyponatremia can lead to medullary washout (the lack of a hypertonic medullary interstitium) so that water is not drawn through the pores of the collecting ducts. Osmotic diuresis, as can occur with diabetes mellitus, decreases the concentration difference between the tubular fluid and medullary interstitium as well as increases the rate of flow through the tubules, resulting in lack of urine concentration. If vasopressin is lacking (central diabetes insipidus), water cannot be reabsorbed across the collecting ducts. Likewise, the kidneys can be resistant to the action of vasopressin, which is thought to contribute to the lack of urine-concentrating ability associated with hyperadrenocorticism, endotoxemia, and hypercalcemia.

Other renal functions

Glomeruli, while allowing many solutes to enter the nephron, are also designed to prevent many blood products from being filtered into the urinary space. Substances about the size of albumin and above do not readily make their way into the glomerular filtrate. In addition to size, the negative charge of the glomerular basement membrane helps maintain the filtration barrier.[15] If this barrier is damaged, substances that normally do not freely filter across, such as albumin, can be lost into the urine, resulting in proteinuria and, eventually, hypoalbuminemia.

An additional function of the kidney is the production of erythropoietin to maintain erythrocyte numbers. Nonregenerative anemia can occur with chronic renal disease due to decreased erythropoietin production.

Urinalysis

Gross evaluation

A full urinalysis is important in the evaluation of the urinary tract. The gross appearance of the urine should be documented, as well as any changes in character of the urine observed during micturition. Evidence of hemorrhage seen only in the early phase of micturition is indicative of urethral hemorrhage, while consistent bloodiness is suggestive of hemorrhage in the bladder or above. Urine often contains more particulates during the end of micturition, as settled sludge within the bladder is often expelled then.[8] Equine urine can normally appear light yellow to dark amber or light brown and is often cloudy, containing crystalline material and mucous (Figure 5.2). Pale, clear urine is associated with polyuria. Urine can appear pink to red with hematuria or hemoglobinuria, red to dark-brown with myoglobinuria or methemoglobinuria, and yellow–brown with bilirubinuria. Normal urine can become darker or even reddish in color over time due to oxidation products present.[14] Ideally urinalysis should be performed within one hour of collection, because objects such as casts can dissolve quickly.

Urine-specific gravity

It is recommended that urine-specific gravity be measured with a refractometer rather than relying on a dipstick reading. Healthy horses typically maintain a urine-specific gravity >1.020. The isosthenuric range of horse urine is 1.008–1.014, indicating that the urine coming out of the bladder has a similar concentration to the glomerular filtrate from the blood, without any significant concentration or dilution. If urine-specific gravity is greater than 1.025 or less

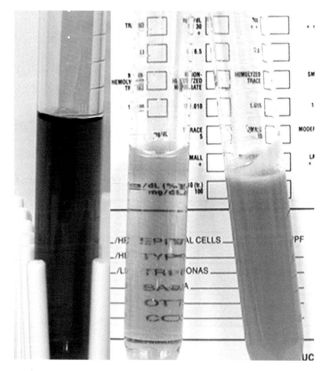

Figure 5.2   Gross evaluation of urine. Equine urine is frequently cloudy, as seen in the right tube. The middle tube contains pale, clear urine, as often seen with polyuria. The reddish brown color of the urine on the left is due to myoglobinuria.

than 1.008, it can be presumed that at least 33% of kidney mass is functioning since dilution of urine, as well as concentration, requires functional tubules.

Pre-renal azotemia is usually due to dehydration, and properly functioning kidneys will conserve water, resulting in concentrated urine, before an animal will become azotemic. Therefore, isosthenuric urine in the face of azotemia is always abnormal. Isosthenuria without azotemia could indicate a lack of ability to concentrate urine, but this would have to be confirmed by some other means.

Concentrating ability is tested by a water deprivation test. This needs to be done carefully, so that an animal will not become dangerously dehydrated if it is not able to concentrate its urine. An animal may also need time to reestablish hyperosmolarity of the medullary interstitium if there has been medullary washout. If urine concentration occurs only after administration of vasopressin, this confirms that a deficit of endogenous vasopressin is the reason for the lack of concentration and not renal disease.

Hyposthenuric urine typically implies interference with or lack of vasopressin or, possibly, water overload. Nursing foals frequently have dilute urine because of their diet, but they normally have the ability to concentrate urine >1.030 from the time of birth.[1]

Reagent test strips

The pH of urine from healthy adult horses is alkaline, usually between 7.5 and 8.5, largely as a result of a herbivorous diet. Bacteriuria, high grain diets, intravenous fluids, strenuous exercise, and starvation can result in acid urine. Healthy suckling foals have acidic urine due to their milk diet. Metabolic acidosis is a common cause of acid urine in adult horses, and paradoxical aciduria can also be seen with metabolic alkalosis, especially when combined with hypokalemia (Figure 5.3).

Equine urine does not normally contain glucose, ketones, or bilirubin. It is thought that the renal threshold for serum glucose is around 150 mg/dl. If glucosuria is present and the serum glucose concentration is less than 150 mg/dl, this is an indication of renal tubular dysfunction. Ketonuria is uncommon as horses are poorly ketogenic. The presence of bilirubinuria should be correlated with the serum chemistry panel and CBC for detection of liver disease, post-hepatic biliary obstruction, or hemolytic anemia.

Equine urine should contain very little protein. In concentrated urine (>1.035), normal protein concentrations may produce a trace to 1+ reaction on the dipstick. False elevations in protein concentration can be expected in horses since alkaline urine may cause false positives on reagent pads. Any increase in urine protein as indicated by a dipstick should be verified; this is often done using the semiquantitative sulfosalicylic acid precipitation test.

Glomerular diseases are often associated with marked proteinuria, while tubular lesions can result in milder proteinuria. Hemorrhage into the urinary tract and inflammation can also result in high urine protein concentrations.

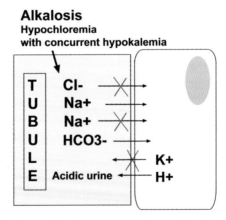

Alkalosis
Hypochloremia
with concurrent hypokalemia

T	Cl-
U	Na+
B	Na+
U	HCO3-
L	K+
E	Acidic urine H+

Figure 5.3 Paradoxical aciduria. In horses with metabolic alkalosis, chloride is less available for reabsorption with sodium into proximal tubular epithelial cells, so there is decreased sodium resorption in the proximal tubule. Depletion of chloride results in resorption of bicarbonate with sodium, exacerbating the alkalosis. If there is a metabolic alkalosis with concurrent volume depletion, sodium resorption is increased in the distal tubule via aldosterone by exchange with a cation, usually potassium, but also hydrogen. With concurrent hypokalemia, potassium is conserved and increased hydrogen is excreted in its place, resulting in aciduria and an exacerbated alkalosis.

Urine protein-to-creatinine (UPC) ratios can be used to assess more accurately the amount of protein in the urine. The UPC ratio should be less than 1.0 in a normal horse.[16] UPC ratios are not indicated if there is evidence of inflammation or hemorrhage in the urinary tract, because protein associated with these processes cannot be differentiated from proteins that may be present due to glomerular or tubular disease. Proteinuria can be transient and not indicative of renal disease, such as can occur post-exercise in horses.[8,10] It is, therefore, important to establish if proteinuria is persistent before further work-up.

The reagent pad for blood measures myoglobin as well as hemoglobin. Therefore, a positive reaction can be due to free hemoglobin from lysed erythrocytes, whole red blood cells, or myoglobin. Some pads help distinguish whole erythrocytes from free hemoglobin. Hemoglobin from intravascular hemolysis may be differentiated from myoglobinuria by examining the color of plasma or serum since hemoglobin can often be visualized while myoglobin will not be. Measuring serum creatine kinase concentration to assess muscle injury, and performing a CBC to look for anemia can also be useful in differentiating the cause of a positive blood pad. Most positive blood reactions are due to hemorrhage within the urinary tract. This can be due to trauma, uroliths, inflammation, neoplasia, vascular defects, or coagulopathy.

Urine sediment exam

The sediment exam is performed by centrifuging 5-10 ml of urine at 1,000-1,500 RPM for 5 minutes and removing the supernatant. After resuspending the sedimented material in the small amount of fluid left over, a drop is placed on a slide and coverslipped. The microscope should be adjusted for high contrast; a sediment stain can also be used to enhance visualization.

At low power (10× objective), casts can be detected and counted and an overall view of the sample obtained. In horses, it is important not to mistake strands of mucous for casts (Figure 5.4). The sample should then be examined at high magnification (40× objective) for erythrocytes, leukocytes, epithelial cells, bacteria, crystals, or any unusual findings. If high numbers of calcium carbonate crystals are obscuring other objects within the sediment, 10% acidic acid can be added to the sediment to dissolve the crystals. If there is uncertainty about what is visualized in a wet-mount, the coverslip can be carefully removed (or a new slide made from the sediment), air-dried, and then stained for cytologic evaluation.

Casts are formed from material within and take the shape of renal tubule lumens. The foundation of all casts is Tamm-Horsfall glycoprotein, which is a normal secretion of renal tubular cells. Hyaline casts contain mostly protein and their number can be increased with renal disease, severe dehydration, and protein-losing nephropathy. Other casts are characterized by what type of cells are trapped within the protein framework (erythrocytes, leukocytes, epithelial cells) or as granular casts if cellular features have degraded so that cells cannot be recognized, or as waxy casts if cellular products are extremely broken down (Figure 5.5). Erythrocytes and leukocytes indicate hemorrhage

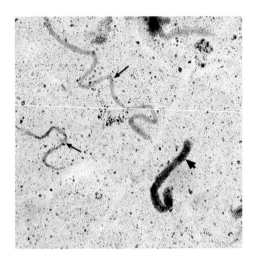

Figure 5.4 Sedimented urine from a horse with rhabdomyolysis. Granular casts indicate renal tubular damage (large arrowhead). Mucous strands are common in equine urine and should not be confused with casts (small arrows). Unstained wet mount, 10× objective.

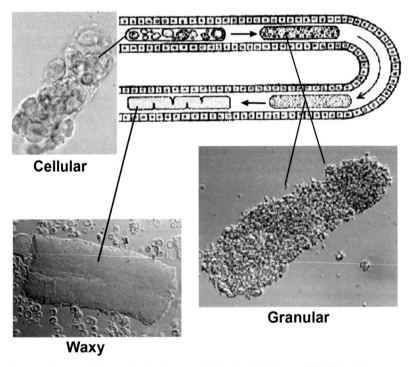

Figure 5.5 Cast formation in the renal tubules. Tubular epithelial cells, leukocytes, and/or erythrocytes sloughed into the tubular lumen form a cast of the tubule. Cellular casts have been immediately flushed from the lumen into urine. In contrast, granular and waxy casts have been retained in the lumen, where they degrade from a cellular to granular and then waxy appearance. Thus, cellular, granular, and waxy casts imply a single process.

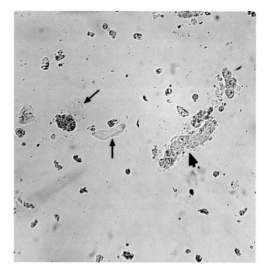

Figure 5.6   Sedimented urine from a severely dehydrated animal. Cellular casts are present, indicating sloughing of renal tubular cells (large arrowhead). A few squamous epithelial cells can be seen in free-catch urine samples (small arrows). Unstained wet mount, 40× objective.

or inflammation within the nephron, respectively. Epithelial cell casts indicate a tubular insult that has caused cell sloughing (Figure 5.6). A few hyaline and rare granular casts may be seen in normal urine, but if increased numbers of casts are present, this is an indication of renal insult.

Urine should contain very few cells. A sediment preparation made from 10 mLs of urine should contain <5-8 erythrocytes or leukocytes per high magnification (40× objective) field.[14] Few epithelial cells should also be present. Squamous epithelial cells may be present within voided samples (Figure 5.6). Increased numbers of transitional epithelial cells may be seen with inflammation, neoplasia, or trauma. Dysplastic changes occur within transitional epithelial cells associated with inflammation, therefore a few irregular clusters of epithelial cells should not raise immediate concern for neoplasia if associated with an inflammatory process.

Inflammation is present with >8 neutrophils per high power field (40× objective). Bacterial infection may be present even if bacteria are not seen. For culture, urine should be collected by catheterization; foals also can be collected by cystocentesis. Greater than 8 erythrocytes per high dry field indicates hemorrhage within the urinary tract. This could be due to trauma, uroliths, inflammation, neoplasia, vascular defects, or coagulopathy. Mild hematuria can be seen post-exercise.[11,14]

Crystals are very common in horse urine, particularly calcium carbonate crystals (Figure 5.7). Calcium phosphate, triple phosphate, and low numbers of calcium oxalate crystals can also be seen. If urine is carefully collected, it should contain very few or no bacteria. Other substances that may be seen

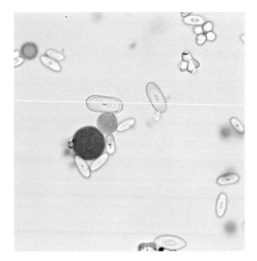

Figure 5.7 Calcium carbonate crystals. Note the concentric lamellar structure and the range of possible shapes of the crystals. Wright-Giemsa stain, 100× objective.

in urine include sperm from stallions, plant or other particulate matter in a voided sample, parasite eggs, or lymphoma cells.

Laboratory abnormalities associated with different disease states

Acute renal failure

In acute renal failure (ARF), the horse will be azotemic with isosthenuria. BUN-to-creatinine ratios are typically <10:1. Hypermagnesemia is often associated with the decrease in GFR. Hyponatremia and hypochloremia are often present and the FE of sodium is > 1.0. Serum calcium and phosphorous concentrations can be variable, from low to normal to high. Phosphaturia is typically present early in the disease process. Enzymuria and glycosuria are also often present.

There is typically a mild to moderate proteinuria associated with acute renal failure. Results of the urine sediment examination may vary with disease process. With acute interstitial nephritis there may be pyuria, WBC casts, eosinophiluria and eosinophilia, and/or hematuria. With acute tubular necrosis, either associated with ischemia or nephrotoxins, granular casts are often present but hematuria is less common.

Chronic renal failure

Horses with chronic renal failure (CRF) will be azotemic and have a urine-specific gravity <1.020. BUN-to-creatinine ratios are often >10:1, likely due to variable distribution of these nitrogenous compounds within body fluids.

It is also thought that urinary excretion of creatinine occurs in chronic renal failure. Serum creatinine concentration can be used as a rough guide to the prognosis of CRF, keeping in mind that there are other factors that also influence creatinine levels. In general, a doubling of creatinine roughly equals a 50% decline in GFR.[9] Horses with creatinine concentrations below 5 mg/dL can do fairly well, at least short term and possibly long term, with management, while creatinine concentrations between 5 and 10 mg/dL are associated with declining renal function. Creatinine concentrations >15 mg/dL indicate a grave prognosis.[13] Monitoring creatinine concentrations over time can be useful in monitoring disease progression.

Hypercalcemia and hypophosphatemia are common in equine CFR. The degree of hypercalcemia is related to the amount of calcium in the diet, as the kidney normally plays a large role in excreting excess calcium.[6] Mild hyponatremia and hypochloremia may be present due to decreased tubular reabsorption, although fractional excretion values may not be abnormal. Most horses with CRF have a normal acid-base status or may be slightly alkalotic. Metabolic acidosis typically occurs in the terminal stages of CRF. Horses with CRF may also be hyperkalemic due to decreased excretion or to metabolic acidosis. Because of decreased erythropoietin production associated with CRF and, possibly, decreased erythrocyte lifespan with exposure to uremic toxins, a mild non-regenerative anemia is often associated with CRF. Horses with CRF can also develop hypercholesterolemia and hypertriglyceridemia, occasionally severe enough to be seen as lipemia.[13] Glycosuria and enzymuria are less common in CRF than in ARF, as are elevated FEs, despite urinary electrolyte losses.[13]

There is typically a degree of proteinuria associated with CRF, and horses are commonly mildly hypoalbuminemic. UPC ratios can be used to assess protein loss more quantitatively. Because urine is isosthenuric and the animals are polyuric, urine sediment is typically devoid of crystals and mucous. Pyuria may also be nonexistent even with infection of the urinary tract. Occasionally, erythrocytes or leukocytes may be seen in urine, depending on the underlying disease process.

Urinary tract rupture

Uroperitoneum secondary to rupture of the urinary bladder is not always easy to diagnose based on serum biochemical changes. The presence of azotemia is variable. The most consistent serum biochemical finding is hyponatremia. Hyperkalemia and hypochloremia are the next most common serum biochemical abnormalities, although all of these changes are less likely if there has been prior fluid administration.[2,4,5,7] Since other disease processes can manifest similarly, collection of abdominal fluid and comparing the concentration of creatinine in the fluid to the serum creatinine concentration is a valuable diagnostic tool. A fluid creatinine concentration >2× the serum concentration confirms uroperitoneum.[7] Presence of calcium carbonate crystals in the peritoneal fluid cytology is also diagnostic for uroperitoneum (see Chapter 11).

"Early" renal disease

Horses are considered to be in renal failure when there is azotemia and isosthenuria, but these are relatively insensitive markers for renal disease. In general, approximately 75% of renal function is lost by the time an animal becomes azotemic and approximately 67% is lost before urine can no longer be concentrated. Ideally, it would be advantageous to be able to diagnose renal disease before 67-75% of the functional kidney is lost so that appropriate therapies or preventative measures can be taken in a timely manner. Direct measurement of GFR is a good way to detect renal dysfunction early in the disease course, but this is not routinely performed, and readers are encouraged to look elsewhere for information on this technique.[8,10]

If a horse presents with isosthenuria without azotemia, it should be determined whether this is because of intrinsic renal disease or due to some other reason. In this scenario, if a cause for the isosthenuric urine is not evident on the CBC, biochemical panel, or urinalysis, one may wish to determine first if the horse can concentrate its urine by rechecking at a later date. If the horse is persistently isosthenuric, one should consider performing a water deprivation test.

Other tests of renal functional ability or injury include FE of sodium and assessment of enzymuria. Elevations in FE indicate that the renal tubules are not functioning properly and the presence of enzymuria indicates damage to the renal tubular cells. Serial assessments may be more useful than a one-time test, and negative findings do not necessarily rule out intrinsic renal diseases.

The urine enzymes that have shown some utility in assessing equine renal insult are GGT, NAG, ALP (all proximal tubular), and LDH (distal tubular).[10] Enzyme activity is typically compared to creatinine concentrations and reported as a ratio. Activities for these enzymes in healthy horse urine are reported to be 0-25 IU GGT/g creatinine, <1 IU NAG/g creatinine, 0-28 IU ALP/g creatinine, and 0-12 IU LDH/g creatinine.[10] Clinically significant thresholds of increased enzymatic activity have not been defined; therefore, caution must be used in the interpretation of results. For GGT, a ratio >100 IU/g is likely clinically significant.[8,10] Many conditions can affect enzymatic activity; therefore, measurements should be assessed within 72 hours of collection and, if not immediately analyzed, the sample should be refrigerated but not frozen.[10] NAG activity is affected by alkaline urine and is most useful when urine pH is acidic to neutral.

Glomerular disease

Renal amyloidosis is rare in horses, but diseases of renal glomeruli are typically characterized by moderate to marked proteinuria. With glomerular disease, animals may become azotemic but can still concentrate urine if the distal tubules are not involved in the disease process. With acute glomerulonephritis, red cell casts may be seen on urinalysis.

Strenuous exercise

Exercise has been associated with transient proteinuria, hematuria, hemoglobinuria, and myoglobinuria.[8,10,14] It is important to keep in mind the timing of urine collection with respect to exercise or to confirm persistence of abnormal findings at a later date.

References

1. Axon JE, Palmer JE. 2008. Clinical pathology of the foal. *Vet Clin North Am Equine Pract* 24:357-385.
2. Behr MJ, Hackett RP, Bentinck-Smith J, et al. 1981. Metabolic abnormalities associated with rupture of the urinary bladder in foals. *J Am Vet Med Assoc* 178:263-266.
3. Chaney KP, Holcombe SJ, Schott HC II, et al. 2010. Spurious hypercreatininemia: 28 neonatal foals (2000-2008). *J Vet Emerg Crit Care* 10:244-249.
4. Dunkel B, Palmer JE, Olson KN, et al. 2005. Uroperitoneum in 32 foals: Influence of intravenous fluid therapy, infection, and sepsis. *J Vet Intern Med* 19:889-893.
5. Higuchi T, Nonao Y, Senba H. 2002. Repair of urinary bladder rupture through a urethrotomy and urethral sphincterotomy in four postpartum mares. *Vet Surg* 31:344-348.
6. LeRoy B, Woolums JW, Davis E, et al. 2011. The relationship between serum calcium concentration and outcome in horses with renal failure presented to referral hospitals. *J Vet Intern Med* 25:1426-1430.
7. Richardson DW, Kohn CW. 1983. Uroperitoneum in the foal. *J Am Vet Med Assoc* 182:267-271.
8. Savage CJ. 2008. Urinary clinical pathologic findings and glomerular filtration rate in the horse. *Vet Clin North Am Equine Pract* 24:387-404.
9. Schott HC II. 2004. Chronic renal failure. In *Equine Internal Medicine*, 2nd ed., pp. 1231-1253. St Louis: Saunders.
10. Schott HC II. 2004. Examination of the Urinary System. In *Equine Internal Medicine*, 2nd ed., pp. 1200-1220. St Louis: Saunders.
11. Schott HC II. 2004. Hematuria. In *Equine Internal Medicine*, 2nd ed., pp. 1270-1276. St Louis: Saunders.
12. Schott HC II. 2004. Renal Physiology. In *Equine Internal Medicine*, 2nd ed., pp. 1184-1199. St Louis: Saunders.
13. Schott HC II. 2007. Chronic renal failure in horses. *Vet Clin North Am Equine Pract* 23:593-612.
14. Schumacher J. 2007. Hematuria and pigmenturia of horses. *Vet Clin North Am Equine Pract* 23:655-675.
15. Toribio RE. 2007. Essentials of equine renal and urinary tract physiology. *Vet Clin North Am Equine Pract* 23:533-561.
16. Uberti B, Eberle DB, Pressler BM, et al. 2009. Determination of and correlation between urine protein excretion and urine protein-to-creatinine ratio values during a 24-hour period in healthy horses and ponies. *Am J Vet Res* 70:1551-1556.

Chapter 6

Acid-Base and Electrolytes

Andrea A. Bohn

Evaluation of electrolyte concentrations and acid-base balance is typically used more to assess severity of disease and to guide treatment rather than as a diagnostic tool, although certain changes can aid in the diagnosis of some disorders. Abnormalities in electrolyte concentrations and acid-base balance are often associated with diarrhea, colic, rhabdomyolysis, prolonged exercise and sweating, renal disease, and endocrine abnormalities. This chapter focuses on electrolyte and acid-base changes commonly seen in horses and their causes.

Acid-base

Maintaining the proper pH of blood and tissues is important for maintaining optimal enzymatic and cellular function. The normal pH range for horse blood is approximately 7.38-7.44. Below this range the blood is acidemic and above the range it is alkalemic. Various processes are in place to help maintain normal pH. These involve the respiratory system, in which carbon dioxide (CO_2) is exhaled, the kidneys, where excess acids or bases can be excreted, and buffer systems, the most important of which for our purposes of evaluation is bicarbonate (HCO_3). An abnormality in acid-base balance is not a disease, but a reflection of many possible disease processes. Evaluation of the acid-base status can give an indication that a serious problem exists.

Acid-base abnormalities are traditionally described as being either a respiratory acidosis or alkalosis or a metabolic acidosis or alkalosis. A primary disorder within one of these systems typically results in a compensatory response in the other. Since the respiratory system is concerned with CO_2, which is weakly acidic, and the metabolic system handles HCO_3, which is a weak base, the movement of the compensatory response should be in the same direction (up or down) as the primary disorder. To determine which is the primary disorder, one must look at the blood pH. If the blood is acidemic, the system that is moving in the acidic direction is the source of the primary disorder. If the blood is alkalemic, the system that is moving in the alkaline direction

Equine Clinical Pathology, First Edition. Edited by Raquel M. Walton.

has the primary disorder. If both branches are moving in an alkaline or acidic direction, there is a mixed acid-base disorder. Likewise, if the compensatory side has shifted more than expected for a compensatory response, there is likely a mixed acid-base disorder. In those cases, the pH may be normal, even with marked acid base abnormalities.

Steps to evaluating acid-base status

The following six-point approach to acid-base status is very useful for a complete characterization:

1. What is the blood pH? Is there an acidemia (<7.38 pH) or alkalemia (>7.44 pH)?
2. Is pCO_2 high (acidic) or low (alkalotic)?
    Is this contributing to the pH change?
    Is this a compensatory response?
3. Is HCO_3 low (acidic) or high (alkalotic)?
    Is this contributing to the pH change?
    Is this a compensatory response?
4. What is the anion gap?
5. What is the corrected chloride concentration?
6. What is the albumin concentration?

Bicarbonate and chloride (Cl) concentrations as well as anion gap (AG) are routinely provided within a serum biochemistry panel, which provides important information in regards to the acid-base status of a horse. A complete characterization of acid-base status, however, requires a full blood gas panel (preferably on arterial blood). Anion gap, when increased, is always an indication of metabolic acidosis. Bicarbonate and Cl concentrations also reflect acid base status, but whether abnormalities in these substances are due to primary metabolic derangements, compensatory mechanisms in response to respiratory acid-base imbalances, or there is a mixed acid-base disturbance often cannot be determined without also knowing the pH and pCO_2 of the blood. Table 6.1 describes expected results for uncomplicated acid-base abnormalities.

Bicarbonate

Bicarbonate is an important buffer in the blood and its concentration therefore reflects the acid-base status of an animal. Changes in HCO_3 concentration can be due to metabolic derangements or compensation for respiratory acidosis or alkalosis. Bicarbonate concentration is typically reported either as total CO_2 (TCO2), which is normally about 5% higher than HCO_3, or as HCO_3 concentration. In this chapter, bicarbonate will be designated as HCO_3.

Exposure of blood or serum to air can result in CO_2 release, which causes underestimation of HCO_3. In contrast, allowing blood to stand without exposure

Table 6.1   Uncomplicated acid-base abnormalities and their expected changes

Acid-Base abnormality	pH	pCO$_2$	HCO$_3$	Cl	AG
High anion gap metabolic acidosis with respiratory compensation	L	L	L	N	H
Hyperchloremic metabolic acidosis with respiratory compensation	L	L	L	H	N
Hypochloremic metabolic alkalosis with respiratory compensation	H	H	H	L	N
Respiratory acidosis with metabolic compensation	L	H	H	L	N
Respiratory alkalosis with metabolic compensation	H	L	L	H	N

H, high; L, low; N, normal.

to air may result in overestimation of HCO$_3$ due to metabolic processes. Therefore, appropriate handling of blood samples is an important step in laboratory analysis.

Metabolic acidosis and alkalosis

Chloride-associated acid-base abnormalities

With primary metabolic acid-base abnormalities, when AG is normal (no increase in organic acids), changes in HCO$_3$ concentration are associated with a converse shift in Cl concentration. In this instance, the pH should reflect the HCO$_3$ and Cl concentrations, and if there is respiratory compensation, the pCO$_2$ will have moved in the same direction (increased or decreased) as HCO$_3$. To determine that there is a primary metabolic acidosis or alkalosis with respiratory compensation or vice versa, it is, again, necessary to evaluate the pH and pCO$_2$. Hypochloremic metabolic alkalosis occurs when HCO$_3$ is retained in the blood as Cl is lost from or sequestered within the upper GI tract or lost from excessive sweating. Hyperchloremic metabolic acidosis occurs when Cl is retained in response to HCO$_3$ loss from the intestinal tract or the kidneys (renal tubular acidosis).

Anion gap

Bicarbonate is a very important buffer for endogenous and exogenous acids. Endogenous acids include lactic acid and uremic acids; ketoacids are common in other species, but horses are poorly ketogenic. Exogenous acids include metabolites of ethylene glycol and salicylate. An increase in any of these acids results in a decrease in HCO$_3$ concentration as it buffers the hydrogen ion. While there are methods to measure many of the acids that cause a metabolic acidosis, an easy way to determine their presence is by calculating the AG. The AG is based on the fact that the numbers of negative and positive charges in plasma are equal. We do not routinely measure all substances in the blood and there are, therefore, many unmeasured anions and cations present. The commonly measured cations are sodium (Na) and potassium (K) and the commonly measured anions are Cl and HCO_3. Because the sum of unmeasured and measured cations must equal the sum of unmeasured and measured anions in blood, we can determine the difference between the unmeasured components (AG) by calculating the difference between the measured components. And since the number of unmeasured cations usually does not change significantly, any abnormality in AG is related to the number of anions.

A decrease in AG is associated with hypoalbuminemia since the predominant unmeasured anion in health is albumin. An increased AG indicates the presence of additional unmeasured anions in the blood; after HCO_3 buffers the hydrogen ion from excess endogenous or exogenous acids, the corresponding anion is left in circulation. Chloride concentration does not change with high AG metabolic acidosis since the decrease in negative charge from HCO_3 buffering is offset by the negative charge of the unmeasured anion present. Hypoalbuminemia can offset and mask the presence of other unmeasured anions when determined by AG.

Respiratory acidosis and alkalosis

Respiratory acidosis typically occurs with respiratory depression or pulmonary disease and the resulting decrease in the amount of CO_2 exhaled. Respiratory alkalosis occurs with hyperventilation (due to pain, anxiety, or iatrogenic means) as the result of increased amounts of CO_2 being exhaled.

The evaluation of the respiratory components of acid-base balance requires knowledge of blood pH and pCO_2. Since pCO_2 is acidic and HCO_3 is basic, a primary increase in pCO_2 is compensated by an increase in HCO_3 and a primary decrease in pCO_2 is compensated by a decrease in HCO_3. When there is a primary respiratory acidosis (increased pCO_2), HCO_3 is retained by the kidneys to compensate for the acidemia. When there is a primary respiratory alkalosis (decreased pCO_2), the kidneys increase HCO_3 excretion in compensation. As HCO_3 concentrations shift to compensate for respiratory acid-base imbalances, Cl concentrations shift in the opposite direction to maintain electrical neutrality.

Compensatory mechanisms

If there are abnormalities in the acid-base balance from metabolic processes, the respiratory system can act quickly to blow off either more or less CO_2 to help maintain blood pH. This compensation can take place within minutes to hours. In general, for every 1 mEq of HCO_3 abnormality, the respiratory system is able to adjust by about 0.7 mmHg CO_2. The lungs blow off extra CO_2 to compensate for metabolic acidosis and they retain CO_2 to compensate for metabolic alkalosis.

Several hours to days are needed for the kidneys to respond to respiratory acidosis or alkalosis. The kidneys eventually excrete an increased amount of HCO_3 to compensate for respiratory alkalosis or retain an increased amount for respiratory acidosis. In respiratory acidosis, for every 10 mmHg increase in PCO_2 the HCO_3 concentration is expected to increase by 1-2 mEq in the acute phase and by 3-4 mEq if chronic. In respiratory alkalosis, for every 10 mmHg decrease in PCO_2 the HCO_3 concentration is expected to decrease by 2-3 mEq in the acute phase and by 4-6 mEq if chronic.

Base excess

Other buffers in the blood besides HCO_3 include sulfates, phosphates, and hemoglobin, thus the concentration of HCO_3 does not always reflect the total buffering capacity of the blood. Base excess (BE) is a reported value that indicates how far off from the normal total buffering capacity an animal is. Another way to think of it is that BE indicates how much acid needs to be added in order to bring the pH back to normal. In health, the reference interval of BE is about -4 to $+4$. Numbers less than -4 indicate a deficiency in anionic buffers (a negative base excess) and therefore an acidosis, while numbers greater than $+4$ indicate an excess of anionic buffers and the presence of an alkalosis that may require addition of acid to bring the pH back to normal.

Electrolytes

Sodium

Sodium concentration and water balance are dependent on each other, therefore when considering reasons for abnormalities in serum Na concentrations, one must also take into consideration water balance. Hydration status is typically determined by a combination of physical examination and laboratory assessments. Decreased skin turgor, increased capillary refill time, and tacky mucous membranes are subjective assessments of dehydration. Hemoconcentration is a result of dehydration that may be evidenced by detecting an increase in PCV and plasma protein concentration. Overhydration in horses is rare and typically does not occur unless there is decreased water excretion from the kidneys, which can be associated with renal, cardiac, or liver disorders. Psychogenic polydypsia can potentially lead to overhydration, but the renal system can usually handle increased water intake.

Hypernatremia

Hypernatremia occurs if there is excess Na (rare) or decreased water content (Table 6.2). The potential for excess Na exists if animals have access to and ingest salt without having access to fresh water. Inappropriate administration of hypertonic fluids can also lead to Na excess. Most causes of hypernatremia include either pure water loss or loss of hypotonic fluids where water loss is greater than electrolyte loss.

Table 6.2   Common causes of electrolyte abnormalities in horses

Sodium
  Hypernatremia
    Dehydration
      Insensible water loss
      Diabetes insipidus (central or nephrogenic)

  Hyponatremia
    Hypertonic fluid loss or isotonic loss with water repletion
      Gastrointestinal disease
      Renal disease
      Sweat loss
    Electrolyte and fluid shifts due to third-spacing of fluids
      Uroperitoneum
      Severe hypoalbuminemia
      Severe hepatic disease
      Severe cardiac disease

Chloride
  Hyperchloremia
    See hypernatremia
    Metabolic acidosis
      HCO_3 loss or sequestration
        Intestinal disease
        Renal loss
    Metabolic compensation for respiratory alkalosis

  Hypochloremia
    See hyponatremia
    Metabolic alkalosis
      HCO_3 retention with Cl loss/sequestration
        Upper GI obstruction
        Sweat loss
    Metabolic compensation for respiratory acidosis

Pure water loss occurs with insensible water loss associated with evaporation from lungs and skin as well as fecal and urine water excretion. If insensible water losses are greater than water intake, serum Na concentration will increase. Increased water loss can occur with strenuous exercise resulting in hypernatremia immediately post-exercise. Decreased water intake can be due to an animal not having access to water or to a defective thirst response as has been seen in horses with debilitating brain disease.[18] It must be remembered that serum Na concentration is related to the ratio of Na to water within vascular plasma and does not necessarily reflect the body's Na content. Hypernatremia may be present when there is decreased water intake and/or increased water loss, even though total body Na concentrations may be depleted from excessive loss during sweating.[14,21,25]

With renal disease there is often loss of electrolytes along with decreased urine concentrating ability, but when there is a defect primarily associated with concentration, as with either central or nephrogenic diabetes insipidus (lack of ADH activity), hypotonic fluid loss and hypernatremia can occur.

Hyponatremia

Hyponatremia most commonly occurs with loss of isotonic fluid and subsequent water repletion or, possibly, with loss of hypertonic fluid (more Na lost than water; Table 6.2). Loss of isotonic fluid can result in hypovolemia, which stimulates renal water retention and thirst. Common sites of isotonic fluid loss include body cavities, the intestinal tract, kidneys, or the skin (sweating).

Many different digestive system disorders cause isotonic fluid loss, including diarrhea, sequestration of fluid in the gastrointestinal tract with ileus or obstruction, gastric reflux, or esophageal obstruction and loss of saliva. Renal failure or diuresis can lead to sodium wasting into the urine. Hyponatremia is also often seen with uroperitoneum since the urine leaking into the abdominal cavity is of low Na concentration, which rapidly equilibrates with plasma Na.[7] Third-space fluid accumulation can lead to hyponatremia because of electrolyte and fluid shifts; hyponatremia can become pronounced with repeated removal of isotonic fluid from body cavities. If there is increased water intake and an antidiuretic hormone (ADH) response, dilutional hyponatremia may ensue. Severe hypoalbuminemia, liver disease, or cardiac disease leading to third-spacing of fluids (edema) may result in mild hyponatremia due to water retention in excess of Na retention, especially if total body Na stores are decreased. Equine sweat contains a Na concentration that is equal to or slightly higher than that of blood.[30] Therefore, sweat can be a source of significant Na loss, particularly with exercise. At high ambient temperatures, horses at rest are typically able to maintain normal Na levels. But after an endurance race, plasma sodium concentrations were shown to drop.[39]

Less common reasons for hyponatremia include iatrogenic hypoadrenocorticism, excess administration of Na-poor fluids, excessive water consumption, syndrome of inappropriate ADH secretion, and pseudohyponatremia. Pseudohyponatremia can occur if there are other substances causing hyperosmolality and drawing water into the vascular space, such as marked hyperglycemia or mannitol. Marked hyperlipidemia or hyperproteinemia can also result in pseudohyponatremia on some chemistry analyzers by taking up space within the plasma volume; using an ion-specific electrode to measure serum Na concentration will avoid this problem since it is not affected by protein or lipid content.

Chloride

Hyperchloremia and hypochloremia with water imbalance

To maintain electrical neutrality, Cl typically moves either with Na or opposite to HCO_3. The factors that lead to hypernatremia and hyponatremia similarly affect Cl levels. To determine if the cause of hypochloremia or hyperchloremia is due to the same process affecting Na concentration, one can perform an easy calculation to "correct" Cl for the concentration of Na. This is done by dividing "normal" Na (typically a value from the middle of the reference interval) by the actual Na concentration and multiplying this result by the actual Cl concentration:

$$\frac{Na_{Reference}}{Na_{Measured}} \times Cl_{Measured} \qquad (6.1)$$

This corrects for any water imbalance that is similarly affecting Na concentration. The corrected Cl is then interpreted in the context of the Cl reference interval. If Cl concentration does not correct into the reference interval (or if Na and Cl abnormalities are obviously disproportional), this suggests that there is an acid-base imbalance that should be reflected by a HCO_3 concentration that is inversely related to the Cl concentration.

Hyperchloremia associated with acid-base abnormalities

Hyperchloremia may be associated with metabolic acidosis or with metabolic compensation for respiratory alkalosis (see Table 6.2). Hyperchloremic metabolic acidosis is seen when there is HCO_3 loss from the intestinal tract or kidneys or sequestration of HCO_3 in the gut. Bicarbonate loss from the kidneys occurs in renal tubular acidosis, which is a rare condition in horses, in which there is decreased reabsorption of HCO_3 by renal tubules.[3]

Hypochloremia with acid-base abnormalities

Hypochloremia may be associated with metabolic alkalosis or metabolic compensation for respiratory acidosis (see Table 6.2). Metabolic alkalosis is often due to loss or sequestration of stomach contents. Since horses cannot vomit, hypochloremia with hyperbicarbonatemia should alert one to a possible upper GI obstruction, either physical or functional. Equine sweat contains up to twice as much Cl as in plasma and more Cl than Na.[30] Therefore, hypochloremia can become more severe than hyponatremia from sweat loss, leading to a metabolic alkalosis. Chloride losses are also greater than Na losses with furosemide diuresis.[22]

Potassium

Potassium (K) is an important intracellular ion and less than 2% of total body K is free within plasma. Therefore, plasma concentrations of K are often not an accurate reflection of the whole body content of K. Normally, the horse's diet is high in K and the kidneys are very efficient in excreting the excess.[22] Some K is also lost from the gastrointestinal tract and in sweat. In addition, K can shift between the intracellular and extracellular compartments, resulting in higher or lower serum concentrations. Because equine erythrocytes contain a high concentration of K, serum concentrations of K may be erroneously high with hemolysis; this pseudohyperkalemia should be considered before other causes of hyperkalemia.

Hyperkalemia

Hyperkalemia is usually due either to the shifting of K from the intracellular to extracellular compartments or to decreased excretion from the urinary system (see Table 6.3). Decreased excretion is most commonly associated with anuric or oliguric renal failure or uroperitoneum. The extracellular movement of K is often a result of metabolic acidosis. Potassium is also released from muscle cells during exercise, and hyperkalemia may be seen during and shortly after strenuous exercise.[16,17,33] Severe rhabdomyolysis can result in hyperkalemia because of release from damaged cells.[36]

Hyperkalemic periodic paralysis (HYPP) is a genetic disease in quarter horses and some horses with quarter horse blood in which there is a mutation in a sodium channel; HYPP attacks are associated with high serum K levels.[2]

Hypokalemia

Hypokalemia can result from decreased intake as well as increased loss of K (see Table 6.3). Decreased intake may be due to a number of different causes associated with the quality or the amount of food ingested. Loss of K occurs from the kidneys, gastrointestinal tract, or sweat.

Alkalosis and insulin (often associated with IV administration of glucose-containing fluids) cause the intracellular movement of K and may result in hypokalemia regardless of whole body potassium content.

Table 6.3 Common causes of electrolyte abnormalities in horses

Potassium
Hyperkalemia
  Decreased renal excretion
  Metabolic acidosis
  Release from muscle cells
    Exercise
    Rhabdomyolysis
  HYPP attack

Hypokalemia
  Dietary insufficiency
  Loss
    Gastrointestinal disease
    Renal disease
    Sweat loss

Calcium

Calcium (Ca) is a very important electrolyte that is under tight hormonal control. Calcitonin, vitamin D, and parathyroid hormone (PTH) all act to maintain a narrow plasma Ca concentration from what is ingested, absorbed, and excreted by the gastrointestinal tract, reabsorbed and excreted by the kidneys, and stored within the skeletal system.

Calcium concentration can be measured as total Ca (tCa) or as the ionized form (iCa). The concentration of Ca in its ionized form is what is physiologically relevant and under hormonal control. It is, therefore, preferable to measure the ionized form, which has become more available with point of care analyzers. The remaining Ca in circulation is either bound to albumin or complexed with anions, and therefore the concentration of tCa can fluctuate depending on the amount of these other substances. Abnormalities in iCa concentration are typically related to dysregulation of hormonal control or of excretion. The amount of iCa in circulation is also pH dependent since the pH determines how much Ca binds to proteins. Acidosis results in higher iCa concentrations and alkalosis results in lower iCa concentrations.

Hypercalcemia

Hypercalcemia (see Table 6.4) is common in horses with chronic renal failure and is thought to be associated with the high Ca content of the equine diet. The kidneys normally excrete a large amount of Ca, and tCa concentration was higher in CRF horses fed an alfalfa diet.[28] Reports of iCa in horses with CRF are limited, but in one study, three out of three horses with CRF had high concentrations of iCa and low PTH.[11]

Hypercalcemia associated with neoplastic processes occurs in horses, as in other species, and has been reported with a variety of tumors including lymphoma, multiple myeloma, and some carcinomas.[5,6,9,12,13,23,29,31,37] Humoral hypercalcemia of malignancy is often associated with PTHrP, a protein with PTH-like activity. Neoplasms that cause bony lysis can also result in hypercalcemia.

Less common causes of hypercalcemia include the ingestion of calcinogenic plants (Cestrum diurnum) or other means of vitamin D toxicosis, granulomatous disease, and primary hyperparathyroidism.[26,32,40] Primary hyperparathyroidism is associated with increased levels of PTH from a parathyroid adenoma or parathyroid hyperplasia, which results in hypercalcemia from increased absorption and hypophosphatemia due to a strong phosphaturic effect. Primary hyperparathyroidism has been reported in horses, ponies, and a mule.[15,35,45]

Hypocalcemia

Hypocalcemia (see Table 6.4) is only relevant physiologically if pertaining to iCa. One of the more common causes of hypocalcemia is hypoalbuminemia, but this only affects tCa concentration; iCa concentration is unaffected. Clinical hypocalcemia, when acute, can be associated with synchronous diaphragmatic

Table 6.4 Common causes of Ca, Phosphorus, and Mg abnormalities

Calcium
  Hypercalcemia
    Chronic renal failure
    Humoral hypercalcemia of malignancy

  Hypocalcemia
    Hypoalbuminemia (only tCa, not iCa)
    Lactation or transport tetany
    Inflammatory mediators
      Colic
      Sepsis
    Heavy exercise
    Canthardin toxicity
    Acute renal failure

Magnesium
  Hypermagnesemia
    Renal failure
    Iatrogenic overdose

  Hypomagnesemia
    See hypocalcemia
    Long-term parenteral or enteral support with low Mg

Phosphorous
  Hyperphosphatemia
    Acute renal failure
    Release from damaged cells
    Phosphate-containing enema
    Dietary excess

  Hypophosphatemia
    Chronic renal failure
    Humoral hypercalcemia of malignancy
    Intracellular shifts

flutter, tetany, or ileus. Chronic hypocalcemia can lead to skeletal abnormalities. Hypocalcemia causing metabolic tetany most often occurs in horses that are lactating.[43] Metabolic tetany also can occur in horses that have been transported long distances.[43] In these horses, it is usually a combination of decreased feed intake associated with stress, as corticosteroids decrease activity of vitamin D and decrease Ca absorption.

Horses with colic are often hypocalcemic.[43] The pathogenesis is likely associated with endotoxemia and activation of inflammatory mediators that impair parathyroid gland function. Sepsis is also commonly associated with hypocalcemia, most often seen in foals.[43] The mechanism of hypocalcemia with sepsis includes parathyroid gland dysfunction, but is likely multifactorial.

Heavily exercised horses can become hypocalcemic via an unknown mechanism. Sweat contains Ca, so excessive sweating may be a factor.[24] In addition, metabolic alkalosis associated with exercise and sweating can result in lower concentrations of iCa due to increased binding to albumin and other anions. It has also been hypothesized that parathyroid gland dysfunction may play a role in exercise-induced hypocalcemia, although most horses participating in endurance rides had elevated levels of PTH in conjunction with low iCa concentrations.[1]

Cantharidin (blister beetle) toxicity is associated with severe hypocalcemia.[19,38] While the underlying mechanism is not known, it is likely related to toxin-induced damage to mucosal surfaces of the gastrointestinal and urinary systems.[43] Tissue damage associated with severe rhabdomyolysis may also cause hypocalcemia.[36] Although rare in horses, pancreatitis may cause hypocalcemia, likely due to saponification of peripancreatic fat.[4,34] Oxalate toxicity can cause chronic hypocalcemia by decreasing the absorption of calcium from the gastrointestinal tract through binding to oxalates.[27] Oxalate binding of dietary calcium is one potential cause of nutritional secondary hyperparathyroidism, resulting in dietary phosphate in excess of calcium.[10]

Primary hypoparathyroidism is rare, but has been described in foals and horses.[8,20] Failure of the parathyroid gland to secrete adequate PTH results in hypocalcemia and hyperphosphatemia. Functional or acquired hypoparathyroidism is also associated with decreased excretion of PTH, but as a result of inflammatory mediators or magnesium deficiency and not of a problem with the gland itself.

Iatrogenic hypocalcemia can occur with administration of furosemide or with tetracyclines.[43] Loop diuretics result in calcium wasting in urine. Tetracyclines chelate Ca and can result in a transient hypocalcemia.

Magnesium

Magnesium (Mg) is a cation with a charge similar to calcium and is also present in the plasma in ionized, protein-bound, or complexed forms. Similar to Ca, the ionized form is the physiologically relevant form; the concentration of total Mg is influenced by the amount of albumin and complexing anions in circulation, and the concentration of the ionized form is pH dependent. Most Mg is intracellular with less than 1% of total body Mg in the extracellular fluid, therefore total Mg concentration may not reflect body content. Hemolysis can erroneously increase measured concentrations due to high intracellular Mg concentration.

Magnesium is absorbed from the gastrointestinal tract. The kidneys primarily are responsible for excretion, but there is also some excretion from the gastrointestinal tract and mammary gland, as well as small amounts in sweat and the growing fetus. Magnesium is important in maintaining electrochemical gradients within excitable tissues and is used in hundreds of enzymatic reactions, including those involving ATP. Hypomagnesemia affects PTH production and secretion and can lead to hypocalcemia. Hypokalemia is also associated with hypomagnesemia as Mg is important in the action of the Na+/K+ AT-Pase pump.[42]

Hypomagnesemia

Causes of hypomagnesemia are similar to those of hypocalcemia (see Table 6.4): lactation and transport over long distances (especially with decreased intake), excessive sweating, endotoxemia, sepsis, cantharidin toxicity, and gastrointestinal disorders. Long-term parenteral or enteral support that is deficient in Mg can also result in hypomagnesemia.

Hypermagnesemia

Hypermagnesemia most commonly occurs with either iatrogenic overdose, including with Epsom salts, or with renal failure (see Table 6.4).[42] Given the high intracellular concentration of Mg, severe tissue damage associated with rhabdomyolysis or acute tumor lysis syndrome can result in hypermagnesemia, along with hyperkalemia and hyperphosphatemia.

Phosphate

The concentration of inorganic phosphorous (Pi) is traditionally interpreted along with Ca, although it does not maintain as narrow of a plasma concentration as Ca does. Serum Pi concentration is normally regulated by gastrointestinal absorption and renal reabsorption. Vitamin D increases the intestinal and renal absorption of both Ca and Pi, while PTH acts on the kidney to reabsorb Ca but increase the renal excretion of Pi. In addition, phosphatonin release from the intestine is dependent on the concentration of phosphates within the intestinal lumen and influences the rate of Pi excretion by the kidney. Phosphatonins (e.g., fibroblast growth factor 23 and secreted frizzled related protein 4) are a group of compounds that may act on multiple organs to regulate phosphate metabolism.[41]

Phosphorus is the predominant intracellular anion, and there can be rapid translocation between intracellular and extracellular pools. Therefore, in contrast to Ca, serum fluctuations in Pi concentrations are often associated with diet, age (higher in foals), physiological state, insulin/glucose status, energy utilization, and sample handling.[44]

Hyperphosphatemia

Causes of hyperphosphatemia include acute renal failure, vitamin D toxicosis, and primary hypoparathyroidism (see Table 6.4). Massive tissue damage associated with rhabdomyolysis, acute tumor lysis, devitalized intestine, or hemolysis may result in hyperphosphatemia from release of intracellular Pi. Foals receiving phosphate-containing enemas can become hyperphosphatemic. Excess Pi in the diet or high Pi to Ca ratios can result in nutritional secondary hyperparathyroidism with hyperphosphatemia as the body attempts to maintain normal Ca levels.

Hypophosphatemia

While acute renal failure is more commonly associated with hyperphosphatemia, hypophosphatemia frequently occurs with chronic renal failure and hypercalcemia (see Table 6.4). Because of its phosphaturic action, primary hyperparathyroidism or PTHrP-associated hypercalcemia of malignancy results in hypophosphatemia.

Many causes of hypophosphatemia are due to shifting of the extracellular Pi to the intracellular space. This can occur with sepsis, refeeding syndrome, alkalosis, and hyperinsulinism, which is thought to be the mechanism associated with parenteral nutrition and hyperglycemia-induced hypophosphatemia.[44]

References

1. Aguilera-Tejero E, Estepa JC, López I, et al. 2001. Plasma ionized calcium and parathyroid hormone concentrations in horses after endurance rides. *J Am Vet Med Assoc* 219:488-490.
2. Aleman M. 2008. A review of equine muscle disorders. *Neuromuscul Disord* 18:277-287.
3. Arroyo LG, Stämpfli HR. 2007. Equine renal tubular disorders. *Vet Clin North Am Equine Pract* 23:631-639.
4. Bakos Z, Krajcsovics L, Toth J. 2008. Successful medical treatment of acute pancreatitis in a horse. *Vet Rec* 162:95-96.
5. Barton MH, Sharma P, LeRoy BE, et al. 2004. Hypercalcemia and high serum parathyroid hormone-related protein concentration in a horse with multiple myeloma. *J Am Vet Med Assoc* 225:409-413.
6. Cook G, Divers TJ, Rowland PH. 1995. Hypercalcaemia and erythrocytosis in a mare associated with a metastatic carcinoma. *Equine Vet J* 27:316-318.
7. Dunkel B, Palmer JE, Olson KN, et al. 2005. Uroperitoneum in 32 foals: Influence of intravenous fluid therapy, infection, and sepsis. *J Vet Intern Med* 19:889-893.
8. Durie I, van Loon G, Hesta M, et al. 2010. Hypocalcemia caused by primary hypoparathyroidism in a 3-month-old filly. *J Vet Intern Med* 24:439-442.
9. Esplin DG, Taylor JL. 1977. Hypercalcemia in a horse with lymphosarcoma. *J Am Vet Med Assoc* 170:180-182.
10. Estepa JC, Aguilera-Tejero E, Zafra R, et al. 2006. An unusual case of generalized soft-tissue mineralization in a suckling foal. *Vet Pathol* 43:64-67.
11. Estepa JC, Garfia B, Gao PR, et al. 2003. Validation and clinical utility of a novel immunoradiometric assay exclusively for biologically active whole parathyroid hormone in the horse. *Equine Vet J* 35:291-295.
12. Finley MR, Rebhun WC, Dee A, et al. 1998. Paraneoplastic pruritus and alopecia in a horse with diffuse lymphoma. *J Am Vet Med Assoc* 213:102-104.
13. Fix AS, Miller LD. 1987. Equine adrenocortical carcinoma with hypercalcemia. *Vet Pathol* 24:190-192.
14. Flaminio MJ, Rush BR. 1998. Fluid and electrolyte balance in endurance horses. *Vet Clin North Am Equine Pract* 14:147-158.
15. Frank N, Hawkins JF, Couëtil LL, et al. 1998. Primary hyperparathyroidism with osteodystrophia fibrosa of the facial bones in a pony. *J Am Vet Med Assoc* 212:84-86.

16. Harris P, Snow DH. 1988. The effects of high intensity exercise on the plasma concentration of lactate, potassium and other electrolytes. *Equine Vet J* 20:109-113.
17. Harris P, Snow DH. 1992. Plasma potassium and lactate concentrations in thoroughbred horses during exercise of varying intensity. *Equine Vet J* 24:220-225.
18. Heath SE, Peter AT, Janovitz EB, et al. 1995. Ependymoma of the neurohypophysis and hypernatremia in a horse. *J Am Vet Med Assoc* 207:738-741.
19. Helman RG, Edwards WC. 1997 Clinical features of blister beetle poisoning in equids: 70 cases (1983-1996). *J Am Vet Med Assoc* 211:1018-1021.
20. Hudson NP, Church DB, Trevena J, et al. 1999. Primary hypoparathyroidism in two horses. *Aust Vet J* 77:504-508.
21. Hyyppä S, Pösö AR. 1998. Fluid, electrolyte, and acid-base responses to exercise in racehorses. *Vet Clin North Am Equine Pract* 14:121-136.
22. Johnson PJ. 1995. Electrolyte and acid-base disturbances in the horse. *Vet Clin North Am Equine Pract* 11:491-514.
23. Karcher LF, Le Net JL, Turner BF, et al. 1990. Pseudohyperparathyroidism in a mare associated with squamous cell carcinoma of the vulva. *Cornell Vet* 80:153-162.
24. Kerr MG, Snow DH. 1983. Composition of sweat of the horse during prolonged epinephrine (adrenaline) infusion, heat exposure, and exercise. *Am J Vet Res* 44:1571-1577.
25. Kingston JK, Bayly WM. 1998. Effect of exercise on acid-base status of horses. *Vet Clin North Am Equine Pract* 14:61-73.
26. Krook L, Wasserman RH, Shively JN, et al. 1975. Hypercalcemia and calcinosis in Florida horses: implication of the shrub, Cestrum diurnum, as the causative agent. *Cornell Vet* 65:26-56.
27. Laan TT, Spoorenberg JF, van der Kolk JH. 2000. Hypocalcemia in a four-week-old foal. *Tijdschr Diergeneeskd* 125:185-187.
28. LeRoy B, Woolums A, Wass J, et al. 2011. The relationship between serum calcium concentration and outcome in horses with renal failure presented to referral hospitals. *J Vet Intern Med* 25:1426-1430.
29. Mair TS, Yeo SP, Lucke VM. 1990. Hypercalcaemia and soft tissue mineralisation associated with lymphosarcoma in two horses. *Vet Rec* 126:99-101.
30. McEwan Jenkinson D, Elder HY, Bovell DL. 2006. Equine sweating and anhidrosis Part 1—equine sweating. *Vet Dermatol* 17:361-392.
31. Meuten DJ, Price SM, Seiler RM, et al. 1978. Gastric carcinoma with pseudohyperparathyroidism in a horse. *Cornell Vet* 68:179-195.
32. Muylle E, Oyaert W, De Roose P, et al. 1974. Hypercalcaemia and mineralisation of non-osseous tissues in horses due to vitamin-D toxicity. *Zentralbl Veterinarmed A* 21:638-643.
33. Nostell K, Funkquist P, Nyman G, et al. 2006. The physiological responses to simulated race tests on a track and on a treadmill in standardbred trotters. *Equine Vet J* Suppl 36:123-127.
34. Ollivett TL, Dives TJ, Cushing T, et al. 2012. Acute pancreatitis in two five-day-old Appaloosa foals. *Equine Vet J* Suppl 41:96-99.
35. Peauroi JR, Fisher DJ, Mohr FC, et al. 1998. Primary hyperparathyroidism caused by a functional parathyroid adenoma in a horse. *J Am Vet Med Assoc* 212:1915-1918.
36. Perkins G, Valberg SJ, Madigan JM, et al. 1998. Electrolyte disturbances in foals with severe rhabdomyolysis. *J Vet Intern Med* 12:173-177.

37. Rosol TJ, Nagode LA, Robertson JT, et al. 1994. Humoral hypercalcemia of malignancy associated with ameloblastoma in a horse. *J Am Vet Med Assoc* 204:1930-1933.
38. Schmitz DG. 1989. Cantharidin toxicosis in horses. *J Vet Intern Med* 3:208-215.
39. Schott II HC, Marlin DJ, Geor RJ, et al. 2006. Changes in selected physiological and laboratory measurements in elite horses competing in a 160 km endurance ride. *Equine Vet J* Suppl 36:37-42.
40. Sellers RS, Toribio RE, Blomme EA. 2001. Idiopathic systemic granulomatous disease and macrophage expression of PTHrP in a miniature pony. *J Comp Pathol* 125:214-218.
41. Shaikh A, Berndt T, Kumar R. 2008. Regulation of phosphate homeostasis by the phosphatonins and other novel mediators. *Pediatr Nephrol* 23:1203-1210.
42. Stewart AJ. 2011. Magnesium disorders in horses. *Vet Clin North Am Equine Pract* 27:149-163.
43. Toribio RE. 2004. Calcium disorders. In *Equine Internal Medicine*, 2nd ed., pp. 1295-1326. Saint Louis: Saunders.
44. Toribio RE. 2011. Disorders of calcium and phosphate metabolism in horses. *Vet Clin North Am Equine Pract* 27:129-147.
45. Wong D, Sponseller B, Miles K, et al. 2004. Failure of Technetium Tc 99m sestamibi scanning to detect abnormal parathyroid tissue in a horse and mule with primary hyperparathyroidism. *J Vet Intern Med* 18:589-593.

Chapter 7
Proteins

Koranda Wallace

Plasma proteins

Proteins are a vast array of molecules essential for an abundant variety of biological functions, which include serving as enzymes, antibodies, hormones, and carriers. Proteins are often combined with other substances including triglycerides or polysaccharides. Those that are most relevant for clinical biochemistry of the domestic animal include plasma and serum proteins. These include albumin, globulin, clotting factors, and acute phase proteins such as fibrinogen. In contrast to plasma, serum does not contain fibrinogen or clotting factors.

Major plasma proteins are produced mainly in the liver with some contribution from B-cells (immunoglobulins). B-cells produce immunoglobulins within the marrow, spleen, and lymph nodes after appropriate stimulation in the presence of pathogens. Hepatocytes produce other essential proteins under the influence of various regulatory factors. One example is albumin, whose production is upregulated by low osmotic pressure and can be downregulated during infection or inflammation due to pro-inflammatory cytokines (e.g., IL-1, IL6, tumor necrosis factor-α).[12] These inflammatory cytokines downregulate some proteins, referred to as negative acute phase proteins, while concurrently upregulating the production of acute phase proteins (see below). Other tissues (intestine, lung, adipose tissue, mammary gland, pituitary) are also capable of protein production in certain situations.[10,23] This chapter discusses major acute phase proteins, factors that affect proteins, and interpretation of serum protein profiles.

Albumin

Albumin is a water-soluble protein, synthesized by the liver, which makes up the vast majority of plasma proteins (35–50%).[9] It functions as a main component of colloid osmotic pressure (COP) and acts as a carrier for hormones, fatty acid, metal ions, and pharmaceutical products. Its production is under the

Equine Clinical Pathology, First Edition. Edited by Raquel M. Walton.
© 2014 John Wiley & Sons, Inc. Published 2014 by John Wiley & Sons, Inc.

control of COP as well as hormones such as insulin, thyroxine, and cortisol.[12] The half-life of albumin varies by species and is reported as 19.4 days in the horse.[31]

There are several dye-binding assays available for the measurement of albumin. The most widely used dyes include bromocresol green (BCG) or bromocresol purple (BCP). BCP has been recommended for equine serum albumin.[1] The dye binds to albumin, thereby altering its absorbance and making it measureable via spectrophotometry. Dye-binding methods are considered accurate when albumin is within the reference interval; however, the accuracy decreases when albumin is very low or high.

Globulin

Globulins are comprised of a variety of proteins that can be separated, via protein electrophoresis, into several fractions: α, β, and γ. Alpha and beta globulins are predominantly synthesized by the liver and include acute phase proteins and few gamma globulins, which may extend away from the gamma globulin fraction (i.e., IgM and IgA). The gamma globulin fraction consists predominantly of immunoglobulins, which are produced by B lymphocytes and plasma cells.

The simplest way to estimate the globulin fraction is to measure the total protein content of serum and subtract the albumin concentration. The globulin fraction can then be subdivided and the percentage of each fraction can be determined via electrophoretic methods. Electrophoretic fractionation methods include serum protein electrophoresis (SPE), cellulose acetate, and agarose electrophoresis. The main differences lie in the support material for protein separation. To decrease the complexity of interpretation, serum, rather than plasma, is used, which excludes fibrinogen.

Principles of electrophoresis are discussed in detail in other major texts and are addressed here only briefly.[9] In short, they are based on the movement of charged proteins within an electrical field. Proteins separate depending on their size and charge and on the strength of the electric field. Negatively charged proteins move toward the positively charged electrode and away from the negative electrode. Once proteins are separated, they are stained and the proportion of each protein is estimated by densitometry. Computer software converts absorbance readings from the densitometer to a graphical representation and calculates the percentage of protein per fraction leading to the depiction of peaks for each fraction. Albumin is represented by a large peak on the left (nearest the positive electrode) and is followed by α1, α2, β1, β2, and γ fractions (Figure 7.1). Typically, agarose gel matrix electrophoresis results in six protein fractions in horses.[40]

Acute phase proteins

Acute phase proteins (APPs) are defined as proteins whose plasma concentrations increase or decrease by at least 25% after an inflammatory stimulus.[14]

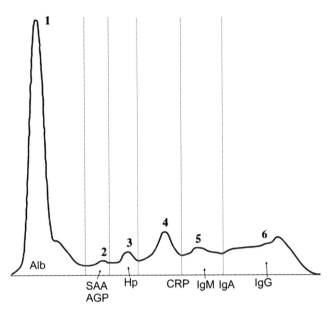

Figure 7.1 Serum electrophoretogram densitometer tracing from a healthy horse. (a) Albumin fraction; (b) α1-globulin fraction; (c) α2-globulin fraction; (d) β1-globulin fraction; (e) β2-globulin fraction; (f) γ-globulin fraction. Abbreviations: Alb, albumin; AGP, α1-acid glycoprotein; CRP, C-reactive protein; Hp, haptoglobin; SAA, serum amyloid A.

They are a key component of an acute phase response (APR). The APR is a highly complex response to inflammation, infection, trauma, stress, and/or neoplasia, which acts as a component of the innate immune system and which serves to minimize tissue damage while enhancing healing and restoring homeostasis (Figure 7.2).[6,7] APPs are generally classified as positive proteins (either major or moderate) and negative proteins depending on whether values increase or decrease in response to a challenge. Positive major proteins have the following characteristics: low to undetectable concentrations in plasma during health; rapid plasma increases (>10-fold in concentration) after

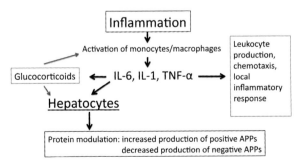

Figure 7.2 Schema depicting the acute phase response.

an APR; a large dynamic range; rapid decreases in concentration once disease has resolved; and increases following secondary infection or disease relapse.[7] Positive moderate APPs are always present in the plasma of healthy horses and have the following characteristics: up to 10-fold increases in concentration in an APR, and slower response (days to weeks) to an APR with a later increase, peak, and return to baseline. The quantification of these proteins may provide valuable diagnostic and prognostic information.

In equine medicine, the most commonly measured positive APPs include fibrinogen (Fb), serum amyloid A (SAA), and haptoglobin (Hp), while the most commonly measured negative APP is albumin.[16] Positive major proteins of the horse include SAA and positive moderate proteins include Hp, Fb, α1-acid glycoprotein (AGP), and C-reactive protein (CRP).

Serum amyloid A

Serum amyloid A (SAA), a small hydrophobic protein produced predominantly by the liver, is found complexed with lipoproteins and is comprised of several different isoforms, designated one through four. In the horse, the major isoform is SAA3, which can also be produced by mammary tissue.[16,23,34,52] The physiological role of SAA is not completely understood, but it is highly conserved among mammals, and may serve basic and essential roles in innate immunity.[6] SAA binds and opsonizes Gram-negative bacteria, participates in leukocyte chemotaxis, inhibits oxidative burst, and may modulate connective tissue remodeling and repair.[15,39,49] SAA is the precursor of amyloid A and is implicated in the pathogenesis of amyloidosis.

In healthy horses, the reference interval has been reported to range from <0.5 mg/L to 20 mg/L with a short half-life and a large dynamic range between resting levels in healthy patients versus those with infection or inflammation.[16,20,37,42] SAA concentrations were highest in horses with colic attributable to inflammatory causes (e.g., colitis, peritonitis, abscesses), and high concentrations appeared to be negatively correlated with survival in one study.[50] A recent study showed that increased concentrations of SAA were positively correlated with body condition score and insulin concentrations, implicating the APR (or SAA) in the pathogenesis of laminitis.[44] High concentrations of SAA have also been shown in association with heaves at early time points post-challenge with respiratory irritants, but SAA was not a good marker for chronic systemic inflammation in heaves.[27]

Several methods have been used to measure equine SAA, including an ELISA, slide-reversed passive latex agglutination test, single radial immunodiffusion, latex agglutination immunoturbidimetric assays, and electroimmunoassays.[3,16,36,38,42,51] Recently a turbidimetric immunoassay (TIA) for human SAA was noted to have excellent reactivity in horses.[21] The assay is based on binding of SAA to a latex conjugated mixture of rabbit polyclonal and mouse monoclonal anti-human SAA antibodies. The mixture causes a precipitate that can be measured turbidimetrically. Automated assays are newly available and are based on an automated latex agglutination turbidimetric immunoassay using monoclonal anti-human SAA antibodies.[4]

Haptoglobin

Haptoglobin (Hp), a glycoprotein produced primarily by hepatocytes, is composed of two α and two β subunits. The physiologic role of haptoglobin is to bind free hemoglobin (Hp-hemoglobin complex), which is then phagocytized by macrophages via the CD163 receptor, ultimately preventing iron loss.[6] Hemoglobin binding reduces the availability of iron and heme groups for bacterial use, contributing to Hp's indirect antibacterial activity. Production of Hp is stimulated by free hemoglobin in the blood.[28] Haptoglobin increases in horses were noted after surgery, noninfectious arthritis, and carbohydrate-induced laminitis.[13,16,24] Haptoglobin was shown to be a marker of both acute and chronic systemic inflammation in horses with heaves.[27]

Equine Hp is time- and effort-consuming to assess and is generally assayed in research laboratories. Automated assays using cyanmethemoglobin are available and are based on Hp's strong affinity for hemoglobin.[41] It is important to note that because Hp functions in binding hemoglobin, it may be consumed in cases of hemolysis.[7] Other assays, based on human haptoglobin immunoturbidimetric assays, have been validated for use in horses.[53]

Fibrinogen

Fibrinogen, a soluble plasma glycoprotein synthesized by the liver, is a large protein composed of a glycoprotein and six polypeptide chains. It is converted to fibrin in the presence of thrombin and is essential for clotting. In addition to its role in clotting, it also binds to cell surface integrins (CD11/CD18) found on phagocytic cells, which initiates cell functions such as phagocytosis, degranulation, and antibody-dependent cytotoxicity.[7] Concentrations of this moderate APP increase up to 10-fold over 24–72 hours during an APR. In healthy horses, the reference range is 200–400 mg/dL. It represents the largest proportion of plasma protein synthesized during an APR. It is considered a fairly insensitive indicator of inflammation due to its wide reference range and long response period.

There are several assays for fibrinogen including quick estimation methods such as refractometry readings before and after heat precipitation, as well as ELISA-based methods.[9,43] More precise methods include the Ratnoff-Menzies assay, clot weight measurement, and anti-fibrinogen antiserum with immunoprecipitate quantification and thrombin time.[7,9]

α1-acid glycoprotein

α1-acid glycoprotein (AGP), one of the most heavily glycosylated proteins in serum, is produced by hepatocytes. It is considered a moderate APP in most species due to its slow increase and prolonged elevation compared with major APPs, and is associated with chronic rather than acute inflammation. In horses, AGP shows a peak value 2–3 days after castration or jejunostomy, with return to baseline by 14 to 28 days post-surgery.[45] Quantitative measurement is performed via single radial immunodiffusion with serum.[45]

AGP has the ability to bind many endogenous metabolites including heparin, histamine, serotonin, steroids, and catecholamines.[9,19] AGP is involved in modulating the immune system reaction by inhibiting phagocytosis, neu-trophil activation, and platelet aggregation and may have some role in T and B lymphocyte maturation.[9,18]

C-reactive protein

C-reactive protein (CRP), composed of five subunits, is a well-documented APP in dogs and, to a lesser extent, horses. It is generally not recognized as an APP in cattle.[39] It functions as an activator of the classical complement pathway, an inducer of pro and anti-inflammatory cytokines, and modulator of phago-cytosis.[7,9,38] Both antibody-based ELISA test and a non-species-dependent assay based on a soybean oil–phosphocholine interaction have been validated in horses and verify that CRP is an acute phase protein in this species.[46,48]

Increases in equine CRP have been reported in arthritis, pneumonia, enteri-tis, and post-castration.[46] In heaves, CRP was not shown to be a good marker of acute or chronic systemic inflammation.[27]

Protein disorders

Protein disorders include dyscrasias (abnormal protein structures) and dys-proteinemias (abnormal concentrations and dyscrasias). Dysproteinemias can be characterized by the following:

1. Nonselective hyperproteinemia (panhyperproteinemia): all proteins are in-creased).
2. Selective hyperproteinemia: total plasma protein is increased, with some proteins increased more than others.
3. Nonselective hypoproteinemia (panhypoproteinemia): total protein is de-creased due to proportional decreases.
4. Selective hypoproteinemia: total protein is decreased due to disproportion-ate decreases of various fractions.

Although proteins may appear to be proportionally decreased or increased, SPE may be needed to evaluate relative concentrations of proteins, especially in the globulin region.[43] Hypoproteinemia can be from dilution of protein by excess fluid, increased loss from the vascular space, or decreased synthesis. Hyperproteinemias can be due to dehydration, inflammation, or neoplasia. In-terpretation of altered protein concentrations depends on determining which fraction of proteins – albumin or globulin – is altered. Causes for alterations in protein concentrations in the horse are summarized below.

Hypoalbuminemia with hypoglobulinemia

Concurrent decreases in both albumin and globulin can be the result of dilu-tion or proportional loss of both constituents. Examples where both are lost proportionally include blood loss, protein losing enteropathy (PLE), exudative skin disease, and effusive disease. In blood loss, albumin and globulins are lost proportionately and then diluted as fluid shifts from the extracellular space to the intracellular space in response to hypovolemia. PLE results from a variety of intestinal lesions including ulceration, parasitism resulting in blood loss, bacterial infection (e.g., Lawsonia intracellularis), neoplasia, and inflammatory infiltrates. In these cases both albumin and globulin leak into the intestinal tract and are lost in the feces or are degraded. Severe exudative skin disease, for example with burns, causes increased vascular permeability and loss of proteins. However, in severe cases, globulins may increase due to severe inflammation. In effusive disease (peritonitis, pleuritis, vasculitis), high-protein fluids may accumulate in body cavities resulting in decreases in albumin and globulin concentrations.

Hypoalbuminemia with normal or increased globulins

Conditions that result in hypoalbuminemia with normal or increased globulins are due either to selective albumin loss or to decreased albumin production. One of the most common causes of selective albumin loss is that which occurs through the glomerulus. In glomerular damage such as in amyloidosis or other types of glomerular nephropathies, albumin molecules, which are smaller than globulins, are selectively lost due to size and charge. This type of hypoalbuminemia is accompanied by proteinuria, increased urine protein/creatinine ratios, and in some cases hypercholesterolemia. Decreased albumin production from the liver can be a result of negative APRs whereby the response downregulates the production of albumin. Changes in negative APPs are not generally greater than 25%. Albumin production can also be decreased due to hepatic failure but typically not until 80% of functional liver mass is compromised (see Chapter 4). This finding should be accompanied by other biochemical changes in liver function values such as low cholesterol, low BUN, increased bilirubin, and/or decreased blood glucose. Starvation and/or malabsorption can lead to deficiencies in amino acids severe enough to compromise albumin production. Chronic gastrointestinal signs usually accompany malabsorption. Amino acid deficiencies are rarely severe enough to result in compromised globulin production.

Hypoglobulinemia with normal to increased albumin

The pattern of decreased globulin and normal to increased albumin is highly associated with decreases in the beta or gamma globulin fractions, typically due to decreased immunoglobulins. This can occur with failure of passive transfer (FPT) or immunodeficiencies. Passive transfer occurs when immunoglobulins (predominantly IgG) are transferred from the mare's colostrum through the semi-permeable intestinal tract of the neonate. Failure to ingest or absorb sufficient colostrum results in FPT. FPT may be masked by concurrent inflammation or dehydration that can increase globulin levels. There are several tests for FPT, including the gold standard radial immunodiffusion assay (RID) for IgG. The majority of neonatal foals have serum IgG concentrations >1000 mg/dL after absorption of sufficient colostrum; foals with concentrations <400 mg/dL are classified as having FPT and those between 800–400 mg/dL have partial FPT.[32,33]

Inherited or acquired immunodeficiency syndromes can result in low concentrations of immunoglobulins and in some cases low globulins. Diseases reported in foals include severe combined immunodeficiency (SCID), selective IgM deficiencies, and agammaglobulinemia.[8]

Hyperalbuminemia

Hyperalbuminemia is primarily and most commonly caused by dehydration. Pseudohyperalbuminemias, however, can result from concentrations determined by bromocresol green dye (BCG) methods.[43] While BCG preferentially binds to albumin, it can also bind some alpha and beta globulins, and can bind fibrinogen in heparinized plasma samples.

Hyperalbuminemia and hyperglobulinemia

The combination of both hyperalbuminemia and hyperglobulinemia is generally a result of dehydration; water loss causes relative increases in both constituents. Other considerations for selective hyperglobulinemia should be considered (see below). In the face of dehydration, concurrent increased or high normal red blood cell volumes should be expected (unless there is a concomitant anemia).

Hyperglobulinemia

The significance of hyperglobulinemia depends on which fraction is increased. The alpha globulins include many of the acute phase proteins. AGP and α1-antitrypsin migrate in the α-1 fraction while Hp, ceruloplasmin, α2-lipoproteins (VLDL), and α2-macroglobulin migrate in the α2 fraction.[9] Therefore, increases in the α1 and α2 fractions may be associated with acute inflammatory disease. Increases in the α2 fraction can also be associated with nephrotic syndrome given that VLDLs can increase with this disease process.

Beta globulins include β2-lipoproteins (LDL), IgM, IgA, CRP, and complement and are rarely increased independently of other fractions.[7,9,45] Beta globulins may increase in nephrotic syndrome due to increases in lipoprotein concentrations.[45] Antigenic responses may increase complement and IgM in the beta fraction. Although most increases are polyclonal, occasionally there are monoclonal spikes, which can signify multiple myeloma, Waldenstrom's macroglobulinemia, or lymphoma.[29] However, monoclonal gammopathies have also been noted in horses infected with intestinal parasites (S. vulgaris, S. westeri) due to an increase in an equine-specific immunoglobulin, IgG(T).[30] Alternatively, the IgG(T) can migrate in the α2 fraction on SPE.[25]

Beta-gamma bridging is the phenomenon whereby there is no clear separation between β2 and γ fractions in conjunction with a decreased albumin to globulin ratio. Although traditionally beta-gamma bridging has been thought to be associated with hepatic disease, a recent paper refutes this finding (see Chapter 4).[2]

Gamma globulins include IgG, IgA, and C-reactive protein. IgA migrates into both the β2 and γ fractions. Gamma globulins with a broad increase are regarded as polyclonal gammopathies while those with a narrow increase are considered monoclonal gammopathies. Polyclonal gammopathies are a result of a heterogeneous group of plasma cells producing a mixture of immunoglobulins. Causes of polyclonal gammopathies include infectious disease, chronic inflammatory disease, and neoplasia such as lymphoma (which can produce either polyclonal or monoclonal gammopathies). Sharp peaks in the beta or gamma region characterize monoclonal gammopathies. The sharpness of a peak can be visually identified by comparing the slope of the peak in question with the slope of either side of the albumin peak. Monoclonal spikes are the result of proliferation of a single plasma cell clone producing a homogenous population of abnormal immunoglobulins or immunoglobulin fragments (paraprotein, M protein, or M component), which migrate together. This type of gammopathy can be produced by neoplastic proliferations (e.g., multiple myeloma, lymphoma, lymphocytic leukemia), infectious disease, and idiopathic conditions.[11, 25, 47]

Hyperfibrinogenemia

The two main differentials for increased fibrinogen concentrations are dehydration and inflammation. The calculation of a plasma protein to fibrinogen ratio can be helpful in distinguishing between the two by eliminating the effect of hydration status. The ratio is simply preformed by dividing the plasma protein value by the fibrinogen value once its units have been converted to g/dl. For the horse, a ratio ≥15 suggests dehydration and a ratio <15 is consistent with a true increase in fibrinogen secondary to inflammation. Concurrent dehydration and inflammation will obscure the clarity of the ratio. The ratio should not be performed on neonatal animals or those with concurrent hypoproteinemia.[43]

Renal disease, especially glomerular disease, is not generally thought to be a cause of hyperfibrinogenemia in the horse. It has been implicated in increased levels in cattle and dogs. Neoplasia has been associated with increases in fibrinogen. Although data is lacking on this point, one study of clinical data associated with equine lymphoma reported that hyperfibrinogenemia was one of the most commonly noted abnormalities.[35]

References

1. Blackmore DJ, Henley MI, Mapp, BJ. 1983. Colorimetric measurement of albumin in horse sera. *Equine Vet J* 15:373–374.

2. Camus MS, Krimer PM, Leroy BE, et al. 2010. Evaluation of the positive predictive value of serum protein electrophoresis beta-gamma bridging for hepatic disease in three domestic animal species. *Vet Pathol* 47:1064–1070.
3. Chavatte, PM, Pepys MB, Roberts B, et al. 1991. Measurements of serum amyloid A protein (SAA) as an aid to differential diagnosis of infection in newborn foals. In *Equine Infectious Diseases VI: Proceedings of the Sixth International Conference*, 7–11 July, Plowright W, Rossdale PD, Wade JF (eds), Newmarket: R and W Publications.
4. Christensen M, Jacobsen S, Ichiyanagi T, et al. 2012. Evaluation of an automated assay based on monoclonal anti-human serum amyloid A (SAA) antibodies for measurement of canine, feline, and equine SAA. *Vet J* 194:332–337.
5. Cray C, Zaias J, Altman NH. 2009. Acute phase response in animals: a review. *Comp Med* 59:517–526.
6. Cray, C. 2012. Acute phase proteins in animals. *Prog Mol Biol Transl Sci* 105:113–150.
7. Crisman MV, Scarratt WK, Zimmerman KL. 2008. Blood proteins and inflammation in the horse. *Vet Clin North Am Equine Pract* 24: 285–297.
8. Crisman MV, Scarratt WK. 2008. Immunodeficiency disorders in horses. *Vet Clin North Am Equine Pract* 24:299–310.
9. Eckersall PD. 2008. Proteins, Proteomics, and the Dysproteinemias. In *Clinical Biochemistry of Domestic Animals*. Kaneko JJ, Harvey JW, Bruss ML (eds). 6th ed. pp. 117–155. Burlington, MA: Elsevier.
10. Eckersall PD, Young FJ, McComb C, et al. 2001. Acute phase proteins in serum and milk from dairy cows with clinical mastitis. *Vet Rec* 148:35–41.
11. Edwards DF, Parker JW, Wilkinson JE, et al. 1993. Plasma cell myeloma in the horse. A case report and literature review. *J Vet Intern Med* 7:169–176.
12. Evans TW. 2002. Albumin as a drug—biological effects of albumin unrelated to oncotic pressure. *Aliment Pharmacol Ther* 16(Suppl 5):6–11.
13. Fagliari JJ, McClenahan D, Evanson OA, et al. 1998. Changes in plasma protein concentrations in ponies with experimentally induced alimentary laminitis. *Am J Res* 9:1234–1237.
14. Gabay C, Kushner I. 1999. Acute-phase proteins and other systemic responses to inflammation. *N Engl J Med* 340:448–454.
15. Hari-Dass R, Shah C, Meyer DJ, et al. 2005. Serum amyloid A protein binds to outer membrane protein A of gram-negative bacteria. *J Biol Chem* 280:18562–18567.
16. Hulten C, Gronlund U, Hirvonen J, et al. 2002. Dynamics in serum of the inflammatory markers serum amyloid A (SAA), haptoglobin, fibrinogen and alpha2-globulins during induced non-infectious arthritis in the horse. *Equine Vet J* 34:699–704.
17. Hulten C, Sletten K, Foyn Bruun C, et al. 1997. The acute phase serum amyloid A protein (SAA) in the horse: isolation and characterization of three isoforms. *Vet Immunopathol* 57:215–227.
18. Hulten C, Tumlano RM, Suominen MM, et al. 1999. A non-competitive chemiluminescence enzyme immunoassay for the equine acute phase protein serum amyloid A (SAA)—a clinically useful inflammatory marker in the horse. *Vet Immunol Immunopathol* 68:267–281.
19. Israili ZH, Dayton PG. 2001. Human alpha-1-glycoprotein and its interactions with drugs. *Drug Metab Rev* 33:161–235.
20. Jacobsen S, Andersen PH. 2007. The acute phase protein serum amyloid A (SAA) as a marker of inflammation in horses. *Equine Vet Education* 19:38–46.

21. Jacobsen S, Kjelgaard-Hansen M, Petersen HH, et al. 2006. Evaluation of a commercially available human serum amyloid A (SAA) turbidimetric immunoassay for determination of equine SAA concentration. *Vet J* 172:315-319.
22. Jacobsen S, Niewold TA, Halling-Thomsen M, et al. 2006. Serum amyloid A isoforms in serum and synovial fluid in horses with lipopolysaccharide-induced arthritis. *Vet Immunol Immunopathol* 110:325-330.
23. Jacobsen S, Niewold TA, Kornalijnslijper E, et al. 2005. Kinetics of local and systemic isoform of serum amyloid A in bovine mastitic milk. *Vet Immunol Immunopath* 104:21-31.
24. Kent JE, Goodall J. 1991. Assessment of an immunoturbidimetric method for measuring equine serum haptoglobin concentrations. *Equine Vet J* 23:59-66.
25. Kent JE, Roberts CA. 1990. Serum protein changes in four horses with monoclonal gammopathy. *Equine Vet J* 22:373-376.
26. Lassen ED. 2004. Laboratory evaluation of plasma and serum proteins. In *Veterinary Hematology and Clinical Chemistry*, Thrall MA, Baker DC, Campbell TW, et al. (eds). pp. 401-415. Philadelphia: Lippincott, Williams, and Wilkins.
27. Lavoie-Lamoureux A, Leclere M, Lemos K, et al. 2012. Markers of systemic inflammation in horses with heaves. *J Vet Intern Med* 26:1419-1426.
28. Levy AP, Asleh R, Blum S, et al. 2010. Haptoglobin: basic and clinical aspects. *Antioxid Redox Signal* 12:293-304.
29. Macewen EG, Hurvitz AI, Hayes A. 1977. Hyperviscosity syndrome associated with lymphocytic-leukemia in 3 dogs. *J Am Vet Med Assoc* 170:1309-1312.
30. Mair TS, Cripps PJ, Ricketts SW. 1993. Diagnostic and prognostic value of serum protein electrophoresis in horses with chronic diarrhoea. *Equine Vet J* 25:324-326.
31. Mattheeuws DR, Kaneko JJ, Loy RG, et al. 1996. Compartmentalization and turnover of I^{131}-labeled albumin and gamma globulin in horses. *Am J Vet Res* 27:155-163.
32. McClure JT, DeLuca JL, Miller J. 2002. Comparison of 5 screening tests for the detection of failure of passive transfer in foals. (Abstract) In *Proceedings of the 20th American College of Veterinary Internal Medicine Forum* 20: 770.
33. McClure JT, Miller J, DeLuca JL. 2003. Comparison of two ELISA screening tests and a non-commercial glutaraldehyde screening test for the detection of failure of passive transfer in neonatal foals. *Proc Am Assoc Equine Pract* 49:301-305.
34. McDonald TL, Larson MA, Mack DR, et al. 2001. Elevated extrahepatic expression and secretion of mammary-associated serum amyloid A3 (M-SAA3) into colostrum. *Vet Immunol Immunopathol* 83:203-211.
35. Meyer J, Delay J, Bienzle D. 2006. Clinical, laboratory, and histopathologic features of equine lymphoma. *Vet Pathol* 43:914-924.
36. Nunokawa Y, Fujinaga T, Taira T, et al. 1993. Evaluation of serum amyloid A protein as an acute-phase reactive protein in horses. *J Vet Med Sci* 55:1011-1016.
37. Pepys MB, Baltz ML, Tennent GA. 1989. Serum amyloid A (SAA) in horses: objective measurement of the acute phase response. *Equine Vet J* 21:106-109.
38. Pepys MB. 1981. C-reactive protein fifty years on. *Lancet* 1(8221):653-657.
39. Petersen HH, Nielsen JP, Heegaard PMH. 2004. Application of acute phase protein measurement in veterinary clinical chemistry. *Vet Res* 35:163-187.
40. Riond B, Wenger-Riggenbach B, Hofmann-Lehmann R, et al. 2009. Serum protein concentrations from clinically healthy horses determined by agarose gel electrophoresis. *Vet Clin Pathol* 38:73-77.

41. Skinner JG, Roberts L. 1994. Haptoglobin as an indicator of infection in sheep. *Vet Rec* 134:33–36.
42. Stoneham SJ, Palmer L, Cash R, et al. 2001. Measurement of serum amyloid A in the neonatal foal using latex agglutination immunoturbidimetric assay: determination of the normal range, variation with age, and response to disease. *Equine Vet J* 33:599–603.
43. Stockham SL, Scott MA. 2008. Proteins. In *Fundamentals of Veterinary Clinical Pathology*. Stockham SL, Scott MA (eds). 2nd ed. pp. 370–413. Ames, IA: Blackwell.
44. Suagee JK, Corl BA, Crisman MV, et al. 2012. Relationships between body condition score and plasma inflammatory cytokines, insulin, and lipids in a mixed population of light-breed horses. *J Vet Intern Med* Dec 6. doi: 10.1111/jvim.12021.
45. Taira T, Fujinaga T, Tamura K, et al. 1992. Isolation and characterization of alpha 1-acid glycoprotein from horses and its evaluation as an acute-phase reactive protein in horses. *Am J Vet Res* 53:961–965.
46. Takiguchi M, Fujinaga T, Naiki M, et al. 1990. Isolation, characterization, and quantitative analysis of C-reactive protein from horses. *Am J Vet Res* 51:1215–1220.
47. Traub-Dargatz J, Bertone A, Bennett D, et al. 1985. Monoclonal aggregating immunoglobulin cryoglobulinaemia in a horse with malignant lymphoma. *Equine Vet J* 17:470–473.
48. Tugirimana PL, De Clercq D, Holderbeke AL, et al. 2011. A functional turbidimetric method to determine C-reactive protein in horses. *J Vet Diagn Invest* 23:308–311.
49. Uhlar CM, Whitehead AS. 1999. Serum amyloid A, the major vertebrate acute-phase reactant. *Eur J Biochem* 265:501–523.
50. Vandenplas ML, Moore JN, Barton MH, et al. 2005. Concentrations of serum amylois A and lipopolysaccharide-binding protein in horses with colic. *Am J Vet Res* 66:1509–1516.
51. Wakimoto Y. 1996. Slide reversed passive latex agglutination test. A simple and practical method for equine serum amyloid A (SAA) protein determination. *Japan J Vet Res* 44:43.
52. Weber A, Weber AT, McDonald TL, et al. 2006. Staphylococcus aureus liptechoic acid induces differential expression of bovine serum amyloid A3(SAA3) by mammary epithelial cells: implications for early diagnosis of mastitis. *Vet Immunol Immunopath* 109:79–83.
53. Weidmeyer CE, Solter PF. 1996. Validation of human haptoglobin immunoturbidimetric assay for detection of haptoglobin in equine and canine serum and plasma. *Vet Clin Pathol* 25:141–146.

Chapter 8

Laboratory Assessment of Lipid and Glucose Metabolism

Raquel M. Walton

> ## Acronyms and abbreviations that appear in this chapter:
>
> | | |
> |---|---|
> | DM | diabetes mellitus |
> | GLUT | glucose transporter |
> | HDL | high-density lipoprotein |
> | LCFA | long chain fatty acids |
> | LDL | low-density lipoprotein |
> | LPL | lipoprotein lipase |
> | NaF | sodium fluoride |
> | NEFA | nonesterified fatty acids |
> | PPID | pituitary pars intermedia dysfunction |
> | PSSM | polysaccharide storage myopathy |
> | VLDL | very low density lipoprotein |

Lipids

Lipids perform a variety of roles in the body ranging from energy storage to serving as major cell membrane components and polar solvents for fat-soluble vitamin and hormone transport. Of the many lipids present in mammals only a very few are of clinical and diagnostic relevance. This chapter discusses the primary lipid abnormalities encountered in equids and the methods for their diagnosis. A preliminary discussion of the types of lipids and their role in metabolism is necessary to adequately understand equine lipid disorders. Hyperlipidemias in horses are largely due to hypertriglyceridemia, so triglyceride metabolism will be emphasized.

Equine Clinical Pathology, First Edition. Edited by Raquel M. Walton.
© 2014 John Wiley & Sons, Inc. Published 2014 by John Wiley & Sons, Inc.

Triglyceride metabolism

Triglycerides are synthesized in intestinal enterocytes from three long chain fatty acids (LCFA) and one glycerol molecule that are absorbed following the digestion of dietary fats by pancreatic lipase (Figure 8.1). Within enterocytes, triglycerides are incorporated into chylomicron particles that are made water-soluble by a protein and phospholipid coating. Chylomicrons are released first into lymphatics and then into blood via the thoracic duct. Lipoprotein lipase (LPL), produced by adipocytes and myocytes, translocates to the luminal surface of endothelium where it breaks down plasma triglycerides into LCFA and glycerol, which are extracted into fat and muscle. In nonruminants, glucose is the primary building block for LCFA used in triglyceride synthesis; acetate is used for LCFA synthesis in ruminants.[37]

Insulin is involved in lipid metabolism by facilitating glucose uptake into adipocytes and myocytes and increasing LPL activity in endothelial tissue.

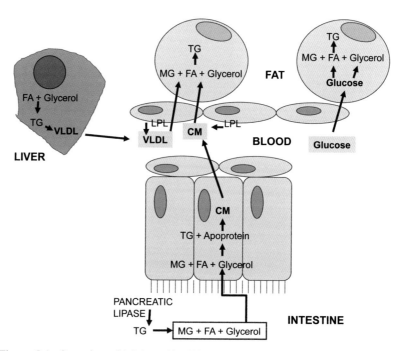

Figure 8.1 Overview of triglyceride (TG) metabolism. TGs are synthesized in enterocytes or in the liver. TGs of dietary origin are synthesized in the intestine from monoglycerides (MG), long-chain fatty acids (FA), and glycerol broken down from dietary fats by pancreatic lipase. Within enterocytes, triglycerides are incorporated into chylomicron (CM) particles that are released first into lymphatics and then into blood via the thoracic duct. In the liver, TGs are synthesized and released as very low density lipoproteins (VLDLs). Lipoprotein lipase (LPL) on the luminal surface of endothelium breaks down plasma triglycerides (in the form of chylomicrons or VLDLs) into FA and glycerol, which are taken up by muscle and fat. In nonruminants, glucose is the primary building block for FAs used in triglyceride synthesis.

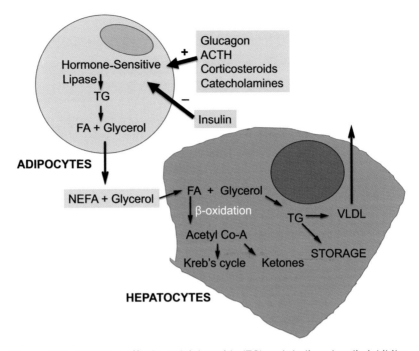

Figure 8.2 Hormone effects on triglyceride (TG) metabolism. Insulin inhibits the breakdown of TGs into nonesterified fatty acids and (NEFA) promotes triglyceride production and increases adipose tissue. Glucocorticoids, ACTH, glucagon, and catecholamines are insulin antagonists that stimulate hormone-sensitive lipase to break down TG into NEFA and glycerol. The increased concentrations of NEFA are taken up by hepatocytes to be oxidized for energy, converted into ketones, or used to synthesize triglycerides that are either stored in the liver or released as VLDL.

Glucagon, corticosteroids, ACTH, and epinephrine stimulate hormone-sensitive lipase in adipocytes to catalyze the hydrolysis of stored triglycerides and release nonesterified fatty acids (NEFA). Hyperinsulinemia promotes triglyceride production and increases adipose tissue, whereas glucagon and corticosteroids counteract these effects. When there is increased release of fatty acids from adipocytes, the NEFA not utilized by peripheral tissues are taken up by hepatocytes to be oxidized for energy, converted into ketones, or used to synthesize triglycerides that are either stored or released as VLDL. Thus, increases in circulating fatty acids contribute to hepatic triglyceride storage and hypertriglyceridemia via hepatic VLDL synthesis (Figure 8.2).

Laboratory characterization of lipid metabolism

Lipids are a class of compounds that are soluble in organic solvents and insoluble in water. Lipid hydrolysis produces fatty acids or complex alcohols than can combine with fatty acids to form esters.[35] Hyperlipidemia and hyperlipemia are used synonymously to denote increases in serum or plasma lipid concentrations. By convention, lipemia refers to the gross appearance of serum or plasma when hypertriglyceridemia is present.

Lipoproteins

The two principal lipids measured in animals are triglycerides and cholesterol. All triglycerides and the majority of cholesterol are carried within lipoproteins. Lipoproteins are classified according to their relative density, which is dependent on their composition. The classes of lipoproteins include very low density (VLDL), low-density (LDL) and high-density (HDL) lipoproteins. The lipoprotein core is hydrophobic and consists of triglyceride and cholesterol ester molecules surrounded by a hydrophilic membrane composed of proteins (apoproteins), phospholipids, and unesterified cholesterol molecules. Lipoproteins are measured after they are separated using electrophoresis or ultracentrifugation.

The predominant lipoprotein in horses is HDL, comprising 61% of the total plasma lipoprotein mass, with VLDL and LDL comprising 24% and 15%, respectively. Similar to humans, VLDL is triglyceride rich, whereas LDL is cholesterol rich and HDL is protein rich. Normal concentrations of VLDL and total triglyceride are reported to be higher in Shetland ponies than Thoroughbred horses.[43] Although lipoprotein fractions are not typically measured in veterinary medicine, they may be of diagnostic utility in metabolic syndrome (discussed below).[15]

Nonesterified fatty acids (NEFA)

Glucose is the most important precursor of long-chain fatty acids (LCFA) in nonruminants, whereas acetate is used in ruminants. As hindgut fermenters, horses absorb volatile fatty acids (acetate, propionate, and butyrate) from insoluble carbohydrates. Horses can readily shift from using glucose-based LCFA synthesis in diets high in soluble carbohydrates to acetate-based synthesis when fed high roughage diets.[2]

Following triglyceride hydrolysis in adipocytes, LCFA are released into circulation as nonesterified fatty acids (NEFA) bound to albumin. Typically NEFA are produced in response to energy demand, thus increased concentrations are considered an indicator of negative energy balance. Concentrations of NEFA increase with stress, exercise, and low blood glucose as a result of hormonal stimulation of adipocyte lipase (Figure 8.2). Accordingly, care should be taken to minimize excitement and exercise should be restricted in the period immediately before sampling.

Serum or plasma can be used for measurement, but heparin anticoagulant should be avoided since it can increase NEFA concentrations during storage. NEFA concentrations are stable in whole blood for 24 hours and in separated serum or plasma for 72 hours as long as the samples are kept at 4°C; storage at room temperature results in increased NEFA concentrations. Because of the instability of NEFA concentrations, NEFAs are best measured in situations in which the sample can be kept cool and submitted to a diagnostic laboratory relatively quickly.

Triglycerides

Circulating triglycerides are present within lipoproteins produced by the liver (VLDL) or intestinal enterocytes (chylomicrons). Triglyceride concentration is preferentially measured in serum and is stable for up to a week at 4°C, for 3 months at −20°C, and for years at −70°C. Triglycerides are made of three LCFAs and a glycerol molecule. Most assays for serum triglycerides use a reaction with a lipase to release glycerol from triglycerides; it is the glycerol that is measured following a coupling reaction with a substance that can be detected spectrophotometrically. Triglycerides should be measured on fasting samples (minimum of 12 hours). Triglycerides are usually reported in mg/dL. To convert into SI units (mmol/L), the concentration in mg/dL is multiplied by a factor of 0.01129.

The gross appearance of lipid in plasma or serum, termed lipemia, is only caused by increased concentrations of triglyceride-rich lipoproteins (chylomicrons and VLDL). Thus, an estimate of triglyceride concentration can be determined visually (Figure 8.3). Serum or plasma that is clear indicates that the triglyceride concentration is <200 mg/dL (2.26 mmol/L); serum with triglyceride concentrations around 300 mg/dL (3.39 mmol/L) appears hazy-turbid, whereas triglycerides >600 mg/dL (6.77 mmol/L) impart an opaque, milky appearance.[35] It is of interest to note that serum triglyceride concentrations exceeding 500 mg/dL (5.65 mmol/L) have been associated with no visible evidence of lipemia in horses.[10] However, the authors may have ignored a hazy-turbid appearance as not consistent with the classic milky appearance associated with lipemia.

The presence of chylomicrons is indicated when a creamy, homogenous layer floating on the surface of plasma or serum appears after refrigeration for several hours. If only chylomicrons are present, the serum below the

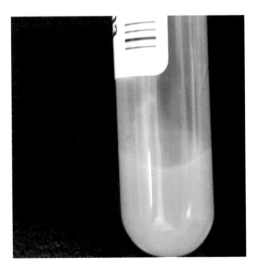

Figure 8.3　Lipemic serum is opaque and white to pink. The pink tinge is common due to mild hemolysis that often occurs with lipemic serum.

floating lipid layer is clear. In contrast, lipemia attributable to increases in VLDL produces turbid or milky serum that persists after refrigeration. Fasting lipemia is due to the presence of VLDL, whereas post-prandial lipemia is associated with chylomicronemia.

Cholesterol

Measurement of cholesterol includes total cholesterol derived mainly from cholesterol-rich lipoproteins LDL and HDL. Like triglycerides, cholesterol can be synthesized in the liver or absorbed from dietary sources in the intestine. Cholesterol concentration is stable for a week at 4°C, for 3 months at −20°C, and for years at −70°C. Measurement involves hydrolysis of cholesterol esters to produce cholesterol. Added cholesterol oxidase produces hydrogen peroxide, which reacts with an indicator dye for spectrophotometric analysis. Cholesterol can be measured in fasted or non-fasted samples.

Equine hyperlipidemias

The laboratory definition of hyperlipidemia is an increase in measurable serum lipids, which in horses are usually triglycerides. Diagnosis of hyperlipidemia is dependent on measurement of serum triglyceride concentration. By convention, equine hyperlipidemias are clinically classified in the following manner: hyperlipidemia is characterized by serum triglyceride concentrations from 100 to 500 mg/dL (1.13 to 5.65 mmol/L) without gross lipemia or clinical signs; hyperlipemia is defined as a serum triglyceride concentration more than 500 mg/dL (5.65 mmol/L) with visible lipemia and fatty infiltration of the liver and/or other organs.[10,23] Hyperlipidemia is usually associated with insufficient food intake and is often unnoticed because it is subclinical.

These categorizations use 100 mg/dL as the cutoff for the lower reference value. Different laboratories and different species under varying conditions will have different cutoff values for hyperlipidemia and hyperlipemia. For example, normal triglyceride concentrations in horses and non-pregnant ponies are often reported as <100 mg/dL, but reference values for ponies during the last trimester of pregnancy concentrations can reach 250 mg/dL (2.83 mmol/L). In one study, concentrations of up to 390 mg/dL (4.4 mmol/L) are reported for healthy donkeys.[5] Thus, hyperlipidemia and hyperlipemia should be defined using the lower end of the reference interval established by the laboratory producing the results.

Hyperlipidemia is typically associated with periods of negative energy balance (e.g., hypophagia, pregnancy, lactation), but is also linked to obesity, stress, sex, and breed. The pathogenesis of equine hyperlipemia lies in disturbances in energy metabolism compounded by insulin resistance. Insulin resistance is the cell's diminished capacity to transport glucose from the blood into peripheral tissues in response to insulin (discussed further in the next section). In the context of insulin resistance, development of a negative energy balance results in excessive and inappropriate mobilization of fatty acids that accumulate in the liver as triglycerides and in the blood as VLDL. The increase in plasma triglyceride and NEFA concentrations can interfere with insulin's inhibition of hormone-sensitive lipase, contributing to increased lipolysis. Cat-echolamines, cortisol, and ACTH, all of which are increased in illness, also stimulate lipoprotein lipase. The hyperlipemia results in accumulation of fatty acid metabolites in myocytes that can interfere with insulin-mediated glucose transport into cells, enhancing insulin resistance.[34] Concomitant azotemia may inhibit lipoprotein lipase activity, further exacerbating the lipidemia.[32] The ensuing self-perpetuating hyperlipemia results in tissue lipidosis and ulti-mately organ dysfunction and failure. Many of the biochemical abnormalities present in hyperlipemia (other than the hypertriglyceridemia itself) can be attributed to either a primary disease process that precipitated hyperlipemia and/or to organ dysfunction/failure caused by lipidosis.

Hyperlipemia in ponies, miniature horses, and donkeys

There is a high prevalence of hyperlipemia in pony breeds, especially Shet-land ponies, as well as in miniature horses and donkeys. Female ponies show a higher prevalence than males, representing 75% or more of cases.[23] In ponies, hyperlipemia is more prevalent in reproductively active mares, with increased incidence in late pregnancy and early lactation. The increased prevalence of hyperlipemia in female miniature breeds and donkeys applies to both repro-ductively active and inactive mares.[5,23] Prevalence reports a range from 3-5% up to 11% in the general population and even higher in hospitalized patients (up to 18%).[5,26]

Hyperlipemia frequently occurs secondary to primary disease processes such as enterocolitis/colitis and colic that produce a negative energy bal-ance and affect insulin sensitivity (see section on insulin resistance below). In miniature horses, hyperlipemia develops consequent to a primary disease in the vast majority of cases. In contrast, ponies and donkeys can present with primary hyperlipemia; stress and obesity are predisposing factors. Both stress and obesity induce decreases in insulin sensitivity, which is considered the primary predisposing factor. There appears to be a genetic predisposition in the case of Shetland ponies.

Horse hyperlipidemias

Hyperlipidemia (triglyceride concentrations above the reference value limit but without gross lipemia or associated illness) is reported in horses, usually as a result of inadequate food intake. Hyperlipidemia/hypertriglyceridemia due to fasting in horses is reported to range from 100 mg/dL to 300 mg/dL.[10] In contrast, hyperlipemia, defined as marked increases in serum triglyceride concentrations (e.g., >500 mg/dL) with gross lipemia and clinical illness, is uncommon in large-breed horses compared to ponies, small breeds, and donkeys.[27,28] A third hyperlipidemic category of marked hypertriglyceridemia (>500 mg/dL) associated with clinical signs but *without* visual evidence of plasma lipemia has been described.[10] The absence of plasma lipemia distin-guishes this disorder from hyperlipemia. It is uncertain why this magnitude of hypertriglyceridemia does not cause visible plasma turbidity or opacity given that triglyceride concentrations >300 gm/dL should cause turbidity and con-centrations >600 mg/dL should impart a milky appearance.[35]

Cases of severe hypertriglyceridemia without visible lipemia were associated with systemic inflammatory response syndrome, which is defined as presence of two or more of the following abnormalities: fever or hypothermia, tachycardia, tachypnea or hypocapnea, leukocytosis, leukopenia, or greater than 10% immature granulocytes (left-shift). All horses had one or more primary disease processes and were off feed, and many were azotemic. Thus, most of the factors contributing to the pathogenesis of hyperlipemia were present. A prevalence of 0.6% over a two-year period was reported.

Equine metabolic syndrome

Metabolic syndrome in horses is primarily a disorder of glucose metabolism and is discussed in this context in the next section. Equine metabolic syndrome (EMS) is not a disease but rather a combination of factors that imply increased susceptibility to laminitis. The primary components defining the syndrome include obesity (generalized or localized), hyperinsulinemia, and insulin resistance with a predisposition to the development of laminitis. Another main component of EMS is mild hypertriglyceridemia (including increased VLDL concentrations). Hypertriglyceridemia is more commonly seen in ponies than horses with EMS.[14] In humans, hypertriglyceridemia with *decreased* HDL-cholesterol concentrations is used as a criterion in the diagnosis of metabolic syndrome. Interestingly, horses with EMS have hypertriglyceridemia (VLDL and VLDL-triglycerides) with *increased* HDL-cholesterol.[15] A positive correlation between plasma HDL and triglyceride concentrations has also been detected in Shetland ponies.[42] It is postulated that this is a result of the near absence of cholesterol ester transfer protein activity in equine blood. Cholesterol ester transfer protein catalyzes transfer of cholesterol from HDL to VLDL in humans. Thus, in humans, triglyceride carried by VLDLs is exchanged for cholesterol when VLDLs interact with HDL in the blood and, as VLDL concentrations increase, interactions with HDL increase and HDL-cholesterol concentrations decrease.

Obese horses with insulin resistance also have increased blood NEFA concentrations.[15] The NEFA concentration increases with obesity because adipose tissues reach their maximum capacity for fat storage and insulin's inhibitory effects on hormone-sensitive lipase are reduced. As a result, the influx of fatty acids into tissues increases, which causes an accumulation of fatty acid metabolites that interfere with insulin receptor signaling, thereby enhancing insulin resistance. Increased uptake of fatty acids by the liver increases the availability of triglyceride for VLDL synthesis, which is part of the mechanism of hypertriglyceridemia associated with insulin resistance. Increased VLDL production has been associated with feed deprivation and hyperlipemia in horses, which are conditions that develop in response to increased mobilization of NEFA from adipose stores.

Glucose

In addition to lipids, the other principal component in energy metabolism in mammals is glucose. Glucose is produced in the liver and, to a lesser extent, in the kidney or is absorbed from dietary sources. Production of glucose is accomplished primarily in the liver through gluconeogenesis and glycogenolysis. In nonruminant species, glucose is manufactured using mainly amino acids. The volatile fatty acid propionate, absorbed in the rumen or hindgut, provides the major building block for *de novo* glucose synthesis in ruminants. As a hindgut fermenter, the horse can use either amino acids or propionate in gluconeogenesis.[13] Equids rely heavily on gluconeogenesis to maintain blood glucose concentrations due to limited stores of glycogen. During negative energy balance, protein catabolism increases to provide amino acids for gluconeogenesis.

Glucose metabolism

There are multiple hormones whose actions result in increases in plasma glucose concentration and one principal hormone that decreases blood glucose. Normoglycemia is the result of the interactions of multiple hormones; however, the two primary processes responsible for glucose homeostasis are insulin secretion by pancreatic β-cells in response to blood glucose concentration and the response of skeletal muscle and adipose tissue to insulin concentrations. Insulin decreases blood glucose concentrations by promoting cellular uptake, utilization, or storage and by inhibiting hepatic gluconeogenesis (Figure 8.4). Glucagon and catecholamines increase blood glucose by stimulating glycogenolysis, glucagon and corticosteroids stimulate gluconeogenesis, and

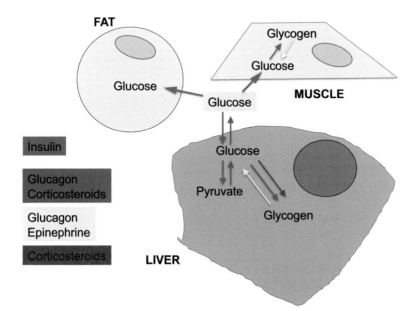

Figure 8.4   The effects of hormones on glucose metabolism. Insulin promotes normoglycemia by increasing glucose uptake, utilization, and storing and inhibiting gluconeogenesis. Glucagon, corticosteroids, and epinephrine cause hyperglycemia through various mechanisms including inhibition of insulin activity and stimulation of gluconeogenesis and glycogenolysis.

glucagon and corticosteroids inhibit insulin activity at the receptor and post-receptor level. Catecholamines inhibit insulin secretion, stimulate glucagon release, and inhibit insulin activity at the post-receptor level. The effects of these hormones on fat metabolism were described previously (Figure 8.2).

After a meal, insulin is released from pancreatic β-cells to facilitate glucose uptake by fat and muscle tissue via the GLUT-4 transporter. Insulin is not required for glucose uptake by the hepatic GLUT-2 transporter, but it affects hepatic glucose metabolism by stimulating hepatic glycolysis, inhibiting glu-coneogenesis, and by facilitating glycogen synthesis. When there is a negative energy balance, normoglycemia is maintained in multiple ways. The metabolic rate slows to limit glucose consumption. Glucagon secretion increases and insulin secretion decreases, resulting in gluconeogenesis, glycogenolysis, and peripheral lipolysis. The metabolism shifts from glucose to fatty acids as a primary energy source. Because the liver uses little fatty acids for energy, and the pathway for ketone body formation is not well developed in horses, if the negative energy balance persists, increasing amounts of triglycerides are produced (Figure 8.2).[25] With time, the hepatocellular triglyceride concentration overwhelms the liver's capacity for synthesizing and exporting VLDL, resulting in increased triglyceride storage and hepatic lipidosis.

Insulin resistance

Insulin resistance is defined as insensitivity to insulin at the cell surface, where glucose entry into the cell is facilitated, or insulin ineffectiveness as a result of the disruption of intracellular glucose metabolism.[24] Glucose and lipid metabolism are intricately linked via insulin, glucagon, and other hormones. Abnormalities in lipid metabolism are therefore associated with dysregulation of glucose metabolism. Increased plasma fatty acid concentrations are associated with several insulin-resistant states in humans through various mechanisms including inhibition of glucose transport or phosphorylation activity.[34] This appears to be a mechanism of insulin resistance in obesity and type II diabetes. Increased concentrations of inflammatory cytokines in humans are reported to be key in the development of obesity-associated insulin resistance. There is evidence that this may also be true in horses.[41]

Insulin resistance in equids has been associated with pasture laminitis, hyperlipidemia, obesity, pituitary pars intermedia dysfunction, type II diabetes mellitus, and equine metabolic syndrome.[11,15,18,39] Specific, quantitative methods of measuring insulin sensitivity are available but are not currently suitable for practical clinical applications.[24,39] The more commonly used tests are indirect methods of assessing insulin sensitivity and include measurement of resting glucose, insulin, and leptin concentrations, the intravenous glucose tolerance test, and the combined glucose-insulin test (discussed below).

Laboratory characterization of glucose metabolism

Although there are multiple methods currently in use to assess insulin sensitivity, many are appropriate only in research situations. This section limits discussion to nonspecific indicators of insulin resistance that are most applicable to clinical practice, rather than specific, quantifiable methods.

Glucose

Blood glucose can be measured in whole blood, serum, or plasma. Because glycolysis continues in blood cells in vitro, serum or plasma should be separated as soon as possible from the blood cells, preferably within an hour after collection. If the sample cannot be separated within an hour, glycolysis can be inhibited with special collection tubes containing sodium fluoride (NaF). If NaF is used for collection, glucose assays based on glucose oxidase cannot be used, becaue NaF inhibits glucose oxidase activity. Glycolysis is reported to decrease glucose concentrations by 5-10% per hour at room temperature; greater decreases can occur if there is marked erythrocytosis or leukocytosis.

The most common glucose assays use glucose oxidase for the initial reaction; other assays are based on glucose reduction of copper or ferricyanide. Because these assays are based on color changes, lipemia, hemolysis, and icterus can interfere with results. Nonphotometric assays rely on the use of oxygen or hydrogen peroxide electrodes to measure consumption or production, respectively, in the glucose oxidase reaction.

Glucose concentrations in serum and plasma are roughly equal; however, whole blood glucose concentrations may vary from plasma or serum concentrations. Most commercially available glucometers use whole blood. Many glucometers were designed for human use and therefore assume a constant stable relationship between plasma and whole blood and equilibration between plasma and erythrocyte glucose concentrations. In humans, this relationship holds true: glucose distribution is 50% within erythrocytes and 50% within plasma. This is not the case in many veterinary species. For example, in dogs and cats, glucose distribution is 12.5% and 7% within erythrocytes and 87.5% and 93% within plasma, respectively.[8] Similarly, in foals and horses, glucose is largely present in plasma, with little measurable glucose in erythrocytes.[19] Whole blood glucose measurements in horses using a point-of-care glucometer designed for human use were poorly correlated with the laboratory analyzer. However, when plasma was separated and tested with the glucometer, there was good agreement.[22] Similarly, in neonatal foals, a point-of-care glucometer designed for human use consistently underestimated blood glucose relative to the clinical laboratory analyzer.[31] In contrast, one study using a veterinary glucometer showed good accuracy and precision in horses relative to the laboratory standard.[20] It is important to note that differences in methodology may yield differences in the reference values. Thus an essential component of test validation is to establish species-specific and instrument-specific reference intervals.

Although point-of-care glucometers use whole blood to measure glucose concentrations, some measure plasma glucose, some measure whole blood glucose, and others calculate the plasma glucose concentration from a whole blood glucose measurement.[36] Glucometers that calculate the plasma glucose concentration from the whole blood glucose concentration may assume a normal hematocrit, which can result in inaccurate results because the erythrocyte concentration can affect the glucose measurement. Few studies have been done on the effects of hematocrit on point-of-care glucometer readings in horses, but one anecdotal report suggests that a high hematocrit does affect accurate glucose measurement by a veterinary glucometer.[20]

Hyperglycemia

Hyperglycemia can present either transiently or persistently (Table 8.1). Transient hyperglycemia may be postprandial, physiologic, or drug-related. Postprandial hyperglycemia, more common with feeds high in simple carbohydrates, can persist for 2–4 hours after feeding. Physiologic hyperglycemia is caused by the insulin-antagonistic actions of catecholamines, glucocorticoids, growth hormone, and glucagon; drug-associated hyperglycemias are often the result of the drug's stimulation or mimicry of these hormones. Glucose homeostatic dysfunction manifesting as hyperglycemia is reported in up to half of adult horses with acute abdominal disease.[21] The hyperglycemia is likely due to a combination of peripheral insulin resistance and increased gluconeogenesis due to the release of epinephrine, cortisol, tumor necrosis factor, and other mediators. Hyperglycemia has negative prognostic significance in colic patients and prognosis worsens with the severity of hyperglycemia.

Pathologic hyperglycemia is associated with glucose metabolic defects stemming from a relative and/or absolute insulin deficiency. In horses, these

Table 8.1 Conditions associated with hyperglycemia

Physiologic
  Postprandial (high simple carbohydrate content)
  Glucocorticoids
    Stress
  Catecholamines
    Pain, exertion, excitement
  Drugs
    Glucocorticoids
    Progesterone
    Xylazine
    Ketamine
    Morphine
  Pathologic
    Diabetes mellitus
    Pituitary pars intermedia dysfunction[a]
    Equine metabolic syndrome[a]
    Colic[a]

[a]Hyperglycemia is not present in all cases.

are most commonly associated with insulin-resistant states such as equine metabolic syndrome and pituitary pars intermedia dysfunction (PPID) that have become uncompensated. Type II diabetes mellitus (DM) is an example of an insulin-resistant disorder with pancreatic β-cell dysfunction. Insulin resistance and associated disorders are discussed in more detail further in the chapter.

Hypoglycemia

Disorders causing hypoglycemia are attributable to increased glucose utilization by tissues and/or decreased glucose production (Table 8.2). Hypoglycemia is associated with sepsis and/or endotoxemia likely as a result of increased tissue glucose utilization and/or impaired gluconeogenesis and glycogenolysis. Extreme exertion in endurance horses can result in hypoglycemia, presumably as a result of decreased glycogen stores, increased glucose utilization, and/or decreased epinephrine responsiveness. Hypoglycemia due to hepatic failure only occurs after a loss of more than 70% of liver function; other clinical signs and laboratory abnormalities support an interpretation of hypoglycemia due to liver failure (see Chapter 4). Neonatal hypoglycemia may occur with poor nursing due to multiple causes (e.g., diarrhea, hypothermia, or agalactia). Foals have comparatively small glycogen and protein reserves as substrates for gluconeogenesis during times of decreased food intake. Hypoglycemia associated with starvation or malabsorption in adult horses and ponies is uncommon and only occurs with long-term decreased glucose availability.

Insulin

Insulin measurement is performed with an immunoassay. Serum or plasma insulin concentration may include proinsulin and is reported in immunoreactive units. Most insulin immunoassays use a commercial radioimmunoassay, but a chemiluminescent immunometric (Siemens, Diagnostic Products Corp.,

Table 8.2   Conditions associated with hypoglycemia

Preanalytic and analytic causes
  Delayed serum/plasma separation from blood cells
  Marked leukocytosis, erythrocytosis[a]
  Assay interference (hemolysis, icterus, lipemia)
Pathologic
  Sepsis/endotoxemia
  Extreme exertion
  Hepatic failure
  Neonatal hypoglycemia
  Starvation, malabsorption[a]
  Glycogen storage disease (Quarter Horse PSSM)

[a]Uncommon. *PSSM*, polysaccharide storage myopathy.

Los Angeles, CA) assay is now available. Equine insulin is stable for 30 days at 6–8°C and for 1 year at −20°C.[29] Serum or heparinized plasma can be used to measure insulin concentration.

Of the tests that evaluate glucose metabolism, measurement of resting insulin concentration is readily available and easy to perform. Resting insulin concentration is a useful screening test for decreased insulin sensitivity because compensatory hyperinsulinemia is a common feature of insulin resistance in horses. However, with mild or early insulin resistance, hyperinsulinemia may not have developed yet or the rise in serum insulin concentration may be too small to be detected using population-based reference values. Moreover, insulin concentration may vary as a result of diurnal variation, stress, or feeding. For these reasons a single blood insulin value is not an accurate indicator of insulin sensitivity.

Reference intervals currently available for horses differ between laboratories as a result of different methodologies and/or reagents. Hyperinsulinemia is defined as a serum insulin concentration above 30 μunits/ml at the University of Tennessee, above 34 μunits/mL at the University of Pennsylvania, and above 43 μunits/ml at the Diagnostic Center for Population and Animal Health at Michigan State University. It is therefore important that results are interpreted using the reference values provided by the diagnostic laboratory supplying the results.

Leptin

The use of leptin concentrations as a diagnostic tool in characterizing equine metabolic syndrome is increasing. The hormone leptin is synthesized by adipocytes in greater quantities when the body is in a positive energy balance and signals the hypothalamus that adipose stores are replete. Serum leptin concentrations have been positively correlated with body condition score in horses, indicating that blood leptin concentrations reflect body-fat mass in horses.[4,15] However, not all obese horses are hyperleptinemic; only about a third of obese mares had high leptin concentrations in one study. Hyperleptinemia has been associated with glucose metabolism disturbances in horses; obese horses with high serum leptin concentrations showed abnormal glucose tolerance test results compared with obese horses that had lower leptin concentrations.[7]

Leptin may decrease as much as 50% with fasting and will rise after feeding up to two times above fasting values.[30] Reference values should clearly state whether they reflect fed or fasting states. Serum and plasma collected in either EDTA or heparin are reported to be acceptable for leptin measurement in horses, but the laboratory offering the test should be consulted before sample submission. In humans, leptin is stable in serum for 2 months at 4°C and for 2 years at −20°C and appears to have similar stability in rodents.[30] Studies in the stability of equine leptin are lacking. Leptin measurement is now being offered at Cornell Animal Health Diagnostic Center (Ithaca, NY), but it is not currently a widely available test.

Glucose tolerance test

Tolerance is typically defined as blood glucose clearance following oral or intravenous glucose administration. Because oral glucose administration is affected by gastrointestinal function, intravenous (IV) administration is a more specific assessment of glucose metabolism. 0.5 g glucose/kg is administered IV. Blood is taken at 0 (baseline), 5, 15, 30, 60, and 90 minutes post-infusion and then hourly for 5–6 hours for measurement of glucose and insulin concentrations. Blood glucose concentrations in horses with normal insulin sensitivity should show an immediate rise, a peak at 15 minutes, and a return to baseline within 1–2 hours. The insulin concentration should parallel the glucose response curve but peak at 30 minutes post-infusion. Horses with insulin resistance will show delayed return to reference values (>2 hours) and a higher blood glucose peak (Figure 8.5).[18]

Combined glucose-insulin test

The combined glucose–insulin test, also known as the frequently sampled intravenous glucose tolerance test, requires collection of a baseline blood sample, infusion of 150 mg/kg 50% dextrose solution, and infusion of 0.10 units/kg regular insulin immediately after the dextrose infusion. Blood samples are collected at 1, 5, 25, 35, 45, 60, 75, 90, 105, 120, 135, and 150 minutes post-infusion. With this method insulin resistance is defined as maintenance of blood glucose concentrations above the baseline value for $\geq$45 min.[12] The test can be shortened to 60 min when used in the field, but the time taken for the blood concentration to return to baseline is important information that should be recorded for future reference. This allows assessment of the response to diet, exercise, or medication.

Care should be taken to minimize stress, exercise, excitement, or pain before and during the testing because of their effect on glucose concentration. Note that there is a small risk of hypoglycemia when performing this test and signs of hypoglycemia should be detected and responded to promptly. Because glucose concentrations are being measured, it is important to separate the plasma or serum from the blood cells within an hour after collection or to use a NaF collection tube. If a glucometer is used for measurement of blood glucose, it should be a veterinary glucometer validated for horses (see earlier section on glucose measurement).

Diseases associated with glucose metabolic defects

Pasture laminitis

Risk factors for the development of pasture laminitis include insulin-resistant states such as pituitary pars intermedia dysfunction (PPID) and obesity (including regional adiposity).[6] Nonstructural carbohydrates (e.g., simple sugars, starches, and fructose polymers) in pasture grass are implicated in the pathogenesis of pasture-associated laminitis, although insulin resistance is thought to be the predisposing factor. Carbohydrate overload is associated with the development and/or exacerbation of insulin resistance that might precipitate

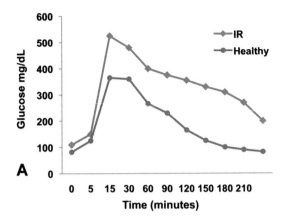

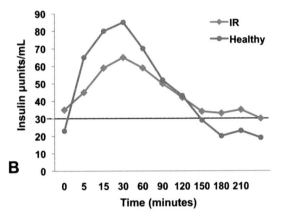

Figure 8.5 Glucose tolerance test. A. Glucose concentration post-administration of intravenous glucose in healthy and insulin resistant (IR) ponies. The blood glucose concentration in the healthy pony shows an immediate rise, a peak around 15 minutes, and a return to baseline within 1-2 hours. In contrast, the IR glucose curve shows a higher peak at 15 minutes without fully returning to reference interval concentrations by the end of the test. B. The insulin concentration parallels the glucose response curve with a peak at 30 minutes post-infusion. The insulin response in the pony with IR is blunted and the insulin concentration remains slightly increased at the end of the testing period.

laminitis by interfering with glucose uptake by hoof keratinocytes or by al-tering blood flow to the hoof. Additionally, carbohydrate overload may alter bacterial flora, causing the release of vasoactive endotoxins, exotoxins, or amines that potentially can alter hoof blood flow. Endotoxin activation of a systemic inflammatory response will also induce insulin resistance, although endotoxemia alone is not sufficient to induce laminitis.[38]

Pasture-associated laminitis follows a seasonal pattern, with increased inci-dence of laminitis in the fall. Pasture grazing increases blood concentrations of glucose and insulin concomitant with seasonal upregulation of ACTH, which may be an important part of the development of laminitis, especially in PPID horses (discussed later in the chapter). There is a positive correlation between insulin concentration and simple sugar content of pasture grass.[16]

Equine metabolic syndrome

In a recent consensus statement regarding the characterization of equine metabolic syndrome (EMS), it was agreed that the three major components of the syndrome comprised obesity (generalized or regional), hyperinsulinemia, and insulin resistance with a predisposition to laminitis.[17] Insulin resistance is defined by hyperinsulinemia or abnormal responses to glucose and/or insulin tolerance tests. It is currently uncertain whether these components alone are responsible for the susceptibility to laminitis or whether there is another, as yet unidentified factor that precipitates laminitis in horses with EMS. Additional characteristics of EMS include hypertriglyceridemia (discussed above), arterial hypertension that is detected in the summer in laminitis-prone ponies, altered reproductive cycling in mares, increased systemic markers of inflammation in association with obesity, and hyperleptinemia.[17] The highest incidence of EMS is seen in pony breeds, Morgan horses, Paso Finos, Arabians, Saddlebreds, Quarter horses, and Tennessee Walking horses.[14]

Current recommendations for screening for EMS include measurement of fasting insulin, leptin, and glucose concentrations. Glucose concentrations may be within reference limits in EMS because hyperinsulinemia often maintains euglycemia. Hyperglycemia in the context of hyperinsulinemia suggests uncompensated insulin resistance (or type II diabetes mellitus). Obese horses with high serum leptin concentrations showed abnormal glucose tolerance test results compared with obese horses that had lower leptin concentrations, suggesting that high leptin concentrations reflect insulin resistance and are a component of EMS.[7] Serum insulin concentrations in conjunction with leptin concentrations and assessment of body condition score are useful in the detection of insulin resistance and EMS. Concurrent hyperinsulinemia, hyperglycemia, and hyperleptinemia are consistent with a diagnosis of EMS. When the patient has physical features of EMS but the screening data are ambiguous, glucose or combined glucose insulin tolerance testing is recommended.[14]

Pituitary pars intermedia dysfunction (PPID)

Pituitary pars intermedia dysfunction is covered fully in Chapter 10 and will only be discussed here in the context of a glucose metabolic disorder. Insulin resistance associated with PPID is a consequence of hypercortisolemia. Cortisol is an insulin antagonist. The net effects of hypercortisolemia include enhanced gluconeogenesis in hepatocytes, increased hormone-sensitive lipase activity resulting in increased NEFA substrate for gluconeogenesis, and inhibition of insulin activity at the receptor and post-receptor level. It is thought that the inhibition of GLUT-4-mediated glucose uptake in the laminar tissue may be integral to the development of laminitis in PPID and other insulin-resistant conditions.

Localized obesity, insulin resistance, and laminitis are recognized components of PPID as well as EMS.[33] These two syndromes may occur alone or in conjunction. Given the clinical similarities, it is important to distinguish between these disorders. Clinical signs supportive of a diagnosis of PPID but not EMS include delayed shedding/retention of winter haircoat, hirsutism, excessive sweating, skeletal muscle atrophy, and polyuria/polydipsia. The patient's age is another distinguishing factor. EMS is generally first identified in younger horses, whereas PPID is commonly diagnosed in older horses. Finally, laboratory results showing inappropriately increased plasma ACTH concentration is a feature of PPID and not EMS.

Diabetes mellitus

Diabetes mellitus (DM) is characterized by persistent hyperglycemia due to reduced insulin secretion and/or insulin resistance. Hyperglycemia in type I DM is attributed to absolute hypoinsulinemia as a result of pancreatic β-cell destruction, and is very rare in horses. Equine type II DM, which is initially a relative insulin deficiency, is gaining increasing recognition.[11] Type II DM is characterized in the early stage by normoglycemia with concurrent hyperinsulinemia (pre-diabetes), but in later stages manifests as hyperglycemia with normo- or hypoinsulinemia as pancreatic β-cell function declines. Type II DM develops in humans as a result of prolonged insulin resistance and subsequent pancreatic β-cell exhaustion. Diagnosis of type II DM requires confirmation of insulin resistance with an evaluation of β-cell function for staging. Low serum insulin concentrations with poor pancreatic β-cell response could indicate either type I or type II DM; quantitative measures of insulin sensitivity are therefore needed to distinguish between the types. Currently, these types of measurements are not feasible in the field and are used mainly in select clinical and research situations. Persistent hyperglycemia with low or normal insulin concentrations and clinical signs of polyuria, polydipsia, and weight loss are strongly suggestive of DM.

Other diseases

While most diseases of equine glucose metabolism are associated with insulin-resistant states, there are two diseases associated with enhanced glucose metabolism: Quarter Horse polysaccharide storage myopathy (PSSM; discussed in Chapter 9) and equine motor neuron disease. Oral and intravenous glucose tolerance testing in PSSM horses reveals increased sensitivity to insulin, which results in increased glucose uptake and storage and hypoglycemia relative to controls.[1,9] Equine motor neuron disease is also associated with increased glucose clearance and decreased blood glucose concentrations relative to healthy control horses during glucose challenge. The mechanism is currently unclear.[3,40]

References

1. Annandale EJ, Valberg SJ, Mickelson JR, et al. 2004. Insulin sensitivity and skeletal muscle glucose transport in horses with equine polysaccharide storage myopathy. *Neuromuscul Disord* 14:666-674.
2. Argenzio RA, Hintz HF. 1972. Effect of diet on glucose entry and oxidation rates in ponies. *J Nutr* 102:879-892.
3. Benders NA, Dyer J, Wijnberg ID, et al. 2005. Evaluation of glucose tolerance and intestinal luminal membrane glucose transporter function in horses with equine motor neuron disease. *Am J Vet Res* 66:93-99.
4. Buff PR, Dodds AC, Morrison CD, et al. 2002. Leptin in horses: tissue localization and relationship between peripheral concentrations of leptin and body condition. *J Anim Sci* 80:2942-2948.
5. Burden FA, Du Toit N, Hazell-Smith E, et al. 2011. Hyperlipemia in a population of aged donkeys: description, prevalence, and potential risk factors. *J Vet Intern Med* 25:1420-1425.
6. Carter RA, Treiber KH, Geor RJ, et al. 2009. Prediction of incipient pasture-associated laminitis from hyperinsulinaemia, hyperleptinaemia and generalised and localised obesity in a cohort of ponies. *Equine Vet J* 41:171-178.
7. Cartmill JA, Thompson DL, Jr., Storer WA, et al. 2003. Endocrine responses in mares and geldings with high body condition scores grouped by high vs. low resting leptin concentrations. *J Anim Sci* 81:2311-2321.
8. Coldman MF, Good W. 1967. The distribution of sodium, potassium and glucose in the blood of some mammals. *Comp Biochem Physiol* 21:201-206.
9. De La Corte FD, Valberg SJ, MacLeay JM, et al. 1999. Glucose uptake in horses with polysaccharide storage myopathy. *Am J Vet Res* 60:458-462.
10. Dunkel B, McKenzie HC, 3rd. 2003. Severe hypertriglyceridaemia in clinically ill horses: diagnosis, treatment and outcome. *Equine Vet J* 35:590-595.
11. Durham AE, Hughes KJ, Cottle HJ, et al. 2009. Type 2 diabetes mellitus with pancreatic beta cell dysfunction in 3 horses confirmed with minimal model analysis. *Equine Vet J* 41:924-929.
12. Eiler H, Frank N, Andrews FM, et al. 2005. Physiologic assessment of blood glucose homeostasis via combined intravenous glucose and insulin testing in horses. *Am J Vet Res* 66:1598-1604.
13. Ford EJ, Simmons HA. 1985. Gluconeogenesis from caecal propionate in the horse. *Br J Nutr* 53:55-60.
14. Frank N. 2011. Equine metabolic syndrome. *Vet Clin North Am Equine Pract* 27:73-92.
15. Frank N, Elliott SB, Brandt LE, et al. 2006. Physical characteristics, blood hormone concentrations, and plasma lipid concentrations in obese horses with insulin resistance. *J Am Vet Med Assoc* 228:1383-1390.
16. Frank N, Elliott SB, Chameroy KA, et al. 2010. Association of season and pasture grazing with blood hormone and metabolite concentrations in horses with presumed pituitary pars intermedia dysfunction. *J Vet Intern Med* 24:1167-1175.
17. Frank N, Geor RJ, Bailey SR, et al. 2010. Equine metabolic syndrome. *J Vet Intern Med* 24:467-475.
18. Garcia MC, Beech J. 1986. Equine intravenous glucose tolerance test: glucose and insulin responses of healthy horses fed grain or hay and of horses with pituitary adenoma. *Am J Vet Res* 47:570-572.
19. Goodwin RF. 1956. The distribution of sugar between red cells and plasma: variations associated with age and species. *J Physiol* 134:88-101.

20. Hackett ES, McCue PM. 2010. Evaluation of a veterinary glucometer for use in horses. *J Vet Intern Med* 24:617–621.
21. Hassel DM, Hill AE, Rorabeck RA. 2009. Association between hyperglycemia and survival in 228 horses with acute gastrointestinal disease. *J Vet Intern Med* 23:1261–1265.
22. Hollis AR, Dallap-Schaer BL, Boston RC, et al. 2008. Comparison of the Accu-Chek Aviva point-of-care glucometer with blood gas and laboratory methods of analysis of glucose measurement in equine emergency patients. *J Vet Intern Med* 22:1189–1195.
23. Hughes KJ, Hodgson DR, Dart AJ. 2004. Equine hyperlipaemia: a review. *Aust Vet J* 82:136–142.
24. Kronfeld DS, Treiber KH, Hess TM, et al. 2005. Insulin resistance in the horse: definition, detection, and dietetics. *J Anim Sci* 83:E22-E31.
25. McKenzie III HC. 2011. Equine hyperlipidemias. *Vet Clin North Am Equine Pract* 27:59–72.
26. Mogg TD, Palmer JE. 1995. Hyperlipidemia, hyperlipemia, and hepatic lipidosis in American miniature horses: 23 cases (1990-1994). *J Am Vet Med Assoc* 207:604–607.
27. Murray M. 1985. Hepatic lipidosis in a post-parturient mare. *Equine Vet J* 17:68–69.
28. Naylor JM, Kronfeld DS, Acland H. 1980. Hyperlipemia in horses: effects of undernutrition and disease. *Am J Vet Res* 41:899–905.
29. Oberg J, Brojer J, Wattle O, et al. 2011. Evaluation of an equine-optimized enzyme-linked immunosorbent assay for serum insulin measurement and stability study of equine serum insulin. *Comp Clin Pathol* DOI: 10.1007/s00580-011-1284-6.
30. Radin MJ, Sharkey LC, Holycross BJ. 2009. Adipokines: a review of biological and analytical principles and an update in dogs, cats, and horses. *Vet Clin Pathol* 38:136–156.
31. Russell C, Palmer JE, Boston RC, et al. 2007. Agreement between point-of-care glucometry, blood gas and laboratory-based measurement of glucose in an equine neonatal intensive care unit. *J Vet Emerg Crit Care (San Antonio)* 17:236–242.
32. Sato T, Liang K, Vaziri ND. 2002. Down-regulation of lipoprotein lipase and VLDL receptor in rats with focal glomerulosclerosis. *Kidney Int* 61:157–162.
33. Schott Jr. HC. 2002. Pituitary pars intermedia dysfunction: equine Cushing's disease. *Vet Clin North Am Equine Pract* 18:237–270.
34. Shulman GI. 2000. Cellular mechanisms of insulin resistance. *J Clin Invest* 106:171–176.
35. Stein EA, Myers GL. 1994. Lipids, lipoproteins and apolipoproteins. In *Tietz Textbook of Clinical Chemistry*, Burtis CA and Ashwood ER (eds), 2nd ed. pp. 1002–1093. Philadelphia: WB Saunders Company.
36. Stockham SL, Scott MA. 2002. Glucose and related regulatory hormones. In *Fundamentals of Veterinary Clinical Pathology*, Stockham SL and Scott MA (eds), pp. 487–506. Ames: Blackwell.
37. Stockham SL, Scott MA. 2002. Lipids. In *Fundamentals of Veterinary Clinical Pathology*, Stockham SL and Scott MA (eds), pp. 521–537. Ames: Blackwell.
38. Toth F, Frank N, Chameroy KA, et al. 2009. Effects of endotoxaemia and carbohydrate overload on glucose and insulin dynamics and the development of laminitis in horses. *Equine Vet J* 41:852–858.
39. Treiber KH, Kronfeld DS, Geor RJ. 2006. Insulin resistance in equids: possible role in laminitis. *J Nutr* 136:2094S-2098S.

40. van der Kolk JH, Rijnen KE, Rey F, et al. 2005. Evaluation of glucose metabolism in three horses with lower motor neuron degeneration. *Am J Vet Res* 66:271-276.

41. Vick MM, Adams AA, Murphy BA, et al. 2007. Relationships among inflammatory cytokines, obesity, and insulin sensitivity in the horse. *J Anim Sci* 85:1144-1155.

42. Watson TD, Burns L, Freeman DJ, et al. 1993. High density lipoprotein metabolism in the horse (Equus caballus). *Comp Biochem Physiol B* 104:45-53.

43. Watson TD, Burns L, Love S, et al. 1991. The isolation, characterisation and quantification of the equine plasma lipoproteins. *Equine Vet J* 23:353-359.

Chapter 9
Skeletal Muscle

Allison Billings

Laboratory evaluation of equine muscle disorders

Most laboratory tests directed to the evaluation of muscle measure the serum activity of enzymes released from muscle tissue after injury. Extraskeletal factors contributing to increases in serum enzyme activity should be considered in interpreting changes in these enzymes. Other constituents released from muscle such as myoglobin and troponin I are also useful biomarkers of muscle injury. The cardiac isoform of troponin I is currently a valuable clinical tool in the assessment of myocardial injury.

General causes of increased serum enzymes

The basis of clinical enzymology of muscle is the measurement of enzyme activities that occur when muscle tissue has been damaged. A range of enzymes and biomarkers are available for use in clinical investigations to monitor the onset or progress of muscle disease. The concentrations of enzymes in serum or plasma can be determined by using the chemical reactions they catalyze or by using an immunoassay.

The concentration of muscle enzymes in serum or plasma is usually low in healthy horses because the enzymes are located within the myofiber. Most of the muscle enzymes are present within the sarcoplasm; however, certain enzymes also have a mitochondrial form. In general, an increase in serum enzyme activity may be secondary to increased production of the enzyme (e.g., hyperplasia) or due to decreased removal of that enzyme from the blood. The major mechanism by which serum enzyme activity increases is through release from damaged myofibers at a rate that exceeds the rate of enzyme inactivation or removal from blood.[16] Cell necrosis and irreversible cell damage lead to release of enzymes and increased serum concentrations. Minor cell injury that causes reversible damage may also create increases in serum enzyme activities through formation of membrane blebs containing cytoplasmic enzymes. These blebs may rupture or be released into blood and lyse, producing an increase in serum enzyme activity.[72]

Equine Clinical Pathology, First Edition. Edited by Raquel M. Walton.
© 2014 John Wiley & Sons, Inc. Published 2014 by John Wiley & Sons, Inc.

The rate of enzyme loss (or its rate of rise in serum) is affected by the severity of tissue damage, the enzyme concentration within the cell, the location of the enzyme within the cell, and how the enzyme enters the blood. Thus, the magnitude of increase does not necessarily correlate with the extent of muscle injury. The common muscle enzymes are cytoplasmic enzymes, and their rate of increase is likely to be greater with more severe muscle damage. Because enzymes from myofibers are released into the interstitial space and enter the plasma via the lymphatics, there is a slower rate of enzyme increase than direct release into blood.[62]

Serum enzymes detecting muscle injury

Aspartate aminotransferase (AST)

Aspartate aminotransferase (AST) was formerly known as glutamic oxaloacetic transaminase (GOT). AST catalyzes the transamination of L-aspartate and 2-oxoglutarate to oxaloacetate and glutamate and requires pyrixidol-5'-phosphate (PP) as a cofactor. The requirement of a cofactor is of note because assays including the cofactor may generate different results from those lacking the cofactor. Poor saturation of serum alanine aminotransferase (ALT) with PP caused underestimation of the total enzyme activity (if PP was not added to the *in vitro* sample) in a study of horses post-exercise; however, the same study showed the majority of AST (94%) was saturated with PP and thus not subject to the same underestimation.[98] The enzyme is reported to be stable for days in serum at room temperature, refrigerated, or frozen.[50] A study of equine clotted blood and serum stored at room temperature revealed significant increases in enzyme activity after 48 hours.[99] Results are reported in international unit per liter (IU/L).

The half-life for equine AST is generally reported to be 7 to 8 days.[18] However, other studies suggest a shorter half-life of 3 to 4 days.[18,85,108] In either case, serum AST has a longer half-life than creatine kinase. Peak values in the horse are reached within 24-48 hours.[22,101,108]

AST is present within the cytoplasm and in larger amounts in the mitochondria. In horses, the ratio of mitochondrial AST (mAST) to cytoplasmic AST (cAST) is greater than in other mammals.[107] It is postulated that severe or irreversible cell injury, which would result in the release of mAST as well as cAST, is likely to lead to a greater magnitude of serum AST increase than minor or reversible cell injury that would only cause the release of cAST. Studies to confirm this suspicion are lacking.

In addition to skeletal muscle, AST is found within cardiac muscle cells, hepatocytes, and erythrocytes. Increases in serum AST activity occur with myocyte injury and hepatocellular injury. Although an increase in AST can reflect some degree of myocyte injury, it can occur with a variety of insults and does not specify a particular disease or disorder. Given the nonspecific nature of AST, assessment of additional organ-specific enzymes is often required to distinguish between myocyte and hepatocellular injury. Hemolysis also causes increases in AST due to its presence in greater concentrations within erythrocytes than plasma.[6]

Serial measurement of AST in conjunction with creatine kinase can often be useful to indicate the time course of muscle injury. CK has a very short half-life, increases very quickly (peaks at 6 to 12 hours), and remains increased only for a couple of days following a muscle injury episode. Continued increases suggest ongoing or active muscle injury. In contrast, AST has a more gradual rise to peak. It can be present for a week to several weeks following an episode of muscle injury and thus may be increased with either persistent or resolved muscle injury. Therefore, serial measurements that initially show an increase in both AST and CK, and later show only an increased AST, indicate that the episode of myonecrosis has resolved (see Figure 9.1).

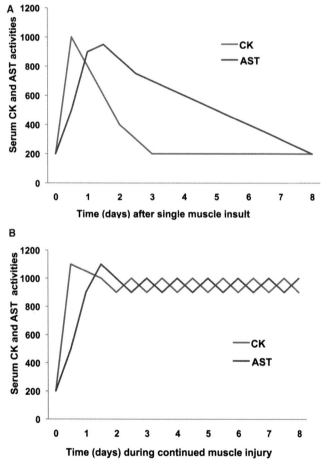

Figure 9.1   Increases in serum CK and AST activities after muscle injury. CK has an earlier rise to peak and shorter half-life than AST. Differences in CK and AST serum activities over time may be helpful in determining the time course of muscle injury. A. After a single insult, both CK and AST are initially increased. If measurements are repeated at day 3 following the insult, CK activity will likely be within or close to normal range while AST will still be increased. B. Continued high levels of both CK and AST suggest repeated or ongoing muscle injury.

Creatine kinase (CK)

Creatine kinase (CK) catalyzes the phosphorylation of creatine by ATP to form phosphocreatine and ADP. In skeletal and cardiac myocytes, this reaction functions to make ATP available for muscle contraction. CK also catalyzes the reverse reaction in the resting myocyte. It is present in negligible amounts in many tissues throughout the body and in high concentrations within skeletal and cardiac muscle.[109] CK is predominantly a cytoplasmic enzyme, although a small amount is present associated with the outer side of the inner mitochondrial membranes.[53] The enzyme is stable for 7 days at 4°C and for 1 month at −20°C in canine serum; however, published studies for refrigerated or frozen stored equine samples are lacking. Equine samples (clotted blood and serum) stored at room temperature resulted in spurious increases in CK after 72 hours.[99] Serum CK is higher than plasma CK in the dog due to release of CK with clot formation, but it is unknown if this is true in the horse as well.[41] Results are reported in international unit per liter (IU/L).

The half-life of CK is relatively short, although specific times vary among studies. Intravenous and intramuscular injections of CK produce half-lives of approximately 2 hours and 12 hours, respectively.[110] The intramuscular administration is expected to be more reflective of actual physiologic conditions as CK must be absorbed from the lymphatics into the blood after muscle injury and release from the myocyte. In more recent studies in horses, CK was shown to peak from 6 to 12 hours.[22] Return of CK to baseline values were reported at 24 hours, 2 to 3 days, and 3 to 4 days in each of the studies.

CK has several isoenzymes. In most tissues, both cytoplasmic CK and mitochondrial CK isoenzymes are co-expressed. Cytoplasmic CK has a dimeric structure made of M (muscle) and B (brain) subunits. There are three cytosolic CK isoenzymes: CK-1 (or CK-BB) is found primarily in the brain and CK-2 (CK-MB) and CK-3 (CK-MM) are found in cardiac and skeletal muscle; CK-2 is present in overall low concentrations in the horse.[9,11] Although it is possible to separate these isoenzymes, CK isoenzyme analysis has not been shown to be diagnostically useful in equine studies.[104]

The majority of serum CK is of muscle origin. Therefore, CK is considered a muscle-specific marker and increases in serum CK activity are considered indicative of muscle injury. However, it is worthy of note that hemolysis can cause increases in CK due to the release of adenylate cyclase from erythrocytes.[6] As discussed above, serial measurements of AST and CK can be utilized to assess the time course of the muscle injury.

Extremely high serum CK activity (>10,000 IU/L) often requires dilution by a technician running the assay. Dilution of the serum results in dilution of endogenous CK inhibitors, thus serial dilution of a sample with high CK activity may result in progressively higher activity levels. Thus, while the true activity level is high, it may be spuriously increased as a result of multiple dilutions to the sample.[58]

Lactate dehydrogenase (LDH)

Lactate dehydrogenase (LDH) is a cytoplasmic enzyme that catalyzes the conversion of pyruvate to lactate at the end of anaerobic glycolysis. It is present in many tissues in the body and is therefore not organ-specific to muscle. However, it is present in higher concentrations in skeletal and cardiac muscle, kidney, and liver.[109] In heparinized equine plasma samples the enzyme is stable when stored at room temperature and remains so for 7 days at −18°C. However, heparinized equine whole blood stored in the same conditions results in a marked increase in LDH activity.[63] In another study, equine clotted blood and serum samples stored at room temperature produce increases in LDH activity after 24 hours.[99] Results are reported in international unit per liter (IU/L).

The half-life of LDH is reported to be 7 days and peak concentrations are expected 24 hours after tissue injury.[108] More recent studies have produced different results for half-life with return to normal values in 3 days in one study and 10-21 days in another.[101,108] Perhaps these variations are due in part to the different half-lives of the LDH isoenzymes, which vary in any one tissue and also between the same isoenzyme in different tissues.[15,27]

LDH is not organ specific and is present in a variety of tissues. Increases in serum LDH activity in the horse can suggest skeletal muscle injury, cardiac muscle injury, or hepatocellular insult; however, in the absence of isoenzyme analysis, utilization of other more muscle and liver-specific enzymes is recommended for interpretation. Erythrocytes contain a greater concentration of LDH than plasma, thus hemolysis can cause increases in LDH as well.[6]

Alanine aminotransferase (ALT)

Alanine aminotransferase (ALT) catalyzes the reversible transamination of L-alanine and 2-oxoglutarate to pyruvate and glutamate. This reaction requires pyrixidol-5′-phosphate (PP) as a cofactor. In horses, a considerable amount of serum ALT is reported to be in the apo-enzyme form (inactive form that is bound to the cofactor), which can generate an underestimation of the total serum ALT activity if PP is not added to the sample. In one study, the increase in serum ALT activity after the addition of PP ranged from an average of 27% in retired, non-Thoroughbred, unexercised horses to 61% in resting Thoroughbred racehorses and 72% in post-exercise Thoroughbred racehorses.[98]

ALT is a cytoplasmic and mitochondrial enzyme, although the mitochondrial form is present in much smaller amounts. ALT activity is found in several organs including muscle and liver in the horse. Based on studies of bovine blood, ALT is stable at room temperature in plasma for 4 days and serum for 2 days, although reports for human blood suggest a shorter stability of 24 hours at room temperature (and up to 7 days at 4°C).[55,118] Plasma ALT half-life in dogs is 2-3 days. Reports for values in the horse are lacking. Results are reported in international unit per liter (IU/L).

Many consider ALT to be a muscle specific enzyme in the horse, as the liver has minimal ALT activity and is expected to contribute little to serum ALT activity.[21] Despite this specificity, it is often absent from large animal biochemical profiles, perhaps due to greater reliance on CK and AST for muscle injury assessment. Hemolysis in equine serum is reported to cause increases in ALT due to both spectral interference and the addition of ALT from erythrocytes.[106]

Additional factors affecting CK and AST enzyme activity

CK and AST changes associated with exercise and training

The effect of exercise and training on serum muscle enzyme activity is difficult to determine. Results vary in the literature due to differences in protocols used by different studies (such as variations in exercise and training duration and intensity), fitness level of the study subjects, and the study interval.

Overall, the majority of studies find minimal to no increases in muscle enzymes during exercise. These studies include protocols of primarily submaximal intensity or short-duration exercise.[18,43,98] In some studies that did report increases in muscle enzyme activity, these increases were attributed to muscle injury. For example, in one study, 3 horses had gluteal muscle injury and 4 had subclinical muscle damage. These horses were exercised on a treadmill at an incline too, which may have predisposed to injury.[102]

In contrast to these results, studies in horses performing maximal or longer-duration (endurance) exercise found significant increases in serum muscle enzymes (CK) activities, but these studies either reported no increase in AST or inconclusive AST results.[8,68] Although CK and AST increases may occur with exercise, values are often not clinically significant and still within normal limits. Generally with exercise there is a 50% increase in enzyme activity. CK increases can be attributed to plasma volume changes and muscle leakage and AST increases can be attributed to plasma volume change.[35]

CK and AST variations with gender and age

Differences in CK and AST due to age and gender are inconsistent in the literature. One study of thoroughbred mares between 2 and 4 years of age found no effects of age on resting CK or AST.[37] However, a separate study of 2- and 3-year-old Thoroughbreds in training revealed that fillies were more likely to have increased CK and AST than colts, and 2-year-olds tended to have higher AST than 3-year olds. Thus, age was a factor for CK and both age and sex were factors for AST.[45] In addition, in another study, 2-year-old Thoroughbred fillies showed more marked fluctuations in AST and CK than 3-year-old Thoroughbred fillies and colts. No relationship was found between elevations in muscle enzymes and the stage of the estrous cycle.[33] Some studies did find evidence that sex differences may be due to the effect of hormones such as progesterone and estradiol on CK and AST release.[7,33] These findings suggest that age- and/or sex-specific reference intervals may be necessary.

CK Changes associated with incorrect venepuncture

Incorrect venepuncture can result in injury to connective tissue surrounding the vein and/or adjacent musculature and subsequent release of CK, which mixes with the sample, thus increasing the CK activity measured. CK can increase more than 125% above those values obtained via normal/correct venepuncture, yielding false positive results.[96]

Other markers detecting muscle injury

Myoglobin

Myoglobin is a heme-containing, oxygen-carrying monomer protein expressed in muscle fibers that may be a useful biomarker of muscle fiber injury. Myoglobin is released immediately into circulation after muscle damage and its concentration peaks shortly (5 to 30 minutes) after muscle injury.[113] Myoglobin is cleared faster from the circulation than CK. Studies of horses with recurrent rhabdomyolysis show decreases to normal levels by 24 to 72 hours after exercise, although a study in humans suggests longer increases (of up to 19 days) may be possible with endurance exercise.[84,113]

Because myoglobin is cleared so quickly from the circulation, measurement of myoglobin in the urine may be of diagnostic value and helpful in situations where blood sampling soon after muscle injury is not possible. Myoglobin causes discoloration of the urine to a reddish-brown (port-wine-like) color (Figure 9.2). Pigmenturia can elicit suspicion for myoglobinuria; however, hematuria and hemoglobinuria must also be considered as possible differentials. Hematuria may be ruled out by sedimentation of erythrocytes after centrifugation of the urine sample for 30 seconds or by microscopic evaluation of the urine sample and detection of erythrocytes. In cases of hemoglobinuria, the plasma will be discolored as well (though it is more of a pink color), whereas myoglobin does not cause a change in plasma color.[13]

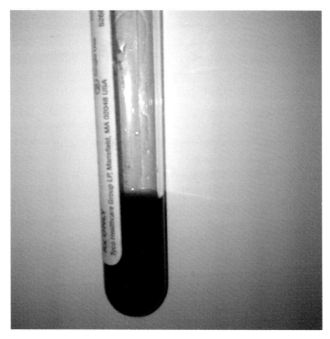

Figure 9.2   Urine sample with myoglobinuria. Unlike hemoglobinuria, a concurrent serum sample will be clear due to the rapid clearance of myoglobin from plasma.

Laboratory methods to detect hemoglobin include urine dipstick tests, ammonium sulfate, spectrophotometric assays, and immunoassays. Cautioned use of urine dipstick tests is recommended as many urine dipstick tests do not distinguish between myoglobin, hemoglobin, and hematuria. Ammonium sulfate, when added to urine, should precipitate out the hemoglobin but not the myoglobin. Hemoglobin precipitates at 80% saturation with ammonium sulfate, whereas myoglobin precipitates at 100% saturation. But because precipitation depends on the pH, temperature, time, and other factors, ammonium sulfate precipitation can give false results and is generally considered unreliable.[42] Spectrophotometric analysis can differentiate hemoglobinuria from myoglobinuria; however, some investigators consider it less reliable due to the rapid degradation of myoglobin to the met-myoglobin form (which changes the spectra). Immunoassays are the most sensitive and specific method of detection for myoglobin in both the blood and urine. Radial immunodiffusion, nephelometry/immunoturbidimetry, and radioimmunoassay have all been described. Radial immunodiffusion and nephelometric methods can detect very low concentrations of myoglobin in urine.

Of particular concern in horses with myoglobinuria is the development of acute tubular necrosis with acute or delayed renal failure due to tubular damage from the excretion of myoglobin. This sequela to muscle injury occurs only in rare cases, and appears to occur in horses with concurrent systemic acidosis and dehydration.[12]

Troponin I

Troponins are proteins that regulate skeletal and cardiac muscle contraction by making actin-myosin interactions sensitive to cytosolic calcium levels. The troponin complex is comprised of three different proteins: troponin C (TnC), which binds calcium; troponin I (TnI), which has an inhibitory function; and troponin T (TnT), which attaches troponin to tropomyosin.[38] The cardiac myocyte contains specific isoforms (cTnI and cTnT) and due to their specificity, they are used as biomarkers for cardiac myocyte injury. Immunoassays have been developed to detect these isoforms for diagnosis of myocardial injury and these are highly selective for the cardiac myocyte isoform in the horse as well.[66,86] Increases in serum cardiac troponin have also been reported in horses after strenuous exercise and renal failure in dogs and cats.[51,92] It is unknown if increases also occur in horses with renal failure.

Skeletal troponin-I (sTnI) is a skeletal muscle specific protein that has been proposed as a marker for skeletal myocyte injury. Significant sequence dissimilarity (40%) exists between sTnI and cTnI isoforms.[88] If this difference is similar in horses, development of a commercial assay to detect skeletal muscle troponin could be useful in assessing muscle specific injury. Studies in humans have shown the utility of sTnI to detect muscle injury and have even been successful differentiating between slow- and fast-twitch muscle isoforms.[103] The enzyme rises in parallel to CK and stays increased for 1 to 2 days. Limited data in rats also shows promise for skeletal muscle troponin as a biomarker for skeletal muscle injury.[115] However, studies in horses are lacking thus far.

Equine muscle diseases

Equine myopathies have many different etiopathogeneses (see Table 9.1). While many result in abnormal increases in laboratory biomarkers of muscle injury, some do not. Most show clinical signs attributable to myopathy that include abnormal function (e.g., tremors and fasciculations), muscle atrophy, and/or pain from muscle necrosis.

Immune-mediated myopathies

Immune-mediated myopathy with muscle atrophy

Immune-mediated myopathy in horses has been reported secondary to infection with or exposure to Streptococcus equi subspecies equi. Both development of a severe infarctive purpura hemorrhagica or an acute, severe rhabdomyolysis has been described secondary to infection with this bacterial agent.[56,105] There are also reports of immune-mediated myositis in horses with a different clinical course (i.e., muscle atrophy). One study in horses with this type of immune-mediated myositis revealed 39% of these horses had a history of exposure to S equi or S zooepidemicus within 3 months prior to the onset of clinical signs; however, the remaining horses had no underlying trigger identified. The same study showed an overrepresentation of the Quarter Horse breed, which raises suspicion for a potential polygenic mode of inheritance in this breed. There appears to be a bimodal age distribution, with horses younger than 8 and older than 17 years more likely to be affected. Clinical signs include rapid onset of muscle atrophy (with the epaxial and gluteal muscles most severely affected), lethargy, stiffness, weakness, and fever. CK and AST levels are often persistently increased (between 1,000 and 10,000 IU/L), although in some cases they remain normal. Histological findings are consistent with immune-mediated myositis with cellular infiltrates of predominantly macrophages and lymphocytes.[60]

Infarctive purpura hemorrhagica

Infarctive purpura hemorrhagica (IPH) has been reported as an uncommon sequela to infection or exposure to Streptococcus equi equi, Corynebacterium pseudotuberculosis, and vaccination against S. equi equi. Rare cases have occurred post-infection with equine influenza virus, equine viral arteritis, equine herpesvirus type I, Streptococcus equi zooepidemicus, and Rhodococcus equi. However, around one-third of cases have no identified underlying etiology. Young to middle-aged horses are most commonly affected. Clinical signs often occur within 2-4 weeks after a respiratory infection. Most common signs include muscle swelling and edema of all the limbs, stiffness, lethargy, anorexia, hemorrhages on mucous membranes, and fever. Increases in CK ranging from 50,000 IU/L to 280,000 IU/L and AST ranging from 1,000 IU/L to 7,000 IU/L are common. Hematological changes include an inflammatory leukogram (leukocytosis characterized by a neutrophilia with left shift and toxic change),

Table 9.1 Equine Myopathies

Immune-mediated	Infectious	Traumatic	Inherited/Congenital
Myopathy with muscle atrophy	Bacterial/rickettsial	Compartment syndrome	Glycogen branching enzyme
Infarctive purpura hemorrhagica	*Anaplasma phagocytophilum*	Postanesthetic myopathy	deficiency
	Clostridial myositis	Extreme exercise	Hyperkalemic periodic paralysis
	Clostridium botulinum		Malignant hyperthermia
	Corynebacterium		Myotonia
	pseudotuberculosis		Polysaccharide storage myopathy
	Streptococcus equi		Recurrent exertional rhabdomyolysis
	Parasitic		
	Otobius megnini		
	Sarcocystis spp.		
	Viral		
	Equine herpesvirus I		
	Equine influenza virus 2		

Toxic	Nutritional	Unknown	Other
Blister beetle	Vit E/selenium deficiency	Acquired motor neuron disease	Pituitary pars intermedia dysfunction
Thiaminase-containing plants		Seasonal pasture myopathy	Aortic iliac thrombosis
Senna occidentalis, obtusifolia		Systemic calcinosis	
Ionophores			
Eupatorium rugosum			

hyperfibrinogenemia and hyperglobulinemia, hypoalbuminemia, and abnormal clotting parameters. Histologic findings show acute coagulative necrosis of affected tissue with leukocytoclastic vasculitis.

Immune complexes in horses with IPH are composed of IgM or IgA and streptococcal M protein. These complexes result in deposition of complement in vessel walls, cell destruction, and vascular occlusion. ELISA for detection of antibodies against Step equi M protein by ELISA may be markedly increased.[56, 93]

Infectious myopathies

Bacterial

Anaplasma phagocytophilum

Rhabdomyolysis associated with Anaplasma phagocytophilum, an obligative intracellular Gram-negative bacterium, has been rarely reported in the literature. Clinical signs include fever, tachycardia, and stiffness. Increases in CK (>100,000 U/L) and AST (>20,000 IU/L) are marked.[49] Microscopic blood smear evaluation may reveal morula (or microcolonies) within neutrophils. Other methods of diagnosis include detection of antibodies via immunofluorescence assay (IFA), western immunoblot (WIB), or enzyme-lined immunosorbent assay (ELISA), which require serial measurement and demonstration of an increasing titer, or detection of antigens in the blood via polymerase chain reaction (PCR).[61]

Clostridial myositis

Clostridium perfringens and C. septicum are the most common species reported in association with myonecrosis in the horse; other, less commonly implicated species include C. chauvoei, C. sordelli, C. novyi and C. fallax. The organisms are large, Gram-positive, anaerobic bacteria that most commonly cause infection in horses by contamination of injection sites or puncture wounds. CK and AST may be mildly to moderately increased if sufficient muscle necrosis is present. Diagnosis may be by microscopic identification of organisms in affected tissue, anaerobic culture, or detection via a fluorescent antibody test.[90, 94]

Clostridium botulinum (botulism)

Clostridium botulinum can also cause myopathy in horses due to type C toxin produced by the Gram-positive anaerobic bacillus. The toxin may be ingested from contaminated feed, produced by ingested bacteria in the intestinal tract, or produced by the bacteria in wounds. Production of toxin within the intestines is the most common cause in foals and usually occurs between 1 week and 6 months of age, while production in wounds is an uncommon cause in horses. The toxin binds irreversibly to presynaptic nerve terminals, prohibiting the release of acetylcholine and causing muscle weakness, tremors, and dysphagia. Signs often progress to generalized flaccid paralysis and recumbency. CK and AST are often normal but may eventually increase due to ischemic myopathy secondary to recumbency. Horses are extremely sensitive to the toxin, and tests to detect and measure toxin levels may not be able to register such low amounts. Diagnosis is based on analysis of stomach contents or feed but is often based on clinical signs and elimination of other possible causes.[36] Equine grass sickness (dysautonomia) is also suspected to be a form of botulism in horses.[76]

Corynebacterium pseudotuberculosis (pigeon fever)

Corynebacterium pseudotuberculosis is a Gram-positive facultative intracellular pleomorphic bacterium. The bacteria may cause a diffuse infection of the limbs and internal or external abscesses. External abscesses are the most common presentation in the western United States. Intramuscular abscesses fall into this external abscess category and are commonly located in the pectoral region and along the ventral midline or abdomen. It is postulated that the bacteria enter the horse through skin abrasions and penetrating wounds. Infections usually occur in the fall and early winter. Both ELISA for detection of antibodies and PCR to identify bacteria isolated from abscesses have been reportedly used for the diagnosis of infection.[4, 94]

Streptococcus equi

Severe acute rhabdomyolysis is a rarely reported but often fatal complication of upper respiratory infections due to Streptococcus equi in the horse. Common signs of infection with this Gram-positive bacterium include myalgia, stiffness, stilted gait (especially in the pelvic limbs), severe swelling and pitting edema of epaxial and gluteal muscles, recumbency, and myoglobinuria. Clinicopathologic findings include a leukocytosis characterized by a neutrophilia, hyperfibrinogenemia, and markedly increased CK (over 100,000 IU/L) and AST. Diagnostic methods include detection of cocci in affected skeletal muscle, bacterial culture of affected tissues, measurement of serum antibody titers to S. equi myosin binding protein via ELISA, immunofluorescent staining of skeletal muscle for S. equi myosin-binding protein, and S. equi PCR.[105]

The exact mechanism of pathogenicity is unknown but may be due to cross-reacting streptococcal antibodies that target skeletal muscle myosin, direct muscle invasion by the bacteria, bacteremia with exotoxin and protease production within skeletal muscle, or nonspecific T-cell stimulation by streptococcal superantigens. Four S. equi superantigens have been identified that elicit immune responses similar to those in humans infected with Streptococcus pyogenes, causing necrotizing myositis and toxic shock.[105]

Parasitic

Otobius megnini (equine ear tick)

Infestation with the equine ear tick (Otobius megnini) is a rare cause of muscle tremors and muscle fasciculations in the horse. CK and AST may be mildly to moderately increased.[71]

Sarcocystis spp

Sarcocystis spp are a common incidental finding in equine skeletal and cardiac muscle; however, infection with Sarcocystis fayeri has been rarely reported as a cause of muscle degeneration and necrosis in the horse.[34,111]

Viral

Equine herpesvirus 1 (EHV-1)

An outbreak of muscle stiffness in Thoroughbreds at a racing yard revealed a significant proportion of horses with antibody levels supportive of EHV-1 infection as well as increases in CK and AST.[44]

Equine influenza virus A2

Equine influenza virus is reported as a rare cause of muscle degeneration in the horse. Clinical signs include upper respiratory infection and myalgia. Clinicopathologic findings can include marked increases in muscle enzymes and myoglobinuria. The disease was rapidly progressive and fatal in all three of the reported cases in one study.[34]

Traumatic myopathies

Accidents or falls can cause significant muscle damage, including diaphragmatic rupture in the horse. Neurological disease can also cause myopathy in the horse, particularly during seizure activity or prolonged recumbency. Illness or trauma that results in prolonged recumbency has the potential to cause ischemic myopathy and rhabdomyolysis. In the horse, the gluteal muscles are often affected in dorsal recumbency and in lateral recumbency muscles such as the triceps group tend to be affected.[54] Trauma to muscle can also occur from medical treatments including surgical incisions and manipulation, injection of medications or irritating substances, and placement of tight casts or bandages. In horses, trauma to specific muscles like the gastrognemius muscle can occur during exercise or while struggling to rise.

Compartment syndrome and postanesthetic myopathy

Compartment syndrome and postanesthetic myopathy develop when accumulation of fluid (edema or hemorrhage) creates high pressure within the enclosed fascia surrounding the muscle. This high pressure results in reduced capillary blood flow to the muscle and ischemic damage. Placement of tight external bandages or casts can also result in a reduction of the compartment size and similar ischemic damage.

Compartment syndrome in horses undergoing anesthesia for surgical or nonsurgical procedures has also been reported and has been referred to as postanesthesia myopathy. The most important contributing factors to development of inadequate muscle perfusion and myopathy are thought to include positioning (with the dependent muscles of recumbent horses often affected), increased intracompartmental muscle pressures, low arterial blood pressure, venous stasis, and a longer length of procedure.[32, 39, 54, 65] Affected muscles may have measured increased intracompartmental pressures and increases in serum muscle enzymes CK and AST are also reported.[64]

Extreme exercise/overexertion

Extreme exercise and overexertion may cause myopathy and rhabdomyolysis in the horse. These cases are considered sporadic, versus the recurrent or chronic exertional rhabdomyolysis discussed later in this chapter. Sporadic exertional rhabdomyolysis occurs most often in cases of extreme exercise, heavy training/exercise after a period of decreased intensity training, or exercise/training in adverse environmental conditions (such as extreme heat). Common clinicopathologic findings include hemoconcentration, lactic acidosis, electrolyte changes, and increases in muscle enzymes (AST, CK, and LDH). Hypochloremia, hypokalemia, and hypocalcemia may all be seen with heavy sweating. Hyponatremia and hypernatremia have both been reported. Case progression may range from subclinical to severe. In more severe cases, moderate to marked increases in muscle enzymes (up to 100,000 times the upper reference limit) and myoglobinuria may be seen. Calcium, magnesium, and potassium depletion can all contribute to stasis of the gastrointestinal tract and related clinical signs. Damage to the kidneys from myoglobin and/or inadequate tissue perfusion can result in renal failure, although this sequela is rare.[19]

Inherited or congenital myopathies

Glycogen branching enzyme deficiency

Glycogen branching enzyme deficiency is a fatal, autosomal-recessive disease of Quarter Horses and American Paint horses caused by a missense mutation of the glycogen branching enzyme I GBE1 gene. Approximately 8% of Quarter Horses and American Paint horses are carriers.[117] The enzyme is essential for the final step of glycogen formation, thus the deficiency results in abnormal glycogen formation and deposition in myocytes (and to a lesser degree hepatocytes). This leads to the inability to store and mobilize glycogen to maintain normal glucose homeostasis. Affected foals may be aborted, stillborn, or weak at birth, with contracted tendons. In surviving foals, rhabdomyolysis or cardiac failure occurs at an early age. Common laboratory findings include leukopenia, intermittent hypoglycemia, and moderate increases in CK, AST, and GGT.

Analysis of peripheral blood or skeletal muscle for reduced activity of the enzyme or histopathologic analysis of myocytes for detection of PAS-positive and amylase-resistant inclusions are supportive of the diagnosis. However, the most accurate method of diagnosis for carriers and affected foals is a DNA test performed on samples from pulled mane or tail hairs.[114]

Hyperkalemic periodic paralysis (HYPP)

Hyperkalemic periodic paralysis (HYPP) is an autosomal-dominant trait found in Quarter Horses, Appaloosas, American Paint horses, and Quarter Horse crossbreeds. Approximately 4% of the Quarter Horse population is estimated to carry the mutation.[14] It is caused by a missense point mutation in skeletal muscle sodium channel gene (SCN4A). Affected horses are either homozygous or heterozygous for the disease.

The HYPP mutation results in an increased resting membrane potential, which is closer to firing than in normal muscle and results in the failure of a subpopulation of sodium channels to inactivate after depolarization. The result is an excessive influx of sodium ions and outflux of potassium ions, which generates a persistent depolarization of the myocyte.[28]

Clinical signs in affected horses vary from asymptomatic to daily muscle fasciculations and weakness that may progress to recumbency. Horses heterozygous for HYPP are often less severely affected, with less frequent episodes than their homozygous counterparts.[81] Respiratory stridor and distress and dysphagia may be evident, with possible obstruction of the upper airway due to pharyngeal collapse or laryngeal paralysis. These clinical signs tend to be seen more frequently in horses homozygous for the trait.[20]

During an episode, clinicopathologic abnormalities often include hyperkalemia (6-9 mEq/L), hemoconcentration, and mild hyponatremia; however, serum potassium concentrations are normal in between episodes and may be normal during mild episodes as well. CK values are usually normal, but mild increases in CK are occasionally seen a few hours after the episode.[28,81]

Episodes are believed to be triggered by a variety of precipitating factors. One of the most important factors is diets high in potassium such as alfalfa, soybean, molasses, electrolyte supplements, and kelp-based supplements.[100] Other precipitating factors include sudden diet change, fasting, anesthesia, sedation, stress, transport, rest after exercise, exposure to cold, pregnancy, and concurrent disease.[20] Diagnosis is now based on a DNA test for the mutation in the SCN4A gene run on submitted mane or tail hairs. The test can distinguish between homozygous affected, heterozygous affected, and normal horses.[28]

Malignant hyperthermia

Malignant hyperthermia in horses is a pharmaco-genetic disease of skeletal muscle. It has been reported in Quarter Horses, Thoroughbreds, Appaloosas, ponies, and Arabs.[48,73]

In Quarter Horses, a genetic basis for disease has been linked to a mutation in the ryanodine receptor 1 gene (RyR1). Because the disease is inherited as an autosomal dominant trait, Quarter Horse–related breeds may also carry the mutation.[3] The mutation causes dysfunction of the sarcoplasmic reticulum calcium release channel of skeletal muscle, resulting in massive release of calcium into the sarcoplasm and a hypermetabolic state characterized by hyperthermia and muscle rigidity.

Clinical signs are triggered by exposure to halogenated anesthetics (halothane, isoflurane), depolarizing muscle relaxants like succinylcholine, and stress.[3] Clinicopathologic abnormalities include respiratory and metabolic acidosis, hyperkalemia, hyponatremia, hypocalcemia, hyperphosphatemia, hyperproteinemia, and azotemia. Marked elevations in CK and AST as well as myoglobinuria may also be noted.[1,3]

Myotonia

This severe, progressive neuromuscular disorder is reported in Quarter Horses, Thoroughbred foals, and Anglo-Arab-Sardinian foals.[46,83,97] The disorder is similar to myotonic dystrophy (myotonia dystrophica) in humans, but less similar to myotonia in the goat. A genetic basis has not yet been established in the horse. Clinical signs of the disease may be apparent as early as 1 month of age and include generalized myotonia, proximal muscle hypertrophy and hypertonicity followed by stiffness, weakness, and atrophy. Horses may have marked exercise intolerance. Testicular hypoplasia, cataract formation, and glucose intolerance have also been reported. Diagnosis is made by percussion dimpling, myotonic EMG discharges, and classic histopathologic findings (sarcoplasmic masses, ringed fibers, internal positioning of sarcolemmal nuclei, and variation in fiber diameter size).

Polysaccharide storage myopathy (PSSM)

Polysaccharide storage myopathy (PSSM) is characterized by accumulation of glycogen and abnormal complex polysaccharide inclusions in skeletal muscle. PSSM has been identified in many breeds. Quarter Horses, American Paint Horses, Appaloosas, Belgian and Percheron Draft Horses, and Warmbloods are the most commonly affected breeds. It is estimated that 5-12% of Quarter Horses and 36% of Belgian Draft horses are affected.[30,52,78]

In many horses, the disease is caused by mutation in the glycogen synthase 1 (GSY1) gene, which encodes the skeletal muscle isoform of glycogen synthase. Though the mutation was first identified in Quarter Horses, it has since been associated with PSSM in several other breeds. Prevalence of the mutation in one study ranged widely among breeds, with approximately 80% of Belgian and Percheron Draft Horses, 50% of Quarter Horses and related breeds, and 8% of Warmbloods with histopathological diagnoses of PSSM demonstrating the mutation. In this same study the mutation was not identified in any of the Standardbred, Thoroughbred, or Arabian Horses with PSSM.[80] A form of PSSM is reported at a lower prevalence in Thoroughbreds, Morgans, Andalusians, Arabians, Standardbreds, and others.[77,169]

Clinical signs range from sporadic or episodic rhabdomyolysis (exertional or nonexertional) to progressive weakness and muscle fasciculations, or less often muscle atrophy.[31,136] Some horses may also be asymptomatic.[30] CK and AST values may range from markedly elevated after an episode of rhabdomyolysis to mildly to moderately increased with exercise or recumbency and possibly at rest. Values are often normal in Draft breeds and Warmbloods.[30] Myoglobinuria may also be seen after episodes of rhabdomyolysis. In rare cases, myoglobin may cause tubular damage and acute or delayed renal failure. Horses that develop renal failure usually have concurrent dehydration and metabolic acidosis.[10]

Recently, members of a family of Quarter Horses with a more severe and occasionally fatal expression of PSSM were demonstrated to have both a mutation in the GYS1 gene and a mutation in the RYR1 gene (previously associated with malignant hyperthermia in Quarter Horses).[79] Diagnosis may be based on histologic evaluation of skeletal muscle biopsy and/or genetic testing for the mutation in GYS1.

Recurrent exertional rhabdomyolysis (RER)

Some sources refer to exertional rhabdomyolysis as an umbrella term that encompasses a variety of myopathies in different breeds, including PSSM in Quarter Horses and RER in Thoroughbreds. Even though these myopathies manifest similarly, they differ in their etiopathogeneses. Recurrent exertional rhabdomyolysis (RER) is a particular form of exertional rhabdomyolysis that is prevalent in Thoroughbred horses and is estimated to affect 5% of the population.[69] In Thoroughbreds, RER is an inherited as an autosomal dominant trait.[70] It is believed to be caused by a defect in intracellular calcium regulation or excitation-contraction coupling leading to excessive muscular contraction and necrosis with exercise.[59] Several risk factors for the disease have been identified and include young age, female gender, high-strung disposition, rest 1 day prior to exercise, gallop during exercise, diets of more than 4.5 kg of grain per day, and concurrent lameness.[69]

Clinical signs include muscle cramping, stiffness, lameness, and sweating. Most affected horses show clinical signs, but in some cases the disease can be hard to detect without analysis of muscle enzyme activity. Classic laboratory abnormalities include increases in serum muscle enzymes after exercise. Horses may also have myoglobinuria with moderate to severe episodes of muscle necrosis. In rare cases, myoglobin may damage renal tubules and lead to acute or delayed renal failure if there is concurrent dehydration and systemic acidosis.[10]

A tentative diagnosis of RER may be based on clinical signs, risk factors, and increased muscle enzymes post-exercise. In some cases a muscle biopsy may be necessary for a definitive diagnosis. Muscle biopsy specimens have been shown to exhibit abnormal *in vitro* contracture response to potassium, caffeine, or halothane compared to control horses.[59]

Toxic myopathies

Blister beetle toxicosis (cantharidiasis)

Blister beetle toxicosis (cantharidiasis) in horses is most often due to ingestion of alfalfa hay or pellets contaminated with blister beetles (Epicauta spp). Blister beetles produce cantharidin, which can exert effects even in absence of the actual blister beetle bodies and can withstand degradation by heating and drying.

Gastrointestinal signs are the most common (colic, irritability, restlessness, and diarrhea), but the toxin may also cause urinary tract signs (hematuria, stranguria, and pollakiuria). Cardiovascular signs and neuromuscular signs (aggressive behavior, seizure-like muscle fasciculations) are less commonly noted. Oral lesions (oral ulcers, profuse salivation) and synchronous diaphragmatic flutter (associated with hypocalcemia and hypomagnesemia) have been reported.[47] Laboratory abnormalities may include hypocalcemia (often marked), hypomagnesemia, hyperglycemia, increases in CK (within 24 hours of ingestion), and hyperglycemia. Urinalysis may reveal hyposthenuria, hematuria, and possibly myoglobinuria. Azotemia may be noted due to dehydration or secondary to toxin-mediated renal tubular necrosis.

The diagnosis can be confirmed via high-pressure liquid chromatography (HPLC) and gas chromatography or mass spectrometry to detect/quantify cantharidin in urine as well as liver, kidneys, and gastric contents.[95]

Thiaminase: Bracken fern (pteridum aquilinum), horsetail (equisetum arvense), rock fern (cheilanthes sieberi)

Thiamine (vitamin B1) is an essential component of energy metabolism and important in maintaining the myelin of peripheral nerves. Thiaminase cleaves the thiamine molecule and renders it inactive. Ingestion of thiaminase produces a thiamine deficiency, which results in metabolic abnormalities as well as myelin degeneration of peripheral nerves. The most common method cause of intoxication in horses is ingestion of contaminated hay.

Clinical signs of thiamine deficiency include anorexia resulting in poor body condition and weight loss, as well as gait disturbances and uncoordinated movements that may progress to loss of muscle control (twitches and tremors).[57]

Senna occidentalis (coffee senna, coffee weed) and Senna obtusifolia (sickle pod, coffee bean, coffee weed)

The toxic effects of Senna occidentalis and Senna obtusifolia are attributed to anthraquinones and their derivatives and alkaloids. Ingestion of the plants may cause liver degeneration, gastrointestinal signs (diarrhea), and muscle necrosis that manifests as muscular weakness that progresses to recumbency and death. Increased serum CK and AST, hyperkalemia, and myoglobinuria are frequent findings.[74]

Ionophore

Horses may suffer ionophore-induced myocardial and skeletal muscle degeneration with ingestion of monensin, lasalocid, maduramicin, narasin, or salinomycin. Ionophores are commonly used as coccidiostats in feed for food animals, and horses may be exposed by access to ruminant feed or by accidental contamination of horse feed. Intoxication may occur with very small doses because horses are highly sensitive to ionophores. The substances increase membrane permeability and cause abnormal movement of ions across cell membranes, thus disrupting normal ionic equilibrium.[2,23,40]

Clinical signs initially include colic and anorexia that rapidly progresses to signs of myopathy/cardiomyopathy, recumbency, and death. Some cases may only present with neurologic signs (ataxia and seizures).[23] Horses that recover from the acute phase may suffer from cardiac damage and present with delayed signs of cardiomyopathy.[2,89] Abnormal laboratory findings may include moderate to marked increases in CK and AST and myoglobinuria. Hypocalcemia and hypokalemia may be seen initially in the first 24 hours after exposure. Some cases report mild hyponatremia, mild hypochloremia, mild hypomagnesemia, and severe hyperglycemia as well.

Diagnosis is usually based on clinical signs, history of exposure, and histopathologic changes. Detection of ionophores may be difficult given the small dose that can cause intoxication; however, feed, stomach contents, and/or affected tissue can be analyzed.

Eupatorium rugosum (white snakeroot)

The toxic principle in this plant is trematone, which can cause depression, muscle weakness and trembling, respiratory difficulty, and dysphagia. Progression of skeletal and heart muscle damage may result in recumbency and signs of cardiac failure. Elevations in CK and AST may be noted.[87]

Nutritional myopathies

Vitamin E/Selenium deficiency

Vitamin E/Selenium deficiency is also referred to as white muscle disease in foals. It is most common in foals (especially from birth up to 2 weeks of age), but cases are also reported in adults. It is caused by a dietary deficiency of selenium and to a lesser extent vitamin E, which results in myodegeneration. In the foal this is commonly due to a selenium-deficient dam. Predisposing factors such as diets high in fat or unaccustomed exercise are reported.[67]

Selenium and vitamin E serve as antioxidants and prevent cellular damage from reactive oxygen species. Foals may present with recumbency, respiratory distress, and muscle pain. Alternatively, they may present with severe weakness, muscle fasciculations, stiffness, muscle pain, and dysphagia. Laboratory abnormalities include marked increase in CK and AST, hyperproteinemia, hyponatremia, hyperkalemia, hypocalcemia, hyperphosphatemia, and myoglobinuria.[91] Whole-blood selenium and glutathione peroxidase activities are low and in some cases plasma vitamin E levels are also decreased. Histologic evaluation of muscle biopsies reveals muscle necrosis and regeneration with histiocytic inflammation.

Myopathies of unknown cause

Acquired equine motor neuron disease (EMND)

Equine motor neuron disease (EMND) is characterized by degeneration of motor neurons in the spinal cord and brainstem that leads to neurogenic muscle atrophy, weight loss, and weakness. Clinical signs may include muscle fasciculations, trembling of the limbs, and frequent episodes of recumbency. Chronic vitamin E deficiency is a major contributing factor, but the etiology is incompletely understood and other factors may contribute to development of the disease.[82] Vitamin E is a known antioxidant that helps in the neutralization of free radicals, and vitamin E deficiency is believed to lead to chronic oxidative stress and death of motor neurons.

Vitamin E deficiency may be attributed to limited access to pasture, access to poor-quality pasture (forage with low vitamin E content), or failure of horses to absorb or retain dietary vitamin E. Other factors that contribute to overall likelihood of EMND include age (older horses are more susceptible to the disease), turnout type and size, predominant type of concentrate fed, and rabies vaccination status.[24,25]

Clinicopathologic abnormalities may include mildly to moderately increased serum muscle enzymes (CK and AST) as well as low plasma vitamin E levels.[26] A tentative diagnosis is based on suggestive clinical, epidemiologic, and laboratory findings. A definitive diagnosis of EMND may be made on examination of muscle biopsy or spinal accessory nerve biopsy.

Seasonal pasture myopathy

Seasonal pasture myopathy is a recently described disease characterized by acute, severe, nonexertional rhabdomyolysis that shares many similarities with outbreaks of atypical myopathy in Europe. The exact cause has not been identified, but there appears to be a seasonal occurrence and link to weather conditions.[29,116]

The primary etiopathogenesis of seasonal pasture myopathy and atypical myopathy remains unclear. Cases of atypical myopathy have been associated with defects in fatty acid oxidation, which causes dysfunctional mitochondrial fatty acid metabolism, and with Clostridium sordellii toxin.[112] Similar associations have not yet been assessed in horses with seasonal pasture myopathy.

Clinical signs include muscle stiffness, fasciculations, and weakness that progress to recumbency. In additional to skeletal muscle necrosis, myocardial degeneration may also occur. Laboratory abnormalities include markedly increased serum CK and AST as well as myoglobinuria. Increases in ALP, GGT, SDH, total bilirubin, and glucose may also be seen. Hyperphosphatemia and hypocalcemia are common; however, other electrolyte abnormalities such as hyponatremia, hyperkalemia, and hypochloremia are less often noted.

Systemic calcinosis

Systemic calcinosis is a well-recognized syndrome of dystrophic calcification in humans, and has more recently been suspected in horses. Affected horses present with lethargy, stiffness, and muscle atrophy. Respiratory signs and severe rhabdomyolysis are occasionally seen. Laboratory abnormalities include increased serum CK and AST, hyperphosphatemia, and hyperfibrinogenemia. Diagnosis is made on post-mortem identification of dystrophic calcification of skeletal and cardiac myofibers, renal tubules, lungs, kidneys, and intestinal vessels.[94]

Other myopathies

Cushing's disease

Equine pituitary pars intermedia dysfunction (PPID) is a common neurodegenerative disease of aged horses and ponies that has an associated myopathy characterized by muscle atrophy and weakness. In horses with PPID there is a loss of dopaminergic inhibitory input to the pituitary pars intermedia that results in increased melanotroph function and oversynthesis of proopiomelanocortin (POMC)-derived peptides and chronic increases in endogenous glucocorticoids. Muscle enzymes are typically within normal range. Results of muscle biopsies demonstrate type 2 myofiber atrophy.[5]

Aortic-iliac thrombosis

Aortic-iliac thrombosis is occasionally reported in horses and causes decreased blood flow and ischemic damage to muscles.

It is most commonly reported in racehorses but can occur in any breed, and males have a higher incidence than females.[75] Horses may have signs of hindlimb lameness (usually unilateral and often exercise-induced) and abdominal distress. The affected limb(s) may be cold and decreased distal pulses (femoral or plantar digital) may be palpated. Decreased blood flow to the hind limbs, internal and external iliacs, and circumflex iliacs are responsible for the clinical signs. The severity of clinical signs varies depending on the degree of vascular occlusion, the presence of collateral circulation, and how long it took the occlusion to form. Diagnosis is based on history, clinical presentation, transrectal palpation, ultrasonography, thermography, and scintigraphy.[17]

References

1. Aleman M, Brosnan RJ, Williams DC, et al. 2005. Malignant hyperthermia in a horse anesthetized with halothane. *J Vet Intern Med* 19:363-366.
2. Aleman M, Magdesian KG, Peterson TS, et al. 2007. Salinomycin toxicosis in horses. *J Am Vet Med Assoc* 230:1822-1826.
3. Aleman M, Nieto JE, Magdesian KG. 2009. Malignant hyperthermia associated with ryanodine receptor 1 (C7360G) mutation in Quarter Horses. *J Vet Intern Med* 23:329-334.
4. Aleman M, Spier SJ, Wilson WD, et al. 1996. Corynebacterium pseudotuberculosis infection in horses: 538 cases (1982-1993). *J Am Vet Med Assoc* 209:804-809.
5. Aleman M, Watson JL, Williams DC, et al. 2006. Myopathy in horses with pituitary pars intermedia dysfunction (Cushing's disease) *Neuromuscul Disord* 16:737-744.
6. Almeida BFM, Zucatto AS, Vieira RFC, et al. 2011. Effect of hemolysis on canine, bovine, and equine serum chemistry. *Medicina Veterinaria (Brasil)* 5:12-17.
7. Amelink GJ, Koot RW, Erich WB, et al. 1990. Sex linked variation in creatine kinase release, and its dependence on oestradiol, can be demonstrated in an in-vitro rat skeletal muscle preparation. *Acta Physiol Scand* 138:115-124.

8. Anderson MG. 1975. The influence of exercise on serum enzyme levels in the horse. *Equine Vet J* 7:160–165.

9. Anderson MG. 1976. The effect of exercise on the lactic dehydrogenase and creatine kinase isoenzyme composition of horse serum. *Res Vet Sci* 20:191–196.

10. Andrews FM. 1994. Acute rhabdomyolysis. *Vet Clin North Am Equine Pract* 10:567–573.

11. Argiroudis SA, Kent JE, Blackmore DJ. 1982. Observations on the isoenzymes of creatine kinase in equine serum and tissues. *Equine Vet J* 14:317–321.

12. Arighi M, Baird J, Hulland T. 1984. Equine exertional rhabdomyolysis. *Compend Cont Educ Pract Vet* 6:S726–S733.

13. Boulton FE, Huntsman RG. 1971. The detection of myoglobin in urine and its distinction from normal and variant haemoglobins. *J Clin Pathol* 24:816–821.

14. Bowling AT, Byrns G, Spier S. 1996. Evidence for a single pedigree source of the hyperkalemic periodic paralysis susceptibility gene in Quarter Horses. *Anim Genet* 27:279–281.

15. Boyd JW. 1967. Rates of disappearance of L-lactate dehydrogenase isoenzymes from plasma. *Biochimica et Biophysica Acta* 132:221–231.

16. Boyd JW. 1983. The mechanisms relating to increases in plasma enzymes and isoenzymes in diseases of animals. *Vet Clin Pathol* 12:9–24.

17. Brama PAJ, Rijkenhuizen ABM, Swieten van HA, et al. 1996. Thrombosis of the aorta and the caudal arteries in the horse; additional diagnostics and a new surgical treatment. *Vet Quart* 18(Suppl 2):85–89.

18. Cardinet GH, Littrell JF, Freedland RA. 1967. Comparative investigations of serum creatine phosphokinase and glutamic-oxaloacetic transaminase activities in equine paralytic myoglobinuria. *Res Vet Sci* 8:219–226.

19. Carlson GP. 1987. Hematology and body fluids in the equine athlete: a review. In *Equine Exercise Physiology*. Gillespie, JR and Robinson NR (eds). 2nd ed. pp. 393–425. Davis, CA: ICEEP Publications.

20. Carr EA, Spier SJ, Kortz GD, et al. 1996. Laryngeal and pharyngeal dysfunction in horses homozygous for hyperkalemic periodic paralysis. *J Am Vet Med Assoc* 209:798–803.

21. Cornelius CE, Bishop J, Switzer J, et al. 1959. Serum and tissue transaminase activities in domestic animals. *Cornell Vet* 49:116–126.

22. Dabareiner RM, Schmitz DG, Honnas CM, et al. 2004. Gracilis muscle injury as a cause of lameness in two horses. *J Am Vet Med Assoc* 224:1605–1606.

23. Dawson DR. 2011. Toxins and adverse drug reactions affecting the equine nervous system. *Vet Clin North Am Equine Pract* 27:507–526.

24. de la Rua-Domenech R, Mohammed HO, Cummings JF, et al. 1997. Association between plasma vitamin E concentration and the risk of equine motor neuron disease. *Equine Vet J* 154:203–213.

25. de la Rua-Domenech R, Mohammed HO, Cummings JF, et al. 1997. Intrinsic, management, and nutritional factors associated with equine motor neuron disease. *J Am Vet Med Ass* 211:1261–1267.

26. Divers TJ, Mohammed HO, Cummings JF, et al. 1994. Equine motor neuron disease: findings in 28 horses and proposal of a pathophysiological mechanism for the disease. *Equine Vet J* 26:409–415.

27. Don M, Masters CJ. 1976. On the comparative turnover rates of the lactate dehydrogenase isoenzymes in rat tissues. *Intnl J Biochem* 7:215–220.

28. Finno CJ, Spier SJ, Valberg SJ. 2009. Equine diseases caused by known genetic mutations. *Vet J* 179:336–347.

29. Finno CJ, Valberg SJ, Wünschmann A, et al. 2006. Seasonal pasture myopathy in horses in the midwestern United States: 14 cases (1998-2005). *J Am Vet Med Assoc.* 229:1134-1141.

30. Firshman AM, Baird JD, Valberg SJ. 2005. Prevalences and clinical signs of polysaccharide storage myopathy and shivers in Belgian draft horses. *J Am Vet Med Assoc* 227:1958-1964.

31. Firshman AM, Valberg SJ, Bender JB, et al. 2003. Epidemiologic characteristics and management of polysaccharide storage myopathy in Quarter Horses. *Am J Vet Res* 64:1319-1327.

32. Franci P, Leece EA, Brearley JC. 2006. Post-anaesthetic myopathy/neuropathy in horses undergoing magnetic resonance imaging compared to horses undergoing surgery. *Equine Vet J* 38:497-501.

33. Frauenfelder HC, Rossdale PD, Rickets SW, et al. 1996. Changes in serum muscle enzyme levels associated with training schedules and stage of the oestrous cycle in thoroughbred racehorses. *Equine Vet J* 18:371-374.

34. Freestone JF, Carlson GP. 1991. Muscle disorders in the horse: a retrospective study. *Equine Vet J* 23:86-90.

35. Freestone JF, Kamerling SG, Church G, et al. 1989. Exercise induced changes in creatine kinase and aspartate aminotransferase activities in the horse: effects of conditioning, exercise tests, and acepromazine. *J Equine Vet Sci* 9:275-280.

36. Gerber V, Straub R, Frey J. 2006. Equine botulism and acute pasture myodystrophy: new soil-borne emerging diseases in Switzerland? *Schweiz Arch Tierheilkd* 148:553-559.

37. Gigli I, Agusee Johnero A, Maizon DO, et al. 1996. Serum muscular enzymes (CPK/AST) and plasma progesterone in Thoroughbred mares in training. *Pferdeheilkunde* 12:496-498.

38. Gordon AM, Homsher E, Regnier M. 2000. Regulation of contraction in striated muscle. *Physiol Rev* 80:853-924.

39. Grandy JL, Steffey EP, Hodgson DS, et al. 1987. Arterial hypotension and the development of postanesthetic myopathy in halothane-anesthetized horses. *Am J Vet Res* 48:192-197.

40. Hall JO. 2001. Toxic feed constituents in the horse. *Vet Clin North Am Equine Pract* 17:479-489.

41. Hall RL, Bender HS. 2011. Muscle. In *Duncan and Prasse's Veterinary Laboratory Medicine: clinical pathology.* Latimer KS (ed), 5th ed. pp. 283-289. Ames, IA: Jon Wiley & Sons, Inc.

42. Hamilton RW, Hopkins III MB, Shihabi ZK. 1989. Myoglobinuria, hemoglobinuria, and acute renal failure. *Clin Chem* 35:1713-1720.

43. Hamlin MJ, Shearman JP, Hopkins WG. 2002. Changes in physiological parameters in overtrained Standardbred racehorses. *Equine Vet J* 34:383-388.

44. Harris PA. 1990. An outbreak of the equine rhabdomyolysis syndrome in a racing yard. *Vet Rec* 127:468-470.

45. Harris PA, Snow DH, Greet TR, et al. 1990. Some Factors influencing AST/CK activities in thoroughbred racehorses. *Equine Vet J* Suppl 9:66-71.

46. Hegreberg GA, Reed SM. 1990. Skeletal muscle changes associated with equine myotonic dystrophy. *Acta Neuropathol* 80:426-431.

47. Helman RG, Edwards WC. 1997. Clinical features of blister beetle poisoning in equids: 70 cases (1983-1996). *J Am Vet Med Assoc* 211:1018-1021.

48. Hildebrand SV, Howitt GA. 1983. Succinylcholine infusion associated with hyperthermia in ponies anesthetized with halothane. *Am J Vet Res* 44:2280-2284.

49. Hilton H, Madigan JE, Aleman M. 2008. Rhabdomyolysis associated with Anaplasma phagocytophilum infection in a horse. *J Vet Intern Med* 22:1061-1064.

50. Hoffman WE, Solter PF. 2008. Diagnostic enzymology of domestic animals. In *Clinical Biochemistry of Domestic Animals*. Kaneko JJ, Harvey JW, Bruss ML (eds), 6th ed. pp. 351-370. Burlington, MA: Academic Press.

51. Holbrook TC, Birks EK, Sleeper MM, et al. 2006. Endurance exercise is associated with increased plasma cardiac troponin I in horses. *Equine Vet J* 38:27-31.

52. Hunt LM, Valberg SJ, Steffenhagen K, McCue ME. 2008. An epidemiologic study of myopathies in Warmblood Horses. *Equine Vet J* 40:171-177.

53. Jacobus WE, Lehninger AL. 1973. Creatine kinase of rat heart mitochondria. Coupling of creatine phosphorylation to electron transport. *J Biol Chem* 248:4803-4810.

54. Johnston GM, Eastment JK, Taylor PM, et al. 2004. Is isoflurane safer than halothane in equine anaesthesia? Results from a prospective multicentre randomised controlled trial. *Equine Vet J* 36:64-71.

55. Jones DG. 1985. Stability and storage characteristics of enzymes in cattle blood. *Res Vet Sci* 38:301-306.

56. Kaese HJ, Valberg SJ, Hayden DW, et al. 2005. Infarctive purpura hemorrhagica in five horses. *J Am Vet Med Assoc* 226:1893-1898.

57. Knight AP, Walter RG. 2001. *A Guide to Plant Poisoning of Animals in North America*. pp. 194-197, 222-224. Jackson, WY: Teton New Media.

58. Lassen ED. 2006. Laboratory evaluation of muscle injury. In *Veterinary Hematology and Clinical Chemistry*. Thrall MA, Baker DC, Campbell TW, et al. (eds), pp. 417. Ames: Blackwell Publishing.

59. Lentz LR, Valberg SJ, Herold LV, et al. 2002. Myoplasmic calcium regulation in myotubes from horses with recurrent exertional rhabdomyolysis. *Am J Vet Res* 63:1724-1731.

60. Lewis SS, Valberg SJ, Nielsen IL. 2007. Suspected immune-mediated myositis in horses. *J Vet Intern Med* 21:495-503.

61. Lillini E, Macri G, Proietti G, et al. 2006. New findings on anaplasmosis caused by infection with Anaplasma phagocytophilum. *Ann N Y Acad Sci* 1081:360-370.

62. Lindena J, Kupper W, Friedel R, et al. 1979. Lymphatic transport of cellular enzymes from muscle into the intravascular compartment. *Enzyme* 24:120-131.

63. Linder A, Hatzipanagiotou A. 1993. Effect of the storage temperature and time and the test sample materials on the LDH isoenzyme activity and protein fractions in equine blood. *Zentrabl Veterinarmed A* 40:128-133.

64. Lindsay WA, McDonnell W, Bignell W. 1980. Equine postanesthetic forelimb lameness: intracompartmental muscle pressure changes and biochemical patterns. *Am J Vet Res* 41:1919-1924.

65. Lindsay WA, Robinson GM, Brunson DB, et al. 1989. Induction of equine postanesthetic myositis after halothane-induced hypotension. *Am J Vet Res* 50:404-410.

66. Lippi G, Targher G, Franchini M, et al. 2009. Genetic and biochemical heterogeneity of cardiac troponins: clinical and laboratory implications. *Clin Chem Lab Med* 47:1183-1194.

67. Löfstedt J. 1997. White muscle disease of foals. *Vet Clin North Am Equine Pract* 13:169-185.

68. Lucke JN, Hall GM. 1980. A biochemical study of the Arab Horse Society's marathon race. *Vet Rec* 107:523-525.
69. MacLeay JM, Sorum SA, Valberg SJ, et al. 1999. Epidemiologic analysis of factors influencing exertional rhabdomyolysis in Thoroughbreds. *Am J Vet Res* 60:1562-1566.
70. MacLeay JM, Valberg SJ, Sorum SA, et al. 1999. Heritability of recurrent exertional rhabdomyolysis in Thoroughbred racehorses. *Am J Vet Res* 60:250-256.
71. Madigan JE, Valberg SJ, Ragle C, et al. 1995. Muscle spasms associated with ear tick (Otobius megnini) infestation in five horses. *J Am Vet Med* Assoc 207:74-76.
72. Mair J. 1999. Tissue release of cardiac markers: from physiology to clinical applications. *Clin Chem Lab Med* 37:1077-1084.
73. Manley SV, Kelly AB, Hodgson D. 1983. Malignant hyperthermia-like reactions in three anesthetized horses. *J Am Vet Med Assoc* 183:85-89.
74. Martin BW, Terry MK, Bridges CH, et al. 1981. Toxicity of Cassia occidentalis in the horse. *Vet Hum Toxicol* 23:416-417.
75. Maxie MG, Physick-Sheard PW. 1985. Aortic-iliac thrombosis in horses. *Vet Pathol* 22:238-249.
76. McCarthy HE, French NP, Edwards GB, et al. 2004. Equine grass sickness is associated with low antibody levels to Clostridium botulinum: a matched case control study. *Equine Vet J* 36:123-129.
77. McCue ME, Ribeiro WP, Valberg SJ. 2006. Prevalence of polysaccharide storage myopathy in horses with neuromuscular disorders. *Equine Vet J* 38(S36):340-344.
78. McCue ME, Valberg SJ. 2007. Estimated prevalence of polysaccharide storage myopathy among overtly healthy Quarter Horses in the United States. *J Am Vet Med Assoc* 231:746-750.
79. McCue ME, Valberg SJ, Jackson M, et al. 2009. Polysaccharide storage myopathy phenotype in Quarter Horse-related breeds is modified by the presence of an RYR1 mutation. *Neuromuscul Disord* 19:37-43.
80. McCue ME, Valberg SJ, Lucio M, et al. 2008. Glycogen synthase 1 (GYS1) mutation in diverse breeds with polysaccharide storage myopathy. *J Vet Intern Med* 22:1228-1233.
81. Meyer TS, Fedde MR, Cox JH, et al. 1999. Hyperkalaemic periodic paralysis in horses: a review. *Equine Vet J* 31:362-367.
82. Mohammed HO, Divers TJ, Summers BA, et al. 2007. Vitamin E deficiency and risk of equine motor neuron disease. *Acta Vet Scand* 49:17.
83. Montagna P, Liguori R, Monari L, et al. 2011. Equine muscular dystrophy with myotonia. *Clin Neurophysiol* 112:294-299.
84. Neubauer O, Konig D, Wagner KH. 2008. Recovery after an Ironman triathlon: sustained inflammatory responses and muscular stress. *Eur J Appl Physiol* 104:417-426.
85. Noonan NE. 1981. Variations of plasma enzymes in the pony and dog after carbon tetrachloride administration. *Am J Vet Res* 42:674-678.
86. O'Brien PJ, Landt Y, Landenson JH. 1997. Differential reactivity of cardiac and skeletal muscle from various species in a cardiac troponin I immunoassay. *Clin Chem* 43:2333-2338.
87. Olson CT, Keller WC, Gerken DF, et al. 1984. Suspected tremetol poisoning in horses. *J Am Vet Med Assoc* 185:1001-1003.
88. Onuoha GN, Alpar EK, Dean B, et al. 2001. Skeletal troponin-I release in orthopedic and soft tissue injuries. *J Orthop Sci* 6:11-15.

89. Peek SF, Marques FD, Morgan J, et al. 2004. Atypical acute monensin toxicosis and delayed cardiomyopathy in Belgian draft horses. *J Vet Intern Med* 18:761-764.

90. Peek SF, Semrad SD, Perkins GA. 2003. Clostridial myonecrosis in horses (37 cases 1985-2000). *Equine Vet J.* 35:86-92.

91. Perkins G, Valberg SJ, Madigan JM, et al. 1998. Electrolyte disturbances in foals with severe rhabdomyolysis. *J Vet Intern Med* 12:173-177.

92. Porciello F, Rishniw M, Herndon WE, et al. 2008. Cardiac troponin I is elevated in dogs and cats with azotaemia renal failure and in dogs with non-cardiac systemic disease. *Australian Vet J* 86:390-394.

93. Pusterla N, Watson JL, Affolter VK, et al. 2003. Purpura haemorrhagica in 53 horses. *Vet Rec* 153:118-121.

94. Quist EM, Dougherty JJ, Chaffin MK, et al. 2011. Equine rhabdomyolysis. *Vet Pathol* 48:E52-E58.

95. Ray AC, Kyle AL, Murphy MJ, et al. 1989. Etiologic agents, incidence, and improved diagnostic methods of cantharidin toxicosis in horses. *Am J Vet Res* 50:187-191.

96. Rayolle P, Lefebvre H, Braun JP. 1992. Effects of incorrect venepuncture on plasma creatine kinase activity in the dog and horse. *Br Vet J* 148:161-162.

97. Reed SM, Hegreberg GA, Bayly WM, et al. 1988. Progressive myotonia in foals resembling human dystrophia myotonica. *Muscle Nerve* 11:291-296.

98. Rej R, Rudofsky U, Magro A, et al. 1990. Effects of exercise on serum aminotransferase activity and pyridoxal phosphate saturation in Thoroughbred racehorses. *Equine Vet J* 22:205-208.

99. Rendle DI, Heller J, Hughes KJ, et al. 2009. Stability of common biochemistry analytes in equine blood stored at room temperature. *Equine Vet J* 41:428-432.

100. Reynolds AJ, Potter GD, Greene LW, et al. 1998. Genetic-diet interactions in the hyperkalemic periodic paralysis syndrome in Quarter Horses fed varying amounts of potassium: III. The relationship between plasma potassium concentration and HYPP symptoms. *J Equine Vet Sci* 18:731-735.

101. Ricketts SW. 2004. Hematologic and biochemical abnormalities in athletic horses. In *Equine Sports Medicine and Surgery: Basic and Clinical Sciences of the Equine Athlete.* Hinchcliff KW, Kaneps AJ, Geor RJ (eds), pp. 949-966. Philadelphia: Saunders.

102. Robertson D, Bolton JR, Mercy AR, et al. 1996. Haematological and biochemical values in 12 Standardbred horses during training. *Aust Equine Vet* 14:72-76.

103. Simpson JA, Labugger R, Collier C, et al. 2005. Fast and slow skeletal troponin I in serum from patients with various skeletal muscle disorders: a pilot study. *Clin Chem* 51:966-972.

104. Slack JA, McGuirk SM, Erb HN, et al. 2005. Biochemical markers of cardiac injury in normal, surviving septic, or nonsurviving septic neonatal foals. *J Vet Intern Med* 19:577-580.

105. Sponseller BT, Valberg SJ, Tennent-Brown BS, et al. 2005. Severe acute rhabdomyolysis associated with Streptococcus equi infection in four horses. *J Am Vet Med Assoc* 227:1753-1754.

106. Stockham SL, Scott MA. 2008. Enzymes. In *Fundamentrals of Veterinary Clinical Pathology.* Stockham SL and Scott MA (eds), 2nd ed, pp. 640-663. Ames, IA: Blackwell.

107. Stokol T, Erb H. 1998. The apo-enzyme content of aminotransferases in healthy and diseased domestic animals. *Vet Clin Pathol* 27:71-78.

108. Teixeira-Neto AR, Ferraz GC, Moscardini ARC, et al. 2008. Alterations in muscular enzymes of horses competing in long-distance endurance rides under a tropical climate. *Arq Bras Med Vet Zootec* 60:543–549.
109. Thornton JR, Lohni MD. 1979. Tissue and plasma activity of lactate dehydrogenase and creatine kinase in the horse. *Equine Vet* 11:235–238.
110. Toutain PL, Lassourd V, Costes G, et al. 1995. A non-invasive and quantitative method for the study of tissue injury caused by intramuscular injection of drugs in horses. *J Vet Pharmacol Ther* 18:226–235.
111. Traub-Dargatz JL, Schlipf JW Jr, Granstro DE, et al. 1994. Multifocal myositis associated with Sarcocystis sp in a horse. *J Am Vet Med Assoc* 205:1574–1576.
112. Unger-Torroledo L, Straub R, Lehmann AD, et al. 2010. Lethal toxin of Clostridium sordellii is associated with fatal equine atypical myopathy. *Vet Microbiol* 144:487–492.
113. Valberg S, Jonsson L, Lindholm A, et al. 1993. Muscle histopathology and plasma aspartate aminotransferase, creatine kinase, and myoglobin changes with exercise in horses with recurrent exertional rhabdomyolysis. *Equin Vet J* 25:11–16.
114. Valberg SJ, Ward TL, Rush B, et al. 2001. Glycogen branching enzyme deficiency in Quarter Horse foals. *J Vet Intern Med* 15:572–580.
115. Vassallo JD, Janovitz EB, Wescott DM. et al. 2009. Biomarkers of drug-induced skeletal muscle injury in the rat: troponin I and myoglobin. *Toxicol Sci* 111:402–412.
116. Votion DM, Linden A, Saegerman C, et al. 2007. History and clinical features of atypical of atypical myopathy in horses in Belgium (2000-2005). *J Vet Intern Med* 21:1380–1391.
117. Wagner ML, Valberg SJ, Ames EG, et al. 2006. Allele frequency and likely impact of the glycogen branching enzyme deficiency gene in Quarter Horse and Paint Horse populations. *J Vet Intern Med* 20:1207–1211.
118. Williams KM, Williams AE, Kline LM, et al. 1987. Stability of serum alanine aminotransferase activity. *Transfusion* 27:431–433.

Chapter 10
Endocrine Evaluation

Jill Beech

> ### Acronyms and abbreviations that appear in this chapter:
>
> | | |
> |---|---|
> | ACTH | Adrenocorticotropin |
> | α-MSH | Alpha-melanocyte stimulating hormone |
> | DST | Dexamethasone suppression test |
> | fT3 | Free triiodothyronine |
> | fT4 | Free thyroxine |
> | fT4D | Free thyroxine dialysis method |
> | L-T4 | Levothyroxine sodium |
> | ODST | Overnight dexamethasone suppression test |
> | PI | Pars intermedia |
> | PPID | Pituitary pars intermedia dysfunction |
> | PTU | Propylthiouracil |
> | rT3 | Reverse T3 |
> | T3 | Triiodothyronine |
> | T4 | Thyroxine |
> | TRH | Thyrotropin releasing hormone |
> | TSH | Thyroid Stimulating Hormone (thyrotropin) |
> | TT3 | Total Triiodothyronine |
> | TT4 | Total Thyroxine |

Testing for pituitary pars intermedia dysfunction (PPID)

Over the years, a number of endocrine tests have been introduced as diagnostic tests for PPID. Although horses with PPID may have anemia, hyperglycemia,

Equine Clinical Pathology, First Edition. Edited by Raquel M. Walton.
© 2014 John Wiley & Sons, Inc. Published 2014 by John Wiley & Sons, Inc.

and other changes in serum biochemical analysis, and measuring nonhormonal blood components may help in managing individual patients with PPID, the data are not specific or sensitive for diagnosis.[40] This chapter presents the individual hormone tests that most commonly have been used, with emphasis on those currently accepted as the most accurate. It is important to remember that most of the tests have been evaluated in small populations, and it is possible that they may not represent large diverse equine populations in different geographic regions.

Cortisol concentrations

Baseline cortisol concentration

Plasma cortisol concentration is usually measured by radioimmunoassay (Diagnostic Products Corp., Los Angeles, CA). Concentrations are affected by stress, including transport, exercise, stage of pregnancy, drugs, and disease states such as colic.[1,20,27,38] Normal horses may have diurnal variation with higher concentrations in the A.M. than in the P.M., but this variation can be eliminated if a horse is moved to a novel environment.[18,28-30] In a study of 50 healthy horses, 64% had less than a 30% difference between the A.M. and P.M. cortisol concentrations.[32] A lack of rhythmicity has also been reported in horses with various health problems.[16]

Basal cortisol concentrations and diurnal variation do not reliably distinguish between normal horses and those with PPID, and horses with PPID may have basal cortisol concentrations that are lower than those in normal horses.[3,5,18,21,43] Cortisol concentrations in donkeys are reported to be similar to those of horses.[17]

Salivary cortisol concentrations

Salivary cortisol concentrations measure free, not total, cortisol concentrations. At present their measurement is not recommended as a diagnostic test for PPID.

Urinary corticoids: Creatinine ratio and cortisol

The urinary cortisol concentration and the cortisol:creatinine ratio have been reported to be higher in horses with PPID compared to normal horses.[10,44] Reports comparing seven healthy normal horses and seven with PPID indicated a 100% sensitivity for the urinary corticoid:creatinine ratio, with ratios greater than 16×10^{-6} seen only in horses with PPID; however, there were also some false negative test results.[44] Another report comparing clinically normal horses with horses with Cushing's disease and with dysautonomia found no difference in the ratios between the groups but reported a diagnostic cutoff in the cortisol:creatinine ratio of $\geq 6.9 \times 10^{-6}$ that gave positive results in 3 out of 12 healthy horses, 12 out of 13 horses with PPID, and 7 out 8 horses with dysautonomia. An increase in the cutoff value to $>12.5 \times 10^{-6}$ (the highest ratio in the normal animals) resulted in positive classification in 8 out of 13 horses with PPID and 6 out of 8 horses with dysautonomia.[10] Low specificity and sensitivity limit the value of the test in diagnosing PPID. The test has not become widely used, especially with the availability of plasma ACTH assays, which are more sensitive and specific.

ACTH stimulation of endogenous cortisol concentration

Administering ACTH elicits cortisol release from the adrenal cortex, the magnitude of which depends on the number of adrenal cortical cells and their activity.[24,25] Responses in horses with PPID have varied.[18,43,45] Although PPID horses as a group have been reported to have a greater response than a group of normal horses, the test does not determine whether an individual horse is affected and the test is not used for diagnosing PPID.

Dexamethasone suppression of cortisol concentrations

For many years the overnight dexamethasone suppression test (DST) was considered the gold standard for diagnosing PPID. Administration of dexamethasone in healthy horses suppresses ACTH secretion, resulting in decreased cortisol concentrations. In 18 out of 18 clinically normal and none out of 43 PPID horses, cortisol concentrations were less than 1 μg/dL (10 ng/ml) 20 to 24 hours following administration of dexamethasone (40 μg/kg by intramuscular [IM] injection). Sixteen hours after dexamethasone, 33 out of 34 control horses and only 5 out of 52 PPID horses had cortisol concentrations <1 μg/dL.[18] However, both false negative and false positive tests subsequently have been reported, and repeated testing can yield varying responses in the same horse. Positive ODST results have been reported in clinically normal horses between May and October, and abnormal cortisol responses have been reported in normal and in previously laminitic ponies in all seasons except spring.[3,7,14,41] Individual horses with PPID can have inconsistent test responses. For these reasons and because of the current availability of an ACTH assay, this author does not advocate the use of ODST for diagnosis of PPID. The potential link between the DST and laminitis is of concern to some, although the test has been widely used without apparent problems; the risk has not been adequately studied.

Thyrotropin releasing hormone (TRH) stimulation

The TRH stimulation test was originally used based on the premise that TRH stimulates the release of ACTH; cortisol was initially measured because of a lack of any commercially available ACTH assay.[5] The initial report of a significant increase in cortisol from baseline following TRH administration was attributed by other investigators to the lower baseline level of cortisol in the PPID horses, and a diminution in response was later reported in PPID horses with high baseline cortisol concentrations.[19,26] The validity of using this test to diagnose PPID was questioned.

Combined dexamethasone suppression and TRH stimulation test

The DST/TRH administration test was reported to have a high specificity and sensitivity in differentiating between normal horses and those with

PPID.[19,21] In this test, blood is obtained before dexamethasone administration (40 µg/kg IV), a blood sample is obtained 3 hours later, and 1 mg of TRH is administered intravenously; blood samples are then obtained at 15, 30, 45, 60, 90 minutes, and 21 hours after TRH administration. The test is considered positive if (1) plasma cortisol concentration is ≥1 µg/dL (10 ng/mL) at 24 hours, or (2) plasma cortisol concentration is increased ≥66% above the 3-hour baseline 30 minutes after TRH. A comparison of 17 PPID horses with 25 clinically normal horses with no pituitary pathology reported a sensitivity of 88%, specificity of 76%, positive predictive value of 71%, and negative predictive value of 90%. Two out of 17 PPID horses had a negative test and 6 out of 25 normal horses had a positive test.[21]

Adrenocorticotropin (ACTH) concentration

With the availability of commercial laboratories measuring ACTH, measuring basal plasma ACTH concentrations has become widely used to test for PPID. Normal reference range depends on the laboratory and methodology. The chemiluminescent immunometric assay (Diagnostic Products Corp., Los Angeles, CA) is commonly used by commercial laboratories in the United States. Veterinarians should determine the basis for the reference range of the laboratory they expect to use. In the United States, generally the same reference range (9-35 pg/mL) is used for both horses and ponies. An early study reported ACTH concentrations were lower in ponies (n=9) compared to horses (n=18), but other studies have not shown a difference.[4,13,14] One study reported ACTH concentrations were more likely to exceed reference range in ponies than in horses in late summer/autumn, which is in contrast to a study in England on ponies, where ACTH concentrations were generally within reference range in summer but above reference range in winter.[2,4] Normal mammoth donkeys (n=45) tested in May/June were reported to have ACTH concentrations that ranged from 36 to 115 pg/mL, which was higher than the laboratory's normal horse range (11.9-25.5 pg/mL).[17] Larger numbers of donkeys in other geographic locations should be tested to further clarify normal ranges. Variable seasonal increases in basal ACTH concentrations in both ponies and horses have been reported from various geographic locations.[4,8,11,14,23,31,35,39,41] Concentrations can exceed reference range from mid-August to mid-October in normal horses and ponies, particularly in the latter. In one study on clinically normal equids, ACTH concentrations sometimes exceeded 200 pg/mL, and in another study several ponies had ACTH concentrations greater than 65 pg/mL between August and mid-October.[4,14] A study in the United Kingdom on circannual variation in ACTH concentrations in normal equids (n=156) and those clinically suspected to have PPID (n=941) suggested a normal upper reference value of 47 pg/mL between August and October and 29 pg/mL from November to July.[11] Another study in the United Kingdom with a smaller group of animals suggested an appropriate cutoff value in March and June of 40 to 50 pg/mL, with a value almost doubled in September and December.[31] Use of the latter reference ranges in equids in areas such as Pennsylvania would result in some individuals being falsely diagnosed as having PPID. As the same chemiluminescent immunoassay was used in these studies, albeit in different laboratories, different populations probably explain the differing results between studies. Although basal concentrations of ACTH can be useful for diagnosing PPID, false negative tests can also occur.[3,4] In one study in the United Kingdom, 556 of 1,497 plasma samples submitted from untreated horses suspected to have PPID were within reference range.[11] Also, some horses with PPID may have basal ACTH concentrations that vary quite widely within a very short time period, and there appears to be greater variability when concentrations are high.[3,4] When measuring basal ACTH concentrations, the author advises obtaining several blood samples separated by at least a 5-10 minute interval. Obtaining several baseline concentrations is especially important if one is using these concentrations for monitoring the horse's status. If a horse suspected to have PPID has normal basal plasma ACTH concentrations, measuring the ACTH concentration change in response to TRH or domperidone administration is advised.

Domperidone stimulation of ACTH

Domperidone is a dopamine (D2) receptor antagonist and its administration should release ACTH and α-MSH secreting cells (melanotrophs) from dopaminergic inhibition, resulting in increased concentrations of these hormones in the blood. An advantage of using domperidone is that its administration per os is approved for treating mares with agalactia and it is more readily available than TRH. Disadvantages are variable blood levels, potentially due to altered gastrointestinal absorption, delayed gastric emptying, and variable food within the stomach.

Both age and pituitary pathology have been reported to correlate with domperidone response.[37] Horses with PPID were reported to have greater increases in ACTH concentration compared to normal horses 4 and 8 hours following administration of doses ranging from 1.25 to 5 mg/kg domperidone per os.[37,42] An increase ≥2-fold basal concentrations was considered a positive response, and it was suggested that the basal and the 4-hour post-domperidone administration samples were best for differentiating between PPID and clinically normal horses.[42] In another study, a ≥2-fold increase in ACTH concentration was seen in 3 out of 15 clinically normal and 4 out of 12 PPID horses at 2 hours and in 4 out of 16 clinically normal and 3 out of 12 PPID horses at 4 hours, leading the authors to conclude that the test did not appear as accurate as measuring ACTH or α-MSH response to TRH administration.[6] If one looked at ACTH concentrations >36 pg/mL as a cutoff for diagnosing PPID, administering domperidone did not increase sensitivity or specificity for making the diagnosis above using baseline ACTH concentrations.[6] Further evaluation of the test using larger numbers of horses is needed to determine its clinical value.

Alpha-melanocyte-stimulating hormone (α-MSH) concentrations

Alpha-MSH is considered a more specific marker of pars intermedia secretion than is ACTH because it is secreted by the melanotropes of the pars intermedia.[33] At the time this chapter was written, the assay was not commercially available; however, as this may change, information on its use as a marker for PPID follows. Studies cited in this chapter reporting its use have quantified the hormone using a radioimmunoassay (American Laboratory Products Co., Windham, NH). A positive correlation has been found between α-MSH and obesity/body mass index in healthy horses greater than 10 years of age, although there was huge individual variation.[15] Concentrations also rise significantly in autumn.[34,35] As the pars intermedia (PI) area, PI/total pituitary ratio, and total pituitary area increase in the fall, the observed increase in α-MSH is not unexpected.[12] A greater seasonal effect was reported for α-MSH than for ACTH.[4,23,32,41] Although greater increases were reported in ponies than in horses in one study, reports are inconsistent, and geographic location and body condition scores could have affected results.[4,12] It is apparent that the range of α-MSH concentration that is considered normal may vary geographically and potentially with the populations being studied. Stabling does not appear to influence seasonal changes.[4,35] Alpha-MSH concentration does not appear to be affected by circadian rhythm.[34] Reports comparing seasonal increases in α-MSH with ACTH have varied, and both geographic location and breed appear influential.[4,35] Whether α-MSH appears superior to ACTH for diagnosing PPID appears unresolved at this time as reports have varied regarding comparative sensitivity and specificity.[4,6,35]

ACTH and α-MSH concentration responses following thyrotropin releasing hormone (TRH) administration

Increases in both ACTH and α-MSH concentration after TRH administration have been documented to be higher in horses with PPID compared to normal horses and can identify horses with PPID that have normal basal hormone concentrations.[3,4,6,33] The protocol is to obtain two baseline plasma samples (5-10 minutes apart), administer 1 mg TRH intravenously, and then obtain a sample 30 minutes later. Although additional samples can be obtained (e.g., at 15 and 45 minutes), sampling at 30 minutes appears to be sensitive and specific for differentiating between clinically normal horses and those with PPID using a cutoff of <36 pg/mL for normal ACTH concentration and ≤50 pmol/L for α-MSH concentration.[4,6] Although concentrations of both hormones increase after administration of TRH, in normal horses they have usually returned to baseline by 30 minutes after TRH administration.

In one study on 53 clinically normal horses and 25 horses with PPID, at baseline 10 out of 60 tests from normal horses and 26 out of 37 tests from PPID horses had ACTH concentrations >36 pg/mL; at 30 minutes post TRH administration, these respective numbers were 16 out of 60 and 36 out of 38. Numbers of clinically normal horses with ACTH >36 pg/mL decreased when the group was limited to horses without pituitary histologic changes; ACTH >36 pg/mL was seen in only 1 out of 23 baseline samples and 2 out of 23 30-minute samples. For α-MSH, a concentration >50 pmol/L was seen in 1 out of 30 baseline samples and 9 out of 30 30-minute samples in clinically normal horses and in 12 out of 18 baseline samples and all 18 30-minute samples in PPID horses. In the clinically normal horses without pituitary changes, no baseline samples and only 1 out of 15 30-minute samples had α-MSH >50 pmol/L.[6] It is unknown whether the TRH stimulation test will identify horses with subclinical PPID that potentially might benefit from early dopaminergic treatment prior to onset of overt signs of PPID.

The advantages of measuring α-MSH or ACTH response to TRH compared to measuring the cortisol response to the combined DST/TRH test are that the hormones of interest being are measured, fewer samples over a shorter period of time during one patient visit are needed, and dexamethasone administration is avoided. Results from one study evaluating cortisol response to the combined DST/TRH test and another evaluating ACTH response to the TRH test showed that 15 out of 17 PPID horses and 6 out of 25 normal horses (with no PI hyperplasia or adenomas) had a positive response to the former test and 36 out of 38 tests in PPID horses and 1 out 23 tests in clinically and pathologically normal horses had a positive response to the latter test.[6,21] However, as different populations comprised each of these studies, further studies would be needed to adequately compare the two tests.

Chemical-grade TRH has been used in published reports of the test, although it is not approved for this use. Acquisition, storage, and preparation of TRH may limit its use among veterinarians. Most studies have not reported side effects, but minor transient to generalized moderate muscle trembling for several minutes after administration of TRH has been seen in a few horses. This response was inconsistent when the test was repeated in the same horses, and the cause of the trembling remains speculative. Transient licking, yawning, and sometimes flehmen have been seen in a few horses.[4,6]

Insulin concentrations

Factors such as diet can explain hyperinsulinemia and insulin resistance (see Chapter 8), and this, combined with highly variable concentrations throughout the day, complicates interpretation of values from single samples. Adiposity associated with insulin resistance has been reported in 15-30% of horses with PPID and hyperinsulinemia has been reported in some horses with PPID.[13,32,35,40] One study reported that although insulin concentrations differed between normal horses and those with PPID, hyperinsulinemia was rare.[22] Normal ponies were reported to have more variable concentrations than horses and more individual clinically normal ponies had insulin concentrations above reference range (24 out of 48 tests in 6 normal ponies versus none of 48 tests in 14 normal horses); however, this could be associated with the greater body condition score in the ponies.[4] When evaluating donkeys, it is important to know that they are reported to have lower concentrations than horses. In one study on 45 healthy donkeys, all but 5 had insulin concentrations below the normal horse reference limit.[17] Non-obese donkeys were reported to have lower insulin concentrations than non-obese horses. Concentrations were significantly higher in obese donkeys and those with a history of laminitis or current laminitis compared to non-obese donkeys. Veterinarians evaluating donkeys should ascertain whether the laboratory they use has reference ranges for donkeys. There has been growing interest in better defining hyperinsulinemia and equine metabolic syndrome and investigating the relationship with PPID (see Chapter 8). It may be useful to monitor insulin concentrations in horses as high concentrations have been predictive for the development of laminitis and low insulin concentrations have been associated with improved survival.[9,36]

In summary, the best screening test for PPID currently is measurement of several basal ACTH concentrations, taking into account the normal seasonal effect. However, if concentrations are normal, a TRH stimulation test should be performed to evaluate whether ACTH concentration rises and remains increased above the normal reference range (Table 10.1).

Table 10.1   Diagnostic Tests

Type of Test	Steps for Testing	Positive Results
Basal ACTH Concentrations	2 EDTA samples 5 to >10 minutes apart	Concentrations above reference interval
TRH Stimulation Test	Baseline plasma samples obtained 1 mg TRH administered IV 30-minute plasma sample obtained	Basal and 30-minute samples above reference interval
Overnight dexamethasone suppression test (DST)	Serum sample obtained 0.04 mg/kg dexamethasone IM @ approximately 5:00 p.m. Serum sample obtained 19-20 hours later	Lack of suppression (cortisol >10 ng/mL)
Combined DST/TRH Test	Serum sample obtained 0.04 mg/kg dexamethasone IV in a.m. Blood sample obtained 3 hours later and 1 mg TRH administered IV Blood samples @ (15), 30, 60 minutes, and 21 hours after TRH	Cortisol concentration ≥10 ng/mL @ 24 hours after DST or cortisol increased >66% @ 30 minutes after TRH

Testing thyroid function in horses

Despite very few documented cases of thyroid dysfunction in horses and the unreliability of single measurements of thyroid hormones, basal serum concentrations of total triiodothyronine (TT3) and total thyroxine (TT4) are frequently evaluated by veterinarians. This section provides information on tests that have been used to evaluate thyroid function and factors that can influence results.

Thyroid dysfunction

There appear to be no studies documenting the prevalence of primary thyroid dysfunction in horses. Naturally occurring hypothyroidism is reported in foals, and there are several case reports of mature/aged horses with hyperthyroidism.[47,49,88,94] Low thyroid hormone concentrations have been measured in horses with various conditions in the absence of evidence of hypothyroidism. Although hypothyroidism has been implicated as a contributing cause of laminitis, it should be noted that no evidence has been found to support measurement of thyroid hormones as a predictor of pasture-associated laminitis in horses, and horses with experimentally induced hypothyroidism have not developed laminitis.[54,57,61,73,90,96] Horses that have been thyroidectomized have shown various clinical signs, most frequently hair coat abnormalities and decreased tolerance to cold.[78] In younger animals, stature is affected. Mares can continue to show normal estrous cycles, conceive and deliver normal foals, and although stallions have decreased libido, they are fertile.[78,81,90] Propylthiouracil (PTU)-induced hypothyroidism has changed serum hormone concentrations in the absence of clinical signs.[54,73] Severe signs have been reported in neonatal foals with naturally occurring hypothyroidism and in foals that have been partially thyroidectomized in utero.[49-51]

Thyroid hormones

Secretion of thyroid hormones is stimulated by thyrotropin (thyroid stimulating hormone [TSH]) released from the anterior pituitary gland. TSH is regulated by thyrotropin-releasing hormone (TRH) secretion from the hypothalamus. The cuboidal to low columnar thyroid epithelial cells secrete thyroglobulin, a glycoprotein containing multiple tyrosine residues. Iodine is oxidized within the gland and bound to tyrosine on thyroglobulin to produce monoiodotyrosine and diiodotyrosine. Thyroxine (T4) and triiodothyronine (T3) result from mono- and diiododtyrosine couplings. Thyroglobulin undergoes proteolysis to release T3 and T4 into the blood. The majority of thyroid hormone released into the blood is in the form of T4 because much more T4 than T3 is formed in the thyroid gland.

Once in the blood, 99% of T4 and T3 are bound to transport proteins (thyroid hormone binding globulin, transthyretin, and albumin). Only the unbound free fractions are metabolically active; free T3 is more metabolically active than T4 because it binds much more avidly to thyroid hormone receptors. The majority of T3 is produced outside of the thyroid gland, via deiodination of T4 in the peripheral tissues by deiodinases. Production of reverse T3 (rT3), a metabolically inactive form of T3, also occurs in peripheral tissues through the action of iodinases, and is important in thyroid hormone regulation.

Extrathyroidal effects on thyroid hormones

One should always inquire whether a horse is receiving medications or supplements and avoid testing if drugs have recently been administered. Drugs that are highly protein bound and could displace thyroid hormones from protein-binding sites are of the greatest concern. Free T3 and T4 (fT3 and fT4) are readily excreted via the kidneys, thus increased concentrations of unbound fT3 and fT4 may result in increases or decreases in thyroid hormone concentrations depending on whether total hormone (TT3 and TT4) or free hormone concentrations are measured. Systemic administration of dexamethasone (0.04 mg/kg SID for 5 days) resulted in significant increases in rT3 and sometimes also fT3, and also blunted response to TSH administration.[80] Topical dexamethasone and neomycin applied on the shaved side of horses' necks (8.5 mg of dexamethasone every 12 hours per 470-660 kg body weight for 10 days) resulted in a significant decline in TT3 by day 2 and this remained less than baseline for at least 20 days after treatment; TT4 concentrations showed a mild but non-significant decrease.[46] Phenylbutazone administration decreases thyroid hormone concentration.[84,85,89] The duration of effect of phenylbutazone treatment (4.4 mg/kg IV BID for 5 days) was reported to last for 10 days for TT4 and 2 days for fT4.[89] However, these dosages of phenylbutazone are rarely used in clinical practice, and the effect of lower or oral dosage regimens has not been reported.

Administration of synthetic thyroid hormone (levothyroxine sodium or L-T4) affects both basal concentrations of thyroid hormones and the response to TRH injections.[92] Dose and duration of treatment with L-T4 affect the magnitude of change in hormones and probably affect the length of drug-free interval required prior to testing a horse that has been receiving L-T4.[92]

Diet can affect thyroid hormone concentration.[57,64,65,82,83] Exercising horses fed high sugar and starch diets were reported to have higher TT3 and fT3 concentrations than horses fed fat and fiber diets.[57] Blood samples should not be obtained close to feeding a high energy and protein meal and an interval of at least 4-6 hours is advised.[57,65] Food deprivation in healthy horses was reported to result in a 42% decrease in TT3 and a 30% decrease in fT3 after 2 days, a 38% decrease in TT4 and 24% increase in fT4 after 4 days, and an increase of 31% in rT3 after 1 day.[82] However, no differences in TT3 and TT4 were reported in weanling horses fed restricted diets.[64]

Age also influences thyroid hormone concentrations.[56,62,71,75,79,83,86] Premature foals have lower serum concentrations of total and free thyroid hormones compared to normal foals. A number of studies have reported that

Table 10.2   Concentrations of Thyroid Hormones in Neonatal Foals

	<12 hrs[a] (n=18)		12 to 36 hrs[b] (n=25)	
	Median	Range	Median	Range
TT4 nmol/L	277	238-337	712	295-012
fT4 pmol/L	78	46-118	NA	NA
fT4D pmol/L	106	78-184	50.2	27-70
TT3 nmol/L	8.2	3.4-10.8	7.9	3.2-9.5
fT3 pmol/L	7.8	2.4-20.3	21.2	6.9-34.3
rT3 pmol/L	NA	NA	6.6	5.2-8.1
TSH ng/mL	0.22	0.12-0.72	NA	NA

[a]Reference 10; [b]Reference 25.

young foals have much higher TT3 and TT4 concentrations than mature horses. Table 10.2 shows concentrations in neonatal foals published in two different reports.[56,70] Concentrations of both TT4 and TT3 are reported to be greatest in foals within 1 hour of birth (prior to colostrum ingestion) and may be 14- and 12-fold greater, respectively, than in blood from mature horses.[71,86] A study on Thoroughbred foals (8 males and 5 females) from 30 to 390 days of age showed an insignificant decrease in TT4 between 1 and 6 months of age but a marked decrease between 7 and 13 months of age. The fT4 decreased significantly by the third month. The TT3 values were more variable, while the fT3 usually decreased over time.[62] Another study on 6 foals reported TT3 and TT4 dropped after 1 month but TT4 remained higher for 12 months.[75] In Standardbred females, plasma TT3 was reported to decline from a mean of 7.9 ng/mL on day 1 to 2.4 ng/mL on day 14, and TT4 declined from 233 ng/mL to 49 ng/mL in the same time period, with insignificant differences reported between samples obtained between 1 month and 22 years.[79] It appears that consensus among the studies exists for changes in young foals, but reports on animals older than 1 month appear variable. If one is evaluating foals for thyroid dysfunction, comparison with age and preferably sex-matched controls is prudent.

The effect of gender on thyroid hormone levels is unclear as reports have been inconsistent. There is usually no gender effect on thyroid hormone concentrations except that males sometimes have significantly higher TT4 concentrations. Estrus and pregnancy do not appear to affect TT3 or TT4.[53,72,74]

Thyroid hormones concentrations are affected by ambient temperature and/or season and these factors should be considered when taking blood samples from horses. A negative relationship for serum TT3 (but not TT4) and temperature has been reported, with significantly higher concentrations in December through May and significantly lower concentrations from July to October.[72] TT4 was reported to have a slight but significant negative association with photoperiod, but this appears unlikely to affect diagnostic testing.

Reports on diurnal variation in TT3 and TT4 vary.[60,75,91] In clinical practice, diurnal rhythm does not appear to be a major influence on deciding when one obtains samples for measuring thyroid hormones.

Exercise can affect thyroid hormone levels. Studies on horses performing endurance exercise have shown no changes or only transient decreases after rides of 40-56 km and decreased concentrations following 160 km rides that return to normal by 24 hours.[67] In one study, training induced increases in fT4 and TT4.[57] In contrast, basal concentrations of TT3 and TT4 were reported to be within reference range for competitive showjumping horses.[59] To avoid any possible influence of exercise, one should avoid measuring thyroid hormone concentrations within several days of strenuous exercise.

Nonthyroidal illness syndrome

Nonthyroidal illness syndrome (NTIS) or euthyroid sick syndrome may result in central hypothyroidism via decreased secretion of TRH by lowering set points for feedback inhibition and inhibition of TSH by glucocorticoids and inflammatory cytokines. Nonthyroidal illness may also decrease thyroid hormone binding protein as well as binding affinity and capacity. The syndrome is characterized by low TT3, increased rT3, and/or low TT4 with normal fT4.[70] With thyroid-dependent hypothyroidism, rT3 is typically decreased, whereas T4 metabolism is altered in NTIS so that the inactivating pathway producing rT3 is upregulated. TSH concentrations are normal, distinguishing NTIS from hypothyroidism in which TSH is increased.

Although nonthyroidal illness syndrome may exist in horses, it has not been well documented except for descriptions of the condition in critically ill foals.[56,70] Critically ill foals were reported to have decreased concentrations of all thyroid hormones except rT3 and concentrations correlated with the sepsis score in septic foals.[70] Another study reported sick term foals had lower TT3 than normal foals but their TT4 concentration was intermediate between premature and normal foals.[56]

Thyroid hormone evaluation

Many commercial laboratories assay TT3 and TT4. Because single measurements of TT3 and TT4 are difficult to interpret as a result of extrathyroidal effects on protein binding, it is important to consider concentrations of free T3 (fT3) and free T4 (fT4). It has been suggested that measuring fT3 and fT4 and fT4 by dialysis (fT4D) is superior to measuring TT3 and TT4, although in normal horses measurement of fT4 (by single RIA) was reported to offer no additional information compared to measuring TT4.[54,55,91] Similar to dogs and humans, measuring fT4 concentrations directly instead of by dialysis appears to underestimate fT4 concentrations in horses. Free T4 by dialysis can be useful to differentiate hypothyroidism from nonthyroidal illness syndrome. With nonthyroidal illness, fT4D is usually within reference limits whereas TT4 and TT3 may be low.[54,55]

Table 10.3 Range of Concentrations of Thyroid Hormones in Mature Horses from Different Diagnostic Laboratories

	A (n = 71)		B	C
	Value Ranges	95% CI	Value Ranges	Value Ranges
TT4 nmol/L	6-46	18-22	7-27	11-31
fT4 pmol/L	6-21	10-12	6-24	NA
fT4D pmol/L	7-47	21-25	8-39	15-23
TT3 nmol/L	0.3-2.9	0.9-1.1	0.7-2.5	0.5-1.2
fT3 pmol/L	0.1-5.9	1.8-2.4	1.7-5.2	NA
TSH ng/mL	0.02-0.97	0.21-0.37	NA	NA

A, Breuhaus;[10] B, Diagnostic Center for Population and Animal Health, Michigan State University, Lansing MI; C, Animal Health Diagnostic Center, Endocrinology Laboratory, Cornell University College of Veterinary Medicine, Ithaca, NY. *NA*, not available.

In a study of PTU-induced hypothyroidism, TT3 and fT3 fell abruptly whereas TT4 and fT4 did not decrease dramatically until weeks 5 and 4 of PTU administration, respectively.[54] This suggests that measuring TT3 and fT3 is superior to measuring TT4 and fT4 in a horse suspected to be acutely hypothyroid.

The use of blood collection tubes with additives (i.e., gel separator and clot activator) should be avoided due to potential interference with test results. Free T4 can be falsely increased if the sample is warmed, so whole blood specimens and processed samples (serum/plasma) should be kept refrigerated, while frozen sample storage is recommended if the time between obtaining the sample and shipping is ≥12 hours. However, veterinarians should consult the laboratory they use to determine the requirements regarding handling of samples and also the source of the laboratory's reference ranges. As shown in Table 10.3, reference ranges vary and results from different laboratories are not interchangeable.

Thyroid stimulating hormone (TSH) concentration

An assay for thyroid stimulating hormone (TSH) has been validated for use in horses but has not become widely available or used.[54,93] TSH has been shown to steadily increase in horses given PTU to induce hypothyroidism, with a dramatic increase by weeks 5 and 6.[73] Concentration decreases in horses receiving L-T4.[92] Concentrations of TSH were reported to be greater in anestrus mares during winter than in estrus mares during summer.[60] To the author's knowledge, further studies on the effect of season and estrus cycle on TSH have not been published. As natural cases of true hypothyroidism or hyperthyroidism appear to be rare, the ranges of serum levels of TSH in these conditions have not been described.

Thyrotropin releasing hormone (TRH) stimulation

Exogenous TRH stimulates release of thyroxine in euthyroid horses.[63,68,72,91] Studies on the TT3 and TT4 responses following administration of intravenous TRH have shown a maximum response at 4 hours for TT4 and 2 hours for TT3. Ponies have responded to 0.5 mg, and the usual dose used in horses is 1 mg. In one study, both TT3 and TT4 remained significantly increased at 6 hours, but in another study TT3 was similar to baseline concentration.[52,58,76] Since both TT3 and TT4 increase significantly from baseline by 2 hours and remain increased for 4 hours, in clinical practice, collecting a second sample within this 2-4 hour period should suffice to show whether the horse has a normal response. A two- to threefold increase from baseline is normal, although individuals may vary especially with regard to T3.[55] In a study of 36 normal mature horses, at 4 hours post TRH administration, TT4 increased 1.3-3.8 times and fT4 and fT4D increased 1.1-2.1 and 1.1-2.8 times baseline, respectively. At 2 hours, TT3 had increased 1.1-10.3 (mean=3) times and fT3 increased 1-53 (mean=4.2) times baseline.[55] These wide variations in response can complicate interpretation of an individual horse's response. It appears that resting baseline levels can affect responses; high resting TT3 or TT4 appeared to have blunted responses or altered the time of peak concentration, and low baseline concentrations were associated with greater responses.[55] An inadequate response can be seen in primary or secondary hypothyroidism.

Other factors may influence response to TRH. Variable effects of exercise on the TRH response test have been reported. A significantly greater increase in TT4 was reported in Thoroughbred horses in training compared to those out of work, but another study in another breed reported no effect.[57,68] Numbers of horses in these studies were small. TT3 and fT3 response were greater in sugar-and-starch-fed horses than fat-and-fiber-fed horses.[57] Obese hyperinsulinemic horses with laminitis were reported to have greater TT3 and fT3 responses compared to horses with chronic lameness due to other musculoskeletal disorders.[66] Medication may also affect response. Administration of oral L-T4 was associated with decreased concentrations of TT4, TT3, fT3, and TSH in response to intravenous TRH, but the fT4 response was unaffected.[92] The chemical form of TRH used in the test is not approved for use in horses, although it has been used in hundreds of horses without significant adverse effects.

TSH stimulation test

There is no equine TSH available and no approved form for use in horses. This test has been evaluated in research but appears less utilized in clinical medicine than the TRH stimulation test.[68,69,84,87] Following 5 IU TSH intravenously, baseline TT3 values were reported to double by 30 minutes, and peak at five times baseline value at 2 hours; TT4 doubled between 2 and 3 hours and peaked at 4 hours (2.4 x baseline concentration).[84] As the TT3 response is of greater magnitude and occurs earlier than the rise in TT4, measurement of TT3 before and 1 hour after 5 IU TSH has been suggested.[69,87]

A greater increase in TT3 than TT4 was documented after IM administration of TSH.[84] Due to variable response to IM administration of TSH, intravenous administration has been advised.[68,69,87] Phenylbutazone decreased baseline TT3 and TT4 but did not decrease response to TSH.[84] In contrast, after 5 days of dexamethasone (0.04 mg/kg IM every 24 hours), the response of thyroid hormones to TSH was blunted.[80]

The clinical value of this test is unclear, and some individual clinically normal horses have failed to respond with a doubling of TT4. In a study in 12 mature horses, only 6 horses' TT4 increased more than twice baseline at 6 hours after TSH, although mean serum concentrations of TT3, TT4, rT3, and fT4 were significantly increased from baseline in all horses. In the group of horses that failed to have a twofold increase in TT4, although the fT3 more than doubled, the increase for the groups was not significant.[80] Currently this test is not recommended for clinical use.

T3 suppression test

This test is performed to confirm hyperthyroidism in a horse with high baseline thyroid hormone concentrations. To the author's knowledge, there are only two published case reports using this test.[47,94] One protocol is to administer T3 (2.5 mg diluted in 5 mL sterile saline) IM at 6 P.M. on day 1, and at 8 A.M. and 6 P.M. on days 2, 3, and 4. Blood samples are taken 5 minutes before each dose of T3, at 8 A.M. and 6 P.M. on days 5 and 7, and at 8 A.M. on day 10.[94] In the other protocol, T3 (2.5 mg diluted in 5 mL sterile saline) is injected IM at 8:30 A.M. and 6 P.M. on days 1, 2, and 3 and at 8:30 A.M. on day 4. Blood samples are obtained 30 and 5 minutes prior to the first injection of T3 and 5 minutes prior to all subsequent T3 injections. Additional blood samples are obtained at 6 P.M. on day 4 and at 8:30 A.M. on days 6, 7, 9, 17, 20, and 22.[47] Hyperthyroid horses fail to show a suppression of thyroid hormones whereas normal horses showed a prompt suppression that persisted for at least 5 days after the last dose of T3.[47,94]

Baseline concentrations of thyroid hormones can be influenced by the many factors described, and low baseline TT4 or TT3 levels by themselves may be inadequate for diagnosis of hypothyroidism. While evaluation of thyroid hormone changes in response to TRH administration are helpful in evaluating thyroid function, the chemical grade of TRH that has most frequently been used is not approved for this use in horses.

References

1. Ayala I, Martos NF, Silvan G, et al. 2012. Cortisol, adrenocorticotropic hormone, serotonin, adrenaline and noradrenaline serum concentrations in relation to disease and stress in the horse. *Res Vet Sci* 93:103-107.

2. Bailey SR, Habershon-Butcher JL, Ransom KJ, et al. 2008. Hypertension and insulin resistance in a mixed-breed population of ponies predisposed to laminitis. *J Vet Res* 69:122–129.

3. Beech J, Boston R, Lindborg S, et al. 2007. Adrenocorticotropin concentration following administration of thyrotropin releasing hormone in healthy horses and those with pituitary pars intermedia dysfunction and pituitary hyperplasia. *J Am Vet Med Assoc* 23:1–10.

4. Beech J, Boston RC, McFarlane D, et al. 2009. Evaluation of plasma ACTH, alpha-melanocyte-stimulating hormone, and insulin concentrations during various photoperiods in clinically normal horses and ponies and those with pituitary pars intermedia dysfunction. *J Am Vet Med Assoc* 235:715–722.

5. Beech J, Garcia M. 1985. Hormonal response to thyrotropin-releasing hormone in healthy horses and in horses with pituitary adenoma. *Am J Vet Res* 46:1941–1943.

6. Beech J, McFarlane D, Lindborg Sue, et al. 2011. α-melanocyte-stimulating hormone and adrenocorticotropin concentrations in response to thyrotropin-releasing hormone and comparison with adrenocorticotropin concentration after domperidone administration in healthy horses and horses with pituitary pars intermedia dysfunction. *J Am Vet Med Assoc* 238:1305–1315.

7. Borer KE, Menzies-Gow NJ, Berthane Y, et al. 2010. Seasonal influence on insulin and cortisol results from overnight dexamethasone suppression tests (DST) in normal and previously laminitic ponies. *J Vet Intern Med* 24:779.

8. Buchanan B, Frank N, Elliot SB, et al. 2010. Effects of season on adrenocorticotropin hormone (ACTH) concentrations in a group of horses located in the state of Texas. *J Vet Intern Med* 24:782.

9. Carter RA, Treiber KH, Geor RJ, et al. 2009. Prediction of incipient pasture-associated laminitis from hyperinsulinemia, hyperleptinemia, and generalized and localized obesity in a cohort of ponies. *Equine Vet J* 41:171–178.

10. Chandler KJ, Dixon RM. 2002. Urinary cortisol:creatinine ratios in healthy horses and horses with hyperadrenocorticism and non-adrenal illness. *Vet Rec* 150:773–776.

11. Copas VE, Durham AE. 2012. Circannual variation in plasma adrenocorticotropic hormone concentrations in the UK in normal horses and ponies, and those with pituitary pars intermedia dysfunction. *Equine Vet J* 44:440–443.

12. Cordero M, McFarlane D, Breshears MA, et al. 2012. The effect of season on the histologic and histomorphometric appearance of the equine pituitary gland. *J Equine Vet Sci* 32:75–79.

13. Couetil L, Paradis MR, Knoll J. 1996. Plasma adrenocorticotropin concentration in healthy horses and in horses with clinical signs of hyperadrenocorticism. *J Vet Intern Med* 10:1–6.

14. Donaldson MT, McDonnell SM, Schanbacher BJ, et al. 2005. Variation in plasma adrenocorticotrophic hormone concentration and dexamethasone suppression test results with season, age and sex in healthy ponies and horses. *J Vet Intern Med* 19:217–222.

15. Donaldson MT, McFarlane D, Jorgensen AJ, et al. 2004. Correlation between plasma alpha-melanocyte stimulating hormone concentration and body mass index in healthy horses. *Am J Vet Res* 65:1469–1473.

16. Douglas R. 1999. Circadian cortisol rhymicity and equine Cushing-like disease. *J Equine Vet Sci* 19:750–753.

17. Dugat SL, Taylor TS, Matthews N, et al. 2010. Values for triglycerides, insulin, cortisol and ACTH in a herd of normal donkeys. *J Equine Vet Sci* 30:141–144.

18. Dybdal NO, Hargreaves KM, Madigan JE, et al. 1994. Diagnostic testing for pituitary pars intermedia dysfunction in horses. *J Am Vet Med Assoc* 204:627–632.

19. Eiler H, Oliver JW, Andrews FM, et al. 1997. Results of a combined dexamethasone suppression/thyrotropin-releasing hormone stimulation test in healthy horses and horses suspected to have a pars intermedia pituitary adenoma. *J Am Vet Med Assoc* 211:79–81.

20. Fazio E, Medica P, Aronica V, et al. 2008. Circulating β-endorphin, adrenocorticotropic hormone and cortisol levels of stallions before and after short road transport: stress effect of different distances. *Acta Vet Scand* 50:6.

21. Frank N, Andrews FM, Sommardahl CS, et al. 2006. Evaluation of the combined dexamethasone suppression/thyrotropin-releasing hormone stimulation test for detection of pars intermedia pituitary adenomas in horses. *J Vet Intern Med* 20:987–993.

22. Frank N, Elliott SB, Chamerou KA, et al. 2010. Association of season and pasture grazing with blood hormone and metabolite concentrations in horses with presumed pituitary pars intermedia dysfunction. *J Vet Intern Med* 24:1167–1175.

23. Funk RA, Stewart AJ, Woolridge AA, et al. 2011. Seasonal changes in plasma adrenocorticotrophic hormone and α-melanocyte stimulating hormone in response to thyrotropin releasing hormone in normal aged horses. *J Vet Intern Med* 25:578–585.

24. Glover CM, Miller LM, Dybdal NO, et al. 2009. Extrapituitary and pituitary pathological findings in horses with pituitary pars intermedia dysfunction: a retrospective study. *J Equine Vet Sci* 29:146–153.

25. Heinrichs M, Baumgarten W, Cape CC. 1990. Immunocytochemical demonstration of proopiomelanocortin-derived peptides in pituitary adenomas of the pars intermedia in horses. *Vet Pathol* 27:419–425.

26. Hillyer MH, Taylor FGR, Mair TS, et al. 1992. Diagnosis of hyperadrenocorticism in the horse. *Equine Vet Educ* 4:131–134.

27. Hinchcliff KW, Rush BR, Farris JW. 2005. Evaluation of plasma catecholamine and serum cortisol concentrations in horses with colic. *J Am Vet Med Assoc* 227:276–280.

28. Hoffsis GF, Murdick PW. 1970. The plasma concentrations of corticosteroids in normal and diseased horses. *J Am Vet Med Assoc* 157:1590–1594.

29. Irvine CH, Alexander SL. 1994. Factors affecting the circadian rhythm in plasma cortisol concentrations in the horse. *Dom Anim Endocrinol* 11:227–238.

30. James VHT, Horner MW, Moss MS, et al. 1970. Adrenocortical function in the horse. *J Endocrinol* 48:319–335.

31. Lee ZY, Zylstra R, Haritou SJ. 2010. The use of adrenocorticotrophic hormone as a potential biomarker of pituitary pars intermedia dysfunction in horses. *Vet J* 185:58–61.

32. McFarlane D. 2011. Equine pituitary pars intermedia dysfunction. 2011. *Vet Clin North Am Equine Pract* 27:93–113.

33. McFarlane D, Beech J, Cribb A. 2006. Alpha-melanocyte stimulating hormone release in response to thyrotropin releasing hormone in healthy horses, horses with pituitary pars intermedia dysfunction, and equine pars intermedia explants. *Dom Anim Endocrinol* 30:276–288.

34. McFarlane D, Donaldson MT, McDonnell SM, et al. 2004. Effects of season and sample handling on measurement of plasma α-melanocyte stimulating hormone concentrations in horses and ponies. *Am J Vet Res* 65:1463–1468.

35. McFarlane D, Paradis MR, Zimmel D, et al. 2011. The effect of geographic location, breed, and pituitary dysfunction on seasonal adrenocortioctropin and α-melanocyte-stimulating hormone plasma concentrations in horses. *J Vet Intern Med* 25:872-881.
36. McGowan CM, Frost R, Pfeiffer DU, et al. 2004. Serum insulin concentrations in horses with equine Cushing's syndrome: response to a cortisol inhibitor and prognostic value. *Equine Vet J* 36:295-298.
37. Miller MA, Pardo ID, Jackson LP, et al. 2008. Correlation of pituitary histomorphometry with adrenocorticotrophic hormone response to domperidone administration in the diagnosis of equine pituitary pars intermedia dysfunction. *Vet Pathol* 45:26-38.
38. Niinistö KE, Korolainen RV, Raekallio MR, et al. 2010. Plasma levels of heat shock protein 72 (HSP72) and beta-endorphin as indicators of stress, pain and prognosis in horses with colic. *Vet J* 184:100-104.
39. Place NJ, McGowan CM, Lamb SV, et al. 2010. Seasonal variation in serum concentrations of selected metabolic hormones in horses. *J Vet Intern Med* 24:650-654.
40. Schott HC. 2006. Pituitary pars intermedia dysfunction: challenges of diagnosis and treatment *Proc Am Assoc Equine Pract* 52:60-73.
41. Shreiber CM, Stewart AJ, Kwessi E, et al. 2012. Seasonal variation in diagnostic tests for pituitary pars intermedia dysfunction in older, clinically normal geldings. *J Am Vet Med Assoc* 241:241-248.
42. Sojka JE, Jackson LP, Moore GE, et al. 2006. Domperidone causes an increase in the endogenous ACTH concentration in horses with pituitary pars intermedia dysfunction (equine Cushing's disease). *Proc Am Assoc Equine Pract* 52:320-323.
43. van der Kolk JH, Wensing T, Kalsbeek HC, et al. 1995. Laboratory diagnosis of equine pituitary pars in intermedia adenoma. *Dom Anim Endocrinol* 12:35-39.
44. van der Kolk JH, Kalsbeek HC, Wensing T, et al. 1994. Urinary concentration of corticoids in normal horses and horses with hyperadrenocorticism. *Res Vet Sci* 56:126-128.
45. van der Kolk JH, Kalsbeek HC, van Garderen E, et al. 1993. Equine pituitary neoplasia: a clinical report of 21 cases (1990-1992). *Vet Rec* 133:594-597.
46. Abraham G, Allersmeier M, Schusser GF, et al. 2011. Serum thyroid hormone insulin glucose, triglycerides and protein concentrations in normal horses: association with topical dexamethasone usage. *Vet J* 188:307-312.
47. Alberts MK, McCann JP, Woods PR. 2000. Hemithyroidectomy in a horse with confirmed hyperthyroidism. *J Am Vet Med Assoc* 217:1051-1054.
48. Alexander SL, Irvine CHG, Evans MJ. 2004. Inter-relationships between the secretory dynamics of thyrotrophin releasing hormone, thyrotrophin, and prolactin in periovulatory mares: effect of hypothyroidism. *J Neuroendocrinol* 16:906-915.
49. Allen AL, Doige CE, Fretz PB, et al. 1994. Hyperplasia of the thyroid gland and concurrent musculoskeletal deformities in Western Canadian foals: reexamination of a previously described syndrome. *Can Vet J* 35:31-38.
50. Allen AL, Fretz PB, Card CE, et al. 1998. The effects of partial thyroidectomy on the development of the equine fetus. *Equine Vet J* 30:53-59.
51. Allen AL, Townsend HGG, Doige CE, et al. 1996. A case-control study of the congenital hypothyroidism and dysmaturity syndrome of foals. *Can Vet J* 37:349-358.

52. Beech J, Garcia M. 1985. Hormonal response to thyrotropin-releasing hormone in healthy horses and in horses with pituitary adenoma. *Am J Vet Res* 46:1941-1943.

53. Berg EL, McNamara DL, Keiser DH. 2007. Endocrine profiles of periparturient mares and their foals. *J Anim Sci* 85:1660-1668.

54. Breuhaus BA. 2002. Thyroid-stimulating hormone in adult euthyroid and hypothyroid horses. *J Vet Intern Med* 16:109-115.

55. Breuhaus BA. 2011. Disorders of the equine thyroid gland. *Vet Clin North Am Equine Pract* 27:115-128.

56. Breuhaus BA, LaFevers DH. 2005. Thyroid function in normal, sick, and premature foals. *J Vet Intern Med* 19:445.

57. Carter RA. 2005. Thyroid status in exercising horses and laminitic ponies. M.S. Thesis, VA Polytechnic Institute and State University: Blacksburg, VA.

58. Chen CL, Li WI. 1986. Effect of thyrotropin releasing hormone (TRH) on serum levels of thyroid hormones in Thoroughbred mares. *Equine Vet Sci* 6:58-61.

59. Cravana C, Medica P, Prestopino M, et al. 2010. Effects of competitive and noncompetitive showjumping on total and free iodothyronines, β-endorphin ACTH and cortisol levels in horses. *Equine Vet J* Suppl 38:179-184.

60. Duckett WM, Manning JP, Weston PG. 1989. Thyroid hormone periodicity in healthy adult geldings. *Equine Vet J* 21:123-125.

61. Frank N, Sojka J, Latour M, et al. 2004. Effect of hypothyroidism on the blood lipid response to higher dietary fat intake in mares. *J Anim Sci* 82:2640-2646.

62. Fazio E, Medica P, Cravana C, et al. 2007. Total and free iodothyronine levels of growing Thoroughbred foals: effects of weaning and gender. *Livestock Sci* 110:207-213.

63. Gentry LR, Thompson DL Jr, Stelzer AM. 2002. Responses of seasonally anovulatory mares to daily administration of thyrotropin-releasing hormone and(or) gonadotropin-releasing hormone analog. *J Anim Sci* 80:208-213.

64. Glade MJ, Gupta S, Reimers TJ. 1984. Hormonal responses to high and low planes of nutrition in weanling Thoroughbreds. *J Anim Sci* 59:658-665.

65. Glade MJ, Reimers TJ. 1985. Effects of dietary energy supply on serum thyroxine, tri-iodothyronine, and insulin concentrations in young horses. *J Endocrinol* 104:93-98.

66. Graves E, Schott HC, Johnson P, et al. 2002. Thyroid function in horses with peripheral Cushing's syndrome. *Proc Am Assoc Equine Pract* 48:178-180.

67. Graves EA, Schott HC, Marteniuk JV, et al. 2006. Thyroid hormone responses to endurance exercise. *Equine Vet J* Suppl 36:32-36.

68. Harris P, Marlin D, Gray J. 1992. Equine thyroid function tests: a preliminary investigation. *Br Vet J* 148:71-80.

69. Held, JP, Oliver JW. 1984. A sampling protocol for the thyrotropin-stimulating test in the horse. *J Am Vet Med Assoc* 184:326-327.

70. Himler M, Hurcombe SDA, Griffin A, et al. 2012. Presumptive nonthyroidal illness syndrome in critically ill foals. *Equine Vet J* Suppl 41:43-47.

71. Irvine CHG, Evans MJ. 1974. Postnatal changes in total and free thyroxine in foal serum. *J Reprod Fert* Suppl 23:709-715.

72. Johnson AL. 1986. Serum concentrations of prolactin, thyroxine and tri-iodothyronine relative to season and the estrus cycle in the mare. *J Anim Sci* 62:1012-1020.

73. Johnson PJ, Messer NT, Ganjam VK, et al. 2003. Effects of propylthiouracil and bromocriptine on serum concentrations of thyrotropin and thyroid hormones in normal female horses. *Equine Vet J* 35:296-301.

74. Katovich M, Evans JW, Sanchez O. 1974. Effects of season pregnancy and lactation on thyroxine turnover in the mare. *J Animal Sci* 38:811-818.
75. Komosa M, Flisinoka-Bojanowska A, Gill J. 1990. Development of diurnal rhythm in some metabolic parameters in foals. *Comp Biochem Physiol A Comp Physiol* 95:549-552.
76. Lothrop CD, Nolan HL. 1986. Equine thyroid function assessment with the thyrotropin-releasing hormone response test. *Am J Vet Res* 47:942-944.
77. Lowe JE, Baldwin BH, Foote RH, et al. 1974. Equine hypothyroidism: the long-term effects of thyroidectomy on metabolism and growth in mares and stallions. *Cornell Vet* 64:276-295.
78. Lowe JE, Baldwin BH, Foote RH, et al. 1975. Semen characteristics in thyroidec-tomized stallions. *J Reprod Fertility* Suppl 23:81-86.
79. Malinowski K, Christensen RA, Hafs HD, et al. 1996. Age and breed differences in thyroid hormones, insulin-like growth factor (IGF)-1 and IGF binding proteins in female horses. *J Anim Sci* 74:1936-1942.
80. Messer NT, Ganjam VK, Nachreine RF, et al. 1995. Effect of dexamethasone administration on serum thyroid hormone concentrations in clinically normal horses. *J Am Vet Med Assoc* 206:63-66.
81. Messer NT, Johnson PJ. 2007. Evidence-based literature pertaining to thyroid dysfunction and Cushing's syndrome in the horse. *Vet Clin North Am Equine Pract* 23:329-364.
82. Messer NT, Johnson PJ, Refsal KR, et al. 1995. Effect of food deprivation on baseline iodothyronine and cortisol concentrations in healthy adult horses. *Am J Vet Res* 56:116-121.
83. Messer NT, Riddle WT, Traub-Dargatz JL. 1998. Thyroid hormone levels in Thoroughbred mares and their foals at parturition. *Proc Am Assoc Equine Pract* 44:248-251.
84. Morris DD, Garcia MC. 1983. Thyroid-stimulating hormone: response test in healthy horses and effect of phenylbutazone on equine thyroid hormones. *Am J Vet Res* 44:503-507.
85. Morris DD, Garcia MC. 1985. Effects of phenylbutazone and anabolic steroids on adrenal and thyroid gland function tests in healthy horses. *Am J Vet Res* 46:359-364.
86. Murray MJ, Luba NK. 1993. Plasma gastrin, somatostatin, and serum thyroxine (T4), triiodothyronine (T3), reverse triiodothyronine (rT3), and cortisol in foals from birth to 28 days of age. *Equine Vet J* 25:237-239.
87. Oliver JW, Held JP. 1985. Thyrotropin stimulation test-New perspective on value of monitoring triiodothyronine. *J Am Vet Med Assoc* 187:931-934.
88. Ramirez S, McClure JJ, Moore RM, et al. 1998. Hyperthyroidism associated with thyroid adenocarcinoma in a 21-year old gelding. *J Vet Intern Med* 12:475-477.
89. Ramirez S, Wolfsheimer KJ, Moore RM, et al. 1997. Duration of effects of phenylbutazone on serum total thyroxine and free thyroxine concentrations in horses. *J Vet Intern Med* 11:371-374.
90. Rowe JE, Foote RH, Baldwin BH, et al. 1987. Reproductive patterns in cyclic and pregnant thyroidectomized mares. *J Reprod Fertil* Suppl 35:281-288.
91. Sojka JE, Johnson MA, Bottoms GD. 1993. Serum triiodothyronine, total thyroxine and free thyroxin concentrations in horses. *Am J Vet Res* 54:52-55.
92. Sommardahl CS, Frank N, Elliott SB, et al. 2005. Effects of oral administration of levothyroxine sodium on serum concentrations of thyroid gland hormones and responses to injections of thyrotropin-releasing hormone in healthy adult mares. *Am J Vet Res* 66:1025-1031.

93. Sticker LS, Thompson Jr DL, Gentry LR. 2001. Pituitary hormone and insulin responses to infusion of amino acids and N-methyl-D, L-aspartate in horses. *J Anim Sci* 79:735-744.

94. Tan RHH, Davies SE, Crisman MV, et al. 2008. Propylthiouracil for treatment of hyperthyroidism in a horse. *J Vet Intern Med* 22:1253-1258.

95. Thompson DL, Nett TM. 1984. Thyroid-stimulating hormone and prolactin secretion after thyrotropin releasing hormone administration to mares: dose response during anestrus in winter and during estrus in summer. *Dom Anim Endocrinol* 1:263-268.

96. Visher CM, Foreman JH, Constable PD. 1999. Hemodynamic effects of thyroidectomy in sedentary horses. *Am J Vet Res Vet* 60:14-21.

Chapter 11

Fluid Analysis

Raquel M. Walton

Acronyms and abbreviations that appear in this chapter:

NCC   nucleated cell count

RBC   red blood cell

TP   total protein

TP_{Ref} total protein by refractometer

TS   total solids

WBC   white blood cell

Pleural and peritoneal fluid

Pleural and peritoneal fluid are ultrafiltrates of plasma that function to reduce friction by lubrication. The constituents of body cavity fluid are affected by the integrity of the mesothelial lining, changes in vascular permeability and lymphatic flow, plasma oncotic pressure, and capillary hydraulic pressure. Thus, changes in the character of the fluid can be attributed to specific disease processes and may yield information in diagnosis, treatment, and/or prognosis. Pleurocentesis and abdominocentesis are valuable clinical tools whose sensitivity and specificity are highest when all components of fluid evaluation are considered together. Fluid evaluations should include assessment of gross appearance, total protein concentration, cell counts (or estimation of cellularity), and cytology. If this is not possible, the minimum testing for fluid evaluation should include measurement of total protein and measurement (or estimation) of cellularity because effusions are defined by these parameters.

Equine Clinical Pathology, First Edition. Edited by Raquel M. Walton.
© 2014 John Wiley & Sons, Inc. Published 2014 by John Wiley & Sons, Inc.

Pathogenetic mechanisms of body cavity effusions

An effusion is defined as an increase in the normal volume of peritoneal or pleural fluid, which may or may not have increased protein or cell concentrations. Pleural effusions within North American equids are most often associated with bacterial pleuropneumonia. Other etiologies include neoplasia, penetrating chest wounds, hemorrhage, and cardiac disease. The majority of abdominal effusions are associated with gastrointestinal disorders, especially those causing colic. The main categories of pleural and peritoneal effusions are formulated to provide insight into the general pathophysiologic mechanism responsible for an increase in the volume of body cavity fluid. Effusions are caused mainly by transudative, exudative, or hemorrhagic processes (Table 11.1). A fourth category, which is uncommon in horses, is lymphorrhagic effusion caused by leakage of lymph from lymphatic vessels (e.g., chylothorax or chyloabdomen).[22]

Transudates

Transudates are caused by increased hydraulic pressure or increased hydraulic and decreased oncotic pressure (Table 11.1). These effusions have low protein concentrations and NCCs. In horses, normal peritoneal and pleural fluids are distinguished from a transudate only by documenting an increase in fluid volume. The most common causes of transudates are the peracute/acute phase of any lesion causing decreased venous/lymphatic drainage in the portal or pulmonary system (e.g., volvulus/torsion, neoplasia, granuloma), lymphatic obstruction, acute uroabdomen, and protein-losing nephropathies and enteropathies. Diagnosis of uroabdomen in the horse is facilitated by the characteristic presence of calcium carbonate crystals in equine urine, which are present extracellularly and within neutrophils and/or macrophages (Figure 11.1). Calcium carbonate crystals should be distinguished from glove starch crystals, which are commonly seen in cytologic preparations (Figure 11.2). Suspicion of uroabdomen should be confirmed by measuring fluid creatinine concentration.

Plasma protein permeability of vessels within the hepatic sinuses is higher than that for vessels elsewhere in the peritoneal cavity. Consequently, increases in hydraulic pressure that involve the hepatic sinuses (i.e., sinusoidal or post-sinusoidal increases) will produce a high protein transudate with a normal NCC. Congestive heart failure and any lesion that produces post-sinusoidal portal hypertension are the most common causes of high protein transudates in the peritoneal cavity. Similarly, the pulmonary vasculature has higher permeability for plasma proteins and high protein transudates may result from increased pulmonary hydraulic pressure.

Exudates

Exudates are characterized by increased vascular permeability due to inflammatory mediators and therefore are attributable to inflammation. Inflammation may be caused by infectious or noninfectious processes (Table 11.1). The

Table 11.1 Classification of Pleural and Peritoneal Effusions

Classification	TP$_{Ref}$	NCC	RBC	Mechanism	Disorder
Transudate	<2.0	$<5 \times 10^3$	$<4 \times 10^4$	Increased hydrostatic and/or decreased oncotic pressure	Nephrotic syndrome Cirrhosis Acute uroabdomen
High-protein transudate	≥2.0	$<5 \times 10^3$	$<4 \times 10^4$	Increased hydrostatic and/or decreased oncotic pressure in post-sinusoidal/sinusoidal hepatic vessels or pulmonary vessels	Congestive heart failure Portal hypertension Neoplasia Acute torsion/volvulus
Exudate	>2.0	$>5 \times 10^3$	$>4 \times 10^4$ $<5 \times 10^5$	Inflammation-mediated increased vascular permeability	Septic: Bacterial, fungal, or parasitic infection Non-septic: Neoplasia Ischemic necrosis Pancreatitis Bile peritonitis Chronic uroabomen
Hemorrhage (acute)	≥2.0	≥ or $≤5 \times 10^3$	$≥1 \times 10^6$	Loss of blood from vessels	Trauma Neoplasia Hemostatic defects Uterine artery rupture

TP$_{Ref}$, total protein by refractometry (g/dL); NCC, nucleated cell count/ul; RBC, red blood cells/ul.

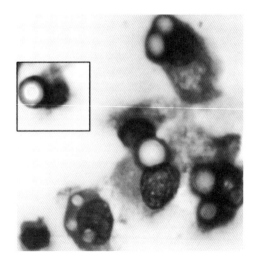

Figure 11.1 Calcium carbonate crystals within macrophages in peritoneal fluid. Note the concentric striations characteristic of the crystal (inset).

absence of microorganisms on cytologic examination does not preclude an infectious process. If clinical findings are suspicious of an infectious process, biochemical evaluation of the fluid (for lactate, glucose, and pH) and bacterial culture are warranted.

Hemorrhagic effusions

Uniformly bloody specimens or consistently bloody specimens from different sites suggest true body cavity hemorrhage, which may be confirmed via

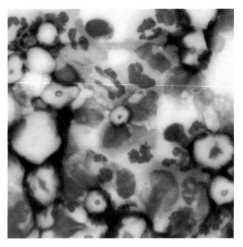

Figure 11.2 Glove talc (starch crystals) in a sample of peritoneal fluid. The crystals are round to rhomboid with a characteristic central divot.

cytology and/or ultrasonographic evaluation of the chest or abdomen. A hemorrhagic effusion is defined by the fluid RBC count (Table 11.1); acute hemorrhagic effusions usually have RBC counts >1,000,000/μL and packed cell
volumes >3%.[22] Erythrocytes and plasma from hemorrhage will be resorbed
by lymphatics so the fluid TP and RBC counts vary with time; in dogs, ~65%
of RBCs are resorbed within 2 days of hemorrhage.[2]

Because platelets (and coagulation factors) are consumed during hemorrhage, hemorrhagic fluid contains no platelets and does not clot, whereas fluid
that contains blood from peripheral or visceral vessels will contain platelets
and will clot. In fluids with high RBC counts, the presence of platelets upon cytologic evaluation indicates a component of blood contamination, since platelets
are not present in hemorrhagic effusions. However, the absence of platelets
does not preclude peripheral blood contamination if the sample was collected
into a non-anticoagulant tube (e.g., red top tube) and subsequently clotted
in vitro. Cytologic findings that support an interpretation of hemorrhage include the presence of erythrocytes and/or hemosiderin within macrophages
(Figure 11.3). Note that if there is a delay in sample processing (>3-4 hours),
RBC phagocytosis can occur *in vitro* in the transport tube. Conversely, erythrophagocytosis can be absent in samples from true hemorrhage if there has
been insufficient time for RBC phagocytosis within the peritoneal cavity (i.e.,
peracute hemorrhage). In general, it takes several hours for erythrophagocytosis to occur; subsequent RBC breakdown into hemosiderin usually takes
at least three days.[8] Thus, cytologic interpretations of bloody fluid should be
undertaken with knowledge of the type of collection tube used, as well as the
amount of time before the sample was processed.

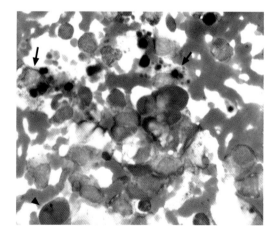

Figure 11.3 Hemorrhagic pleural effusion. Macrophages contain a globular
green-black material consistent with hemosiderin (arrows). Note the presence
of a binucleated mesothelial cell with hemosiderin (arrowhead). Mesothelial
cells with hemosiderin can occasionally be seen in association with chronic
hemorrhage.

Body cavity fluid analysis

One of the first things to consider when evaluating body cavity fluid is whether the sample is representative. Two common causes of nonrepresentative fluid sampling include blood contamination and enterocentesis. Blood contamination may occur when a peripheral vein or abdominal organ (usually the spleen) is punctured. Blood contamination becomes apparent during centesis when the initial sample is clear and then becomes bloody or is bloody then clears. As little as 0.05 mL blood in 1 mL of peritoneal fluid (5% contamination) can result in fluid RBC counts up to 449,000/μL, which is nearly 10 times the upper limit of RBC reference values.[4,18] However, WBC counts and TP concentration remain within reference intervals with up to 17% blood contamination.[18]

Inadvertent enterocentesis has a reported frequency rate of 2-5%.[4] The incidence of complications directly related to inadvertent enterocentesis was reported to be 0.5% (4 cases in 850 abdominocentesis samples) over a 2-year period at one institution.[24] Enterocentesis may manifest grossly as a green to brown discoloration of peritoneal fluid, but contaminated fluid may also appear grossly normal with contamination only evident upon cytologic evaluation. Presence of large ciliated protozoa, plant material, and a mixed bacterial population indicates enterocentesis or intestinal rupture (Figure 11.4). Peritoneal fluid evaluation alone cannot distinguish between enterocentesis

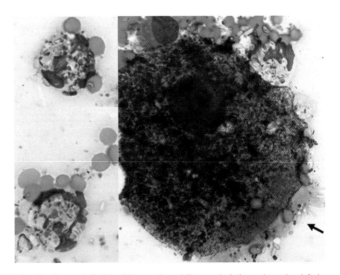

Figure 11.4 Peritoneal fluid with neutrophils containing abundant intracellular bacteria (left panels) and a ciliated protozoal organism (right panel; arrow). The protozoal organism indicates enteric contents are present. Neutrophils with intracellular bacteria suggest intestinal rupture/leakage and peritonitis rather than inadvertent enterocentesis. However, while less likely, these findings could be consistent with enterocentesis if suppurative enteritis were present.

and peracute intestinal leakage or perforation. This distinction is best accomplished in the context of the patient's clinical assessment.

Volume

Peritoneal fluid volume in health typically ranges from 100 mL[1] to 300 mL[1], although it has been estimated that up to 2L may be present.[4] While the equine peritoneal cavity normally contains a large volume of fluid, abdominal paracentesis typically yields <10 mL of fluid and most commonly 3-5 mL.[23] The pleural cavity often yields a similar volume of normal fluid (2-8 mL); however, it may not be possible to retrieve pleural fluid from some healthy horses.[26] The amount of fluid obtained from paracentesis does not necessarily correlate with presence or absence of effusion. In seriously ill horses with effusion confirmed surgically or post-mortem, abdominal paracentesis may yield only a small volume.[23] Diagnosis of mild to moderate effusions in equids, especially adults, can be difficult due to the constraints on palpation and large spaces that accommodate even moderate effusion volumes. Ultrasound is often necessary to diagnose effusion. In horses, it is convention to classify abnormal peritoneal and pleural fluid (i.e., increased protein concentration and/or cell count) as an effusion regardless of whether an increased volume is documented. In contrast, a fluid with a normal cell count and protein concentration is only classified as an effusion if there is a confirmed increase in volume.

Color and clarity

The physical characteristics of body cavity fluid may provide hints as to its cellularity or biochemical composition. Normal body cavity fluid is yellow and transparent. Discoloration of the fluid may reflect hemorrhage (orange to red), enteric rupture (green or brown), bile peritonitis (dark green), infection (yellow-white), or vascular compromise (orange to reddish brown). Abnormal abdominal fluid color has been used in studies to predict the need for surgical treatment. The sensitivity and specificity of subjectively discolored fluid for predicting the need for surgical intervention varies in different reports: 92% and 74%, 78% and 48%, and 51% and 95%, respectively.[10,19,27] Weimann et al. used hemoglobin concentration as an objective measurement of discoloration from hemolysis and found that when peritoneal hemoglobin concentration was >0.01 mmol/L (0.02 g/dL), the test was 80% sensitive and 82% specific for selecting surgical treatment.[27] While discolored peritoneal fluid, especially serosanguineous, supports the need for surgical treatment,[10,19,27] an interpretation of discolored fluid should only be made when the possibility of enterocentesis or blood contamination has been excluded and should be formulated in the context of physical exam findings.

The clarity of body cavity fluid in health reflects low cellularity. Increased turbidity is usually reported in terms of cloudy/hazy or opaque, and suggests increased cellularity, presence of plant material, or, rarely, lipid (i.e., chyloabdomen or chylothorax). While turbidity is abnormal, measurement of cell numbers and cytologic evaluation of the fluid are necessary to determine its cause.

Biochemical evaluation

Fluid protein concentration

Because body cavity fluid is an ultrafiltrate of plasma, protein concentrations are much lower than plasma. Protein can be rapidly and accurately measured by handheld refractometers. Protein measured by refractometer for body cavity fluids is linearly related to protein measured by biochemical methods, and results are accurate to at least to 0.6 g/dL.[13] Pleural fluid protein concentration runs slightly higher than for peritoneal fluid (0.2-4.7 g/dL), but the majority of healthy horses have pleural fluid protein concentrations <2.5 g/dL just as for peritoneal fluid.[26] Many references cite the upper reference value for normal body cavity fluid protein concentration as <2.5 g/dL,[4] which is the lowest protein reading on many refractometers. To report values below the lower end of the protein scale, the value measured using either refractive index, refraction, or urine specific gravity scales can be converted to total protein (TP) with published conversion tables.[12] When abdominal fluid protein was calculated using conversion tables or measured biochemically, normal values were typically ≤2.0 g/dL in many studies.[1,14,17] Increases in fluid protein concentration above reference values indicate either increased permeability of the capillaries due to inflammatory mediators or increased hydraulic pressure within hepatic sinusoids or pulmonary vessels, which have higher permeability to protein. An increase in protein concentration due to inflammatory mediators is typically accompanied by an increase in nucleated cell counts.

Because refractometers measure protein via a total solids-based technique, the total dissolved solids in the sample affect light refraction.[12] In addition to protein, total solids include electrolytes, glucose, urea, and lipids. While the altered refraction of body fluid is mostly due to protein content, increases in lipid, glucose, or urea content interfere with refractometric protein measurements. However, marked increases in urea or glucose (273 mg/dL and 649 mg/dL, respectively) are needed to increase protein measurement by 0.4-0.5 g/dL.[20] Unlike glucose and urea, lipid does not freely diffuse into peritoneal fluid from plasma; increased concentrations of lipid in pleural or peritoneal fluid only occur in cases of chylous effusion.

Another potential cause of erroneous refractometer readings is the addition of EDTA from K_3EDTA anticoagulant tubes. At the standard concentration of EDTA (5 μmol/ml), K_3EDTA by itself has minimal effect on the fluid's refraction (≤0.1 g/dL increase). At higher concentrations of EDTA (10 and 20 μmol/ml), EDTA can increase refractometer total protein (TP_{Ref}) by 0.9-1.0 g/dL. Underfilling of EDTA tubes has the effect of increasing the EDTA concentration and will cause spurious increases in the TP_{Ref}. Some commercial tubes with K_3EDTA anticoagulant may also contain additives to prevent crystallization of the EDTA. Tubes that contain the additive may increase TP_{Ref} readings by up to 0.9 g/dL, even when properly filled.[9] It is recommended that TP_{Ref} readings should be performed on either fluid collected in serum tubes or in properly filled K_3EDTA tubes containing no additives. While sodium heparin anticoagulant has no effect on TP_{Ref},[9] heparin has deleterious effects on cellular morphology and is not recommended for samples that will be evaluated cytologically.

The term "total solids" has caused much confusion in the reporting of refractometric protein results. Total protein (TP) and total solids (TS) are not synonymous. Currently the vast majority of all refractometers incorporate a conversion factor in their design so that the scales report TP and not TS. Contributing to the confusion is the fact that at least one refractometer is named the TS meter (AO Corporation) when it is in fact calibrated to report TP.[12] Today nearly all refractometers report TP and not TS, so comparisons between fluid samples are appropriate.

Specific gravity (SG) has also been used to estimate protein concentration in equine body cavity fluid. However, use of the refractometer SG scale will yield erroneous results because the SG scale is calibrated specifically for urine. Urea, not protein, is the principal constituent of urine, thus SG calibrated for urine gives falsely high results for body fluids.[12] A caveat applies to low protein fluid (<1.0 g/dL); in this instance, the urine SG scale more accurately estimates true SG because the fluid's refractive index is more similar to urine.[22]

Other biochemical tests

Fluid lactate, glucose, and pH

Most biochemical testing of body cavity fluid is performed on peritoneal rather than pleural fluid because of the importance of identifying severely diseased bowel and the ability to assess pulmonary disease via airway evaluation (see Chapter 12). Intestinal ischemia or infarction is one of the most common causes of mortality in colic cases because of subsequent circulatory collapse that can occur. Lactate is the end-product of anaerobic glycolysis and has been used as a marker for ischemia in colic studies. Normal peritoneal fluid lactate concentrations vary with respect to assay methodology, but are usually <1.0 mmol/L.[5,17] Studies of colic cases have shown peritoneal lactate, TP, NCC, and glucose concentrations were significantly increased compared with peritoneal fluid from clinically normal horses.[5,17] When the colic cases were subdivided on the basis of strangulating versus non-strangulating obstructions, peritoneal lactate concentrations were significantly higher in strangulating lesions, with the exception of strangulating small colon obstructions.[5,17] Increases in fluid lactate, decreases in fluid pH, and abnormal fluid color and/or turbidity were most strongly correlated with ischemic strangulating lesions. Peritoneal fluid lactate concentrations were shown to be more sensitive than blood lactate concentrations in detecting early ischemic lesions.[5,17] The prognosis becomes progressively poorer for both strangulating and non-strangulating lesions as peritoneal fluid lactate concentrations increase. One study showed the probability of death in non-strangulating lesions to be 63% for peritoneal lactate concentrations of 12 mmol/L and 82% for lactate concentrations of 16 mmol/L; the same concentrations of peritoneal fluid lactate had 82% and 92% probabilities of death, respectively, in strangulating lesions.[5]

Peritoneal glucose concentrations have been shown to be useful as a relatively rapid test for distinguishing septic from non-septic exudates.[25] Positive bacterial culture or cytologic identification of intracellular bacteria in abdominal fluid is a definitive indicator of abdominal sepsis, but false negatives do occur, especially with antimicrobial therapy. In one study of 36 peritonitis cases, peritoneal fluid glucose concentration and pH were significantly lower in horses with septic versus non-septic peritonitis.[25] Serum to peritoneal fluid glucose concentration differences >50 mg/dL were most diagnostically useful in confirming sepsis.

Fluid D-dimer concentration

Mesothelial cells play a significant role in the initiation and resolution of inflammation by secretion of immunomodulatory mediators, which impact on coagulant and fibrinolytic factors such as D-dimer.[3,6] D-dimer concentrations in normal peritoneal fluid are reported to be <88 ng/mL,[6,7] whereas in horses with colic, median peritoneal fluid D-dimer concentrations ranged from 2,023 to 24,301 ng/mL depending on diagnosis. Among colics, median fluid D-dimer concentrations were highest with enteritis, ischemic lesions, and septic peritonitis (8,028 ng/mL, 16,181 ng/mL, and 24,301 ng/mL, respectively) compared with large colon obstructions (2,023 ng/mL).[6] Blood contamination up to 20% does not alter peritoneal fluid D-dimer concentrations in colic cases.[7] These studies show that peritoneal fluid D-dimer concentration appears to be a useful indicator of fibrinolytic activity, and higher concentrations are correlated with greater disease severity.

Cells and cell counts

Cytologic evaluation of body cavity fluid can yield important information that may even lead to the effusion's etiology (e.g., large cell lymphoma, carcinoma, uroabdomen, or septic inflammation). Cytology should be interpreted in the context of clinical signs, cell counts, and biochemical evaluation.

Erythrocytes

Erythrocytes are not normally present in body cavity fluid in health, but blood contamination during thoracocentesis may produce RBC counts up to 540,000/μL; however, the vast majority of horses have <370,000/μL.[26] Reported counts for paracentesis are less, ranging from <5,000/μL to <43,200/μL in healthy horses.[4,18,22] Visual assessment of discoloration attributable to RBCs was not detected for samples with <40,000 RBCs/μL,[15] thus typical amounts of blood contamination associated with centesis should not change the fluid color. Erythrocyte counts will increase above reference values because of minor blood vessel damage associated with necrosis and/or inflammation; true hemorrhagic effusions are discussed in the section on effusion classifications.

Nucleated cells

Total nucleated cell counts (NCCs) for pleural and abdominal fluid are performed with automated blood count analyzers or manually with a hemocytometer. Reference values for pleural and peritoneal fluids are similar. The total NCC for pleural fluid for most horses is <8000/μL.[26] Generally, total NCC reference values in normal peritoneal fluid are reported as <10,000/μL[4,22] and often are <5000/μL.[1,4,25] Many equine practitioners and clinical pathologists consider values <5,000/μL normal, values between 5,000/μL and 10,000/μL to be ambiguous, and values >10,000/μL as abnormal. Reference values for peritoneal fluid in foals are <1500/μL.[14]

The cells normally present within the pleural and peritoneal cavity comprise leucocytes and mesothelial lining cells. Nucleated cells in cytologic differentials are categorized as neutrophils, lymphocytes, and monocyte/macrophages. Some practitioners will use a large mononuclear cell category that may include monocyte/macrophages and mesothelial cells, but many cytopathologists and practitioners do not include mesothelial cells in the differential count.

In horses, mature neutrophils comprise the predominant cell type in the differential evaluation (typically 50-80% of nucleated cells). Because neutrophils age and die in body cavity fluid, pyknotic and hypersegmented neutrophils are normally noted in a proportion of the population. Increased numbers of neutrophils enter into the body cavity in response to chemotactic inflammatory mediators. During inflammation, the ability of neutrophils to respond to stimuli and migrate into tissue increases with maturation. Consequently, mature neutrophils arrive first and immature forms (i.e., bands, metamyelocytes) are only present in tissue when mature neutrophils have been severely depleted. Thus, the presence of band or earlier forms of neutrophils in fluid indicates severe inflammation; a caveat would be if the immature forms originate from blood and there is significant blood contamination of the sample. If blood contamination is not apparent, the presence of immature neutrophils in peritoneal fluid has been shown to have a poorer prognosis (i.e., need for surgical intervention and increased mortality rates).[11]

Degenerate change in neutrophils is characterized by swollen, pale-staining chromatin and loss of membrane integrity (Figure 11.5). While degenerate change is not pathognomonic for infection, the presence of degenerate neutrophils warrants a more thorough search for organisms. These changes occur *after* the cell has left the blood and indicate release of neutrophil enzymes and/or exposure to bacterial cytotoxins. In contrast, "toxic" neutrophils are characterized by the presence of cytoplasmic basophilia (often with Dohle bodies), foamy cytoplasm, less-condensed chromatin, nuclear hyposegmentation, and larger cell size (see Chapter 2). These changes reflect maturational defects in the bone marrow that are associated with rapid neutropoiesis due to a strong systemic inflammatory stimulus. In contrast to degenerate change, toxic change exists in neutrophils *before* they enter the pleural or peritoneal cavity. Toxic change is often associated with severe bacterial infections or significant tissue necrosis.

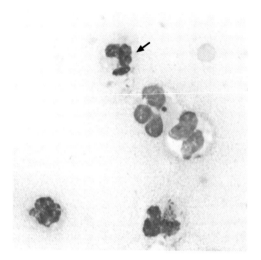

Figure 11.5 Degenerate changes in neutrophils from a suppurative pleural effusion. Two nondegenerate (arrow) and three degenerate neutrophils are present. Degenerate changes are characterized by loss of membrane integrity with nuclear swelling. One of the three degenerate neutrophils contains bacterial rods within the cytoplasm (bottom right).

Large mononuclear cells include both monocytes/macrophages and mesothelial cells. When monocytes exit the vasculature, they differentiate into macrophages; both forms will be present in body cavities (Figure 11.6). Macrophages will occasionally contain senescent neutrophils. As with neutrophils, increases in monocyte/macrophage concentrations in fluid are attributable to inflammation and usually accompany neutrophil increases;

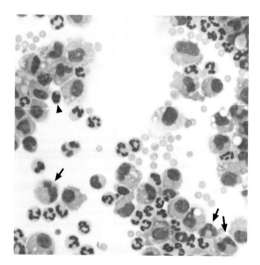

Figure 11.6 Concentrated preparation of normal peritoneal fluid. Monocytes (arrows), macrophages, neutrophils, and a single small lymphocyte (arrowhead) are present.

neutrophil proportions typically exceed those of monocyte/macrophages in acute inflammation, whereas mononuclear cells may predominate with chronic effusions and certain disease processes (e.g., fungal infection).

The lymphocytes in normal fluid are small to medium-sized (7-10 um in diameter) and constitute the smallest proportion of the three main cell types in normal cavity fluid. Increases in lymphocytes may be associated with chronic inflammatory conditions, parasitism, or chylothorax/abdomen. In chronic inflammation, the lymphocyte population is often a mixture of small lymphocytes, medium lymphocytes (prolymphocytes), reactive lymphocytes, and plasma cells. Reactive lymphocytes are usually slightly larger than small lymphocytes (9-11 um in diameter) and are characterized as having deeply basophilic cytoplasm and a mature chromatin. Lymphoblasts are large lymphocytes (12-16 in um diameter) whose nuclei have immature chromatin and usually contain a nucleolus or nucleoli. The presence of lymphoblasts in significant numbers is abnormal and is usually associated with large cell lymphoma. However, in the context of reactive lymphocytes and plasma cells, rare lymphoblasts may be part of the inflammatory response.

Eosinophils, basophils, and mast cells do not contribute to the cellular differential in normal body cavity fluid. The largest increases in eosinophil numbers can be associated with parasitic infections (including larval migration). Before routine deworming programs, it was not uncommon to find *Setaria equina* microfilariae in pleural or peritoneal fluid (Figure 11.7). The adults, however, are harmless inhabitants of the pleural and peritoneal cavities and their presence is not associated with eosinophilia. Smaller increases in eosinophil numbers may be seen with inflammation due to any etiology. Eosinophilia in peritoneal fluid (Figure 11.8) may also be seen with focal eosinophilic enteritis

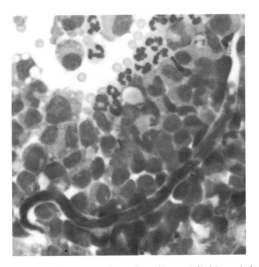

Figure 11.7　Concentrated preparation of peritoneal fluid containing microfilaria of *Setaria* species. The fluid cell count and protein concentration were within reference limits.

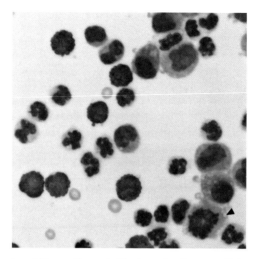

Figure 11.8 Eosinophilic peritoneal effusion of unknown etiology. The horse had a concurrent eosinophilia in the peripheral blood and eosinophilic hyperplasia in the bone marrow.

and, rarely, lymphoma.[16, 21] Basophils and mast cells can increase concurrently with eosinophils, though both are rare findings, even in inflammation.

Mesothelial cells may be present individualized or in small clusters or sheets (Figure 11.9). They are readily identified when they are present in cohesive aggregates and are rare in both normal fluid and effusions. Although sometimes included in the large mononuclear cell group, they comprise only a minor fraction of the large mononuclear cell differential. Mesothelial cells have round

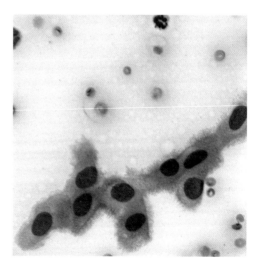

Figure 11.9 Mesothelial cells in pleural fluid. Mesothelial cells are rare in most body cavity samples from horses. Note the eosinophilic brush border, often referred to as a glycocalyx.

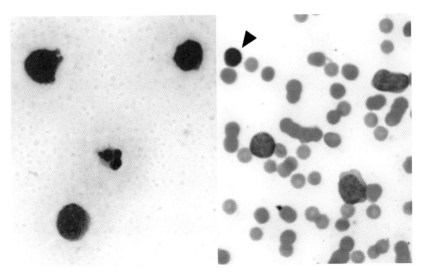

Figure 11.10   Pleural effusion (left panel) from a 14-year-old Thoroughbred horse. Lymphocytes are identified by the scant rim of basophilic cytoplasm. Although the chromatin is difficult to evaluate on this preparation because the cells are not spread out well, the lymphocytes are larger than a neutrophil, indicating that they are immature lymphocytes. The predominance of immature lymphocytes is consistent with an interpretation of lymphoma. The peripheral blood also contained large, immature lymphocytes (right panel). The arrowhead points to a small, mature lymphocyte.

to oval nuclei with smooth chromatin, 1-2 small, variably distinct nucleoli, and a moderate rim of basophilic cytoplasm. Mesothelial cells may have a pink to red brush border that is variably prominent (Figure 11.9).

Neoplastic cells can occasionally be found in body cavity fluid. Lymphoma (Figure 11.10) and carcinoma (Figure 11.11) are the most common neoplasms identified in cavity effusions. Since mesothelial cells are rarely noted in body cavity fluid, the presence of significant numbers of cohesive cells in body cavity effusions indicates either carcinoma or mesothelioma. It is difficult to distinguish between mesothelial and epithelial cells using morphology alone, but carcinoma occurs with more frequency than mesothelioma. Immunohistochemical staining of carcinoma is positive for cytokeratin markers and negative for vimentin, whereas staining of mesothelioma is positive for both cytokeratin and vimentin. Criteria of malignancy are often present with mesothelioma or carcinoma and include variability in nuclear size and shape (anisokaryosis), variability in cell size (anisocytosis), prominent and/or bizarre nucleoli, and multinucleation. The absence of criteria of malignancy does not preclude the possibility of carcinoma. The mere presence of epithelial cells in an effusion is diagnostic of carcinoma because epithelial cells are not normally present in body cavity fluid. The presence of mesothelial cells in body cavity fluid can be normal, however, so a very large number (especially with atypical morphology) must be present to permit an interpretation of mesothelioma.

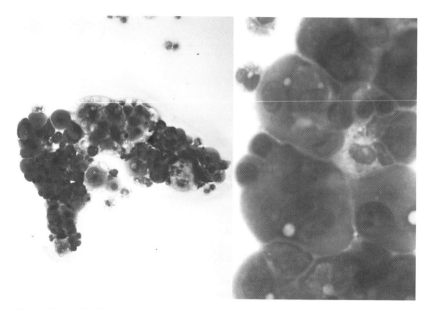

Figure 11.11 Peritoneal effusion from a 20-year-old Standardbred horse. The cytology showed many large aggregates of cohesive round cells (left panel). High-magnification evaluation of the cells shows moderate to marked anisokaryosis and marked anisocytosis. Note the prominent basophilic nucleoli in many nuclei. Differential interpretations for the cytology would include carcinoma or mesothelioma. Immunohistochemical staining of the neoplastic cells was positive for cytokeratin and negative for vimentin, consistent with a diagnosis of carcinoma.

An interpretation of lymphoma in body cavity effusion is based on the presence of significant numbers of large, immature lymphocytes. Criteria of malignancy are not taken into consideration, only the type of lymphocyte (lymphoblast, small lymphocyte, or prolymphocyte). A predominance of lymphoblasts and/or prolymphocytes in body cavity effusion is abnormal and would be consistent with an interpretation of lymphoma. A predominance of small lymphocytes in an effusion could indicate an inflammatory response, chylothorax/chyloabdomen, or a small lymphocytic lymphoma. Identification and histologic evaluation of an enlarged lymph node or mass would be necessary to establish a diagnosis of small cell lymphoma.

Synovial fluid

Synovial fluid serves to both lubricate and nourish the articular cartilage. The fluid is an ultrafiltrate of plasma that is modified by hyaluronate and glycoproteins secreted by the synovial lining cells. The synovial fluid is filtered through the synovial membrane, a thin lining of tissue macrophage A cells, fibroblast-like B cells, and fenestrated capillaries. The cells of the synovium are discontinuous, separated by gaps several microns in width between cells. The extracellular matrix in these gaps contains collagen and other molecules such as hyaluronate (HA) and glycoproteins that permit molecules such as glucose and electrolytes to pass but restrict most proteins.

Fluid analysis

Inflammatory, traumatic, and degenerative arthropathies are reflected in the composition and properties of joint fluid. As with body cavity effusions, a complete fluid evaluation should include assessment of gross characteristics, protein concentration, cell counts, and cytology. When there is a limited quantity of fluid, cytologic examination is the single most useful test. With small sample volumes, the color and turbidity can be noted and the viscosity assessed as the sample is expelled onto a glass slide for preparation of a direct smear for cytologic examination. In the absence of cell counts, an estimation of cellularity may suffice. A mean of 0-2 WBCs per 10 high-power fields (40× objective) corresponds with an actual WBC count <1300/μL.[31]

Synovial fluid should be evaluated and interpreted in the context of physical examination and radiographic and/or MRI findings. The most common application of synovial fluid analysis in horses is to distinguish between septic and degenerative arthropathies. The main categories of equine arthropathies and their associated fluid characteristics are listed in Table 11.2. These values are generally accepted for articular joints as well as for the digital flexor tendon sheath synovial fluid.[34]

Physical characteristics

Color and clarity

In health, synovial fluid varies from colorless to straw-colored and is clear. Changes in color and clarity reflect increases in cell count and decreases in hyaluronate concentration (Table 11.2). Increased turbidity is usually reported in terms of cloudy/hazy or opaque, and suggests increased cellularity. A red color to the fluid reflects the presence of red blood cells, either from hemarthrosis or blood contamination. Blood contamination becomes apparent during arthrocentesis when the initial sample is clear and then becomes bloody or is bloody and then clears. Blood contamination will adversely impact fluid analysis and interpretation and should be avoided.

Viscosity

Viscosity is assessed by the length of the intact string of fluid when suspended between fingertips or pulled with an applicator stick. A fluid with normal viscosity should produce fluid strings 2-3 cm in length before breaking. Synovial fluid may become gelatinous upon standing, a property known as thixotropism. When this occurs, the sample can often be put back into suspension by simple agitation. If there is any blood contamination, the sample should be immediately placed into EDTA to avoid actual clotting. Note that EDTA will interfere

Table 11.2 Synovial Fluid Characteristics[a]

	Normal	Degenerative	Inflammatory	Hemarthrosis
Color, clarity	Colorless to yellow, clear	Colorless, clear	Whitish, turbid to opaque	Red or xanthochromic, cloudy
Viscosity	High	Normal to decreased	Normal to decreased	Decreased
Mucin clot	Good	Normal to poor	Normal to poor	Fair to poor
Cellularity (NCC μl)	<500	<5000	>5000	High RBC count
Neutrophils	<10%	<10%	>10%	Proportional to blood
Mononuclear cells	>90%	>90%	<90%	Proportional to blood

[a]Includes the digital flexor tendon sheath synovial fluid.

with the mucin clot test and heparin should be used if a mucin clot test is desired.

Mucin clot test

Samples for mucin clot evaluation should be submitted in a serum tube or one with heparin anticoagulant because EDTA interferes with the test. The mucin clot test provides a semiquantitative assessment of the degree of hyaluronate polymerization. The test is performed by mixing one part synovial fluid (centrifuged supernatant) with four parts 2.5% glacial acetic acid. Results are categorized as good, fair, poor, and very poor. A good mucin clot is characterized by the presence of a single clot that forms in a clear solution. A fair clot is present in a turbid solution, a poor clot is friable in cloudy solution, and a very poor clot consists of small flecks in a cloudy solution.[48] The mucin clot test is no longer performed as part of the routine synovial fluid analysis in many laboratories.

Protein concentration

Protein can be rapidly measured by handheld refractometers, but the most accurate measurement of synovial fluid protein concentration is measured using chemical methods. Refractometer readings provide values that are useful for clinical classification and interpretation of joint fluids and compare reasonably to biuret or Coomassie blue methods (see Chapter 7). Reference values for healthy synovial fluid using the biuret method range from 0.9 g/dL to 3.1 g/dL; the Coomassie blue method yields similar values.[48] Most reference values for equine synovial fluid are reported to be <2.5 g/dL.

Cells and cell counts

The cells normally present within the joint fluid comprise leukocytes and synovial lining cells. Nucleated cells in cytologic differentials are categorized as neutrophils, small lymphocytes, and large mononuclear cells (Figure 11.12). The large mononuclear cell category includes both macrophages and synovial lining type B cells. Individually, these cells cannot be distinguished morphologically unless the macrophages are activated (cytoplasmic vacuolization and/or phagocytic activity). Synovial type B cells can be readily distinguished when they are present in sheets.

Reference values for most joints in horses are typically <500 cells/μl (Table 11.2). Cell counts may be performed manually or using an automated hematology analyzer. Sample viscosity often makes it difficult to perform cell counts, especially with automated analyzers. Addition of lyophilized hyaluronate helps in liquefying the sample so that counting can be performed. Fewer problems with sample aspiration and flow and more accurate counts were obtained using automated analyzers when samples were pretreated with hyaluronidase. Hyaluronidase is used at a final concentration of 0.01 mg/mL and incubated until the samples are sufficiently fluid (5-30 minutes).[35] Use of automated point-of-care hematology analyzers for determining synovial fluid counts should be undertaken only after the procedure has been properly

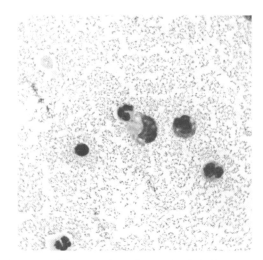

Figure 11.12 High-magnification view of synovial fluid from a horse with a resolving acute injury. Three large mononuclear cells, two neutrophils, and a small lymphocyte are present within a stippled eosinophilic glycosaminoglycan background.

validated by comparing with manual methods currently in use. Evaluation of viscosity and mucin clot should always be performed *before* hyaluronidase is added.

Cytology

Microscopic evaluation of synovial fluid should include assessment of cellularity (normal or increased) and the glycosaminoglycan background (normal or dilute and/or clumped). These evaluations are performed at both low power (10× objective; Figure 11.13) and high power (40× or 100× objective). A differential count is performed at high power. The differential count in healthy synovial fluid is comprised of >90% mononuclear cells, the majority of which are macrophages and type B synoviocytes, with the remaining proportion represented by neutrophils. Increases in the proportion of neutrophils can be seen in both septic and nonseptic synovitis and with blood contamination or hemorrhage. In cases of blood contamination or hemarthrosis, interpretation of the neutrophil proportion can be difficult. The proportion of neutrophils can be compared to the amount of blood present to subjectively assess whether a component of suppurative inflammation exists, but this method requires an experienced observer and knowledge of the peripheral neutrophil concentration, and is highly subjective. It is usually possible to distinguish between blood contamination and hemorrhage (see section on hemarthrosis).

Cellular morphology is evaluated concurrently with the differential count. Neutrophil morphology is evaluated for degenerative changes or evidence of phagocytic activity (Figure 11.14). The presence of degenerative neutrophils is supportive of a septic process, but is not pathognomonic, and the absence of

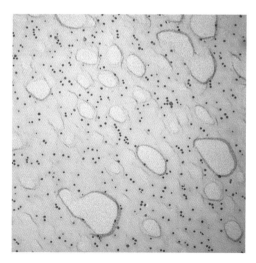

Figure 11.13 Low-magnification view of synovial fluid from a horse with an acute carpal chip injury. Cellularity is markedly increased. Note the presence of crescents in the glycosaminoglycan background, which are characteristic of synovial fluid cytology.

detectable infectious agents does not preclude a septic process. In healthy joint fluid the majority of macrophages are non-phagocytic with few vacuoles. Increased numbers of phagocytic macrophages or the presence of binucleated or multinucleated forms indicates histiocytic inflammation, even in the absence of increased cell counts (Figure 11.15). Some macrophages/synoviocytes may contain few magenta granules.

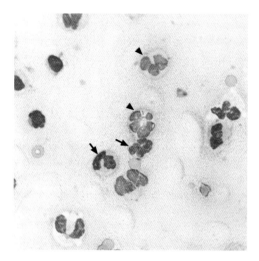

Figure 11.14 Degenerate neutrophils (arrowheads) and nondegenerate neutrophils (arrows) in a septic joint. Note the presence of basophilic bacterial rods within one of the degenerate neutrophils. The glycosaminoglycan background is dilute.

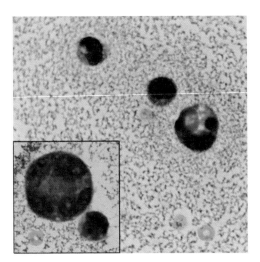

Figure 11.15 High-magnification view of a phagocytic macrophage and a multinucleated cell (inset) in a joint with a degenerative arthropathy subsequent to a chip fracture.

Degenerative arthropathies

Degenerative processes that affect the joint have minimal to no inflammation as reflected in the synovial fluid, but inflammation of the synovium is recognized. The most common types of "degenerative" arthropathies in the horse include osteoarthritis and osteochondritis dissecans, both inflammatory processes. Osteoarthritis (OA) is one of the most common equine arthropathies. Currently, three type of OA are recognized: Type 1 (primary) OA, Type 2 (secondary) OA, and Type 3 (nonprogressive) OA. Synovial fluid cell counts associated with OA are usually <5,000/µL, with total protein concentrations within normal limits or slightly increased and a mononuclear cell predominance. Osteochondritis dissecans (OCD) is a defect in the subchondral bone with secondary effects on the articular cartilage that may result in osteoarthritis. Typical synovial fluid nucleated cells counts in OCD are <1,000/µL, and the total protein concentration is often within reference limits or slightly increased. Similar to OA, the predominant cell type is mononuclear. Conventional synovial fluid analysis in joints affected with OA or OCD may reveal findings that are all within normal limits. However, in the context of clinical signs, this would support an interpretation of a degenerative, noninfectious arthropathy. Distinction between processes such as OA or OCD cannot be made using synovial fluid analysis alone; the fluid findings should be interpreted in the context of imaging findings, signalment, and clinical signs.

Synovial fluid and serum biomarkers show promise in the diagnosis of active cartilage damage; however, most of these tests are not readily available in the clinical setting. Examples of fluid biomarkers include chondroitin and keratan sulfate epitopes, total glycosaminoglycans, matrix metalloproteinases, osteocalcin, and bone-specific alkaline phosphatase (BAP). BAP is an isoform of alkaline phosphatase that can be measured in most diagnostic laboratories. BAP concentrations in the synovial fluid from joints affected with OA or osteochondrosis are increased compared with normal joints.[38,58]

Inflammatory arthropathies

Septic synovitis

Diagnosis of a septic joint can be difficult in the absence of identifiable bacteria on cytologic examination. Only about a quarter of cases demonstrate bacteria on Gram stain. Moreover, the gold standard for the diagnosis of septic synovitis, a positive bacterial culture, is negative in almost half of clinical cases if enrichment medium is not used.[46] Use of an enrichment media greatly improves culture success, but even with enrichment media 27% can still be negative.[53] Prior treatment with antibiotics and/or bacterial sequestration in the synovium may contribute to these results.[54] One study showed blood culture medium enrichment performed significantly better than conventional enrichment media for equine synovial fluid cultures.[33] Blood culture medium enrichment combined with 16S rRNA gene PCR had the highest sensitivity for detection of synovial infection (91.8%).[51]

Identification of intracellular bacterial organisms on cytologic examination is a definitive indicator of septic synovitis, but their absence does not preclude infection. Identification of the organisms as cocci or bacilli with Romanovksy stains can aid in the preliminary antimicrobial treatment. Gram stains, when performed correctly, provide further information for antimicrobial selection. However, experience has shown that when the stain is old or the procedure done incorrectly, the stain may be misleading. Often all organisms will stain as Gram-negative in these instances.

In addition to cytology, fluid cell counts and differential can be helpful in distinguishing septic from nonseptic inflammatory processes. Cell counts in septic joints typically exceed 10,000/μL and are often much higher.[42,53,55] However, septic joints with counts <10,000/μL can be seen in early sepsis, with corticosteroid administration, and with draining lesions.[46] Moreover, traumatic or chemical synovitis can have cell counts up to 90,000/μL and 30,000/μL, respectively, that are predominantly suppurative.[37] Despite the overlap in cell counts and protein concentrations for septic and nonseptic synovitis, cell counts >50,000/μL are highly suspicious for sepsis and >100,000/μL considered diagnostic. Clinical signs, history, and radiographic and cytology findings should be interpreted in context. In cases where the cytology and fluid analysis fall within the "grey zone," the joint should be treated as if it were septic until proven otherwise.

Because synovial fluid is an ultrafiltrate of plasma, fluid glucose and pH are similar to plasma and may be useful in detecting bacterial infection. Glucose concentrations have been shown to be useful as a relatively rapid test for distinguishing septic from nonseptic effusions.[59] Differences between serum and fluid glucose concentrations of >2 mmol/L were reported in experimentally in-duced infectious arthritis. However, measurement of glucose concentrations using handheld glucometers should be undertaken using only veterinary glu-cometers validated for use in horses (see Chapter 8). Synovial fluid glucose concentrations and pH both decrease and lactate increases relative to serum when there is bacterial infection. While these parameters are supportive of a septic process, they are not suitable to serve as primary diagnostic tests. These tests may help in confirming the diagnosis in cases that are clinically and cytologically suspicious for bacterial synovitis but negative upon culture.

Nonseptic suppurative synovitis

Traumatic and chemical synovitis

Synovitis resulting from traumatic or chemical causes may present with sig-nificantly high cell counts (>10,000/μL), with neutrophils as the predominant cell type. Traumatic synovitis usually causes mild mononuclear or suppura-tive inflammation with cell counts <5,000/μL, but infrequently it may cause suppurative inflammation with counts exceeding 10,000/μL.[48,54] Chemical synovitis, also known as a post-injection flare, can occur in response to injec-tion of corticosteroids, local anesthetics, saline, antibiotics, and polysulfated glycosaminoglycans.[34,63,64] Intra-articular injection of 1 mL 0.9% saline alone may increase the nucleated cell count to values up to 14,000/μL.[56] Injection of polysulfated glycosaminoglycans, antibiotics, or anesthetics can produce nucleated cell counts >30,000/μL with a neutrophil predominance.[30,41,43,49] Prior sampling or treatment should be considered in the interpretation of synovial fluid findings. Because there can be overlap with findings for nonsep-tic and septic arthropathies, repeated lameness examination and follow-up sampling are necessary. Chemical synovitis usually occurs within hours after injection and resolves within three to seven days.

Immune-mediated synovitis

Nonseptic inflammation may be immune-mediated, often secondary to infec-tion, gastrointestinal disease, or neoplasia. A noninfectious nonerosive syn-drome has been described in foals with Rhodococcus equi infection and usu-ally resolves as the pneumonia resolves with antimicrobial therapy. Approx-imately a third of foals with R. equi infection develop synovitis.[28,57] These foals have single or multiple joint distention but negative bacterial culture, no or mild lameness or stiffness, and a nucleated cell count of <8,000/μL, with neutrophilic or mixed inflammation.[40,45,50] Synovial membrane biopsies of affected joints showed positive immunofluorescence for immune com-plexes, supporting an immune-mediated etiology. Similar findings have been described in a foal with bacterial endocarditis caused by Escherichia coli.[45]

Lupus erythematosus (LE) is another immune-mediated nonerosive in-flammatory arthropathy that may be present in horses.[29,62] A lupus erythematosus-like syndrome was diagnosed in two horses based on the pres-ence of a positive LE cell preparation and positive antinuclear antibody titers.

Given the uncertainty of the significance of LE cells in horses, a definitive diagnosis of LE is questionable. Reported synovial fluid cell counts ranged from 25,200/μl to 46,000/μL with a predominance of neutrophils. Histologically, there was marked villous proliferation with infiltration of macrophages, lymphocytes, and plasma cells.

An idiopathic polysynovitis in four horses characterized by a suppurative, nonseptic synovitis in at least two different joints has been described.[44,52] Immunoglobulins were detected in a synovial membrane biopsy from the only horse that was evaluated, but the horses were negative for antinuclear antibodies and LE cells. The horses presented with stiffness or lameness, fever, polysynovitis with a nucleated cell count <7,000/μL with increased neutrophils (12%–81%), and TP <3.6 g/dL. The cases showed response to immunosuppressive therapy and a microbial cause could not be identified on culture.

Eosinophilic synovitis

Eosinophils are rare to absent (<1%) in equine synovial fluid in health. Eosinophilic synovitis is rare: there have only been two clinical cases reported to date. In humans, eosinophilic synovitis has been reported postarthography (dye or air) and can be associated with infectious diseases (e.g., Lyme disease, tuberculosis, and parasitism), rheumatoid arthritis, hypereosinophilic syndrome, neoplasia, or may be idiopathic. Eosinophilic synovitis has been experimentally induced in horses via intra-articular injection of streptococcal antigen in horses hyperimmunized with Streptococcus equi M protein vaccine.[47] The first reported equine clinical case was associated with prior intra-articular injections of methylprednisolone acetate into the affected joints.[60] No etiology was determined for the second clinical case.[32] Nucleated cell counts in the reported cases range from 8,300/μL to 12,800/μL with 11% to 76% eosinophils.

Hemarthrosis

A hemorrhagic effusion is defined by the fluid RBC count (Table 11.2); acute hemorrhagic effusions usually have RBC counts >1,000,000/μL. In one study, discoloration attributable to RBCs was not detected visually with <40,000 RBCs/μL.[39] Accordingly, a reddish synovial fluid should have >40,000 RBCs/μL. Erythrocytes and plasma from hemorrhage will be resorbed by lymphatics so fluid TP and RBC counts vary with time.

Hemarthrosis in horses is most often associated with joint trauma (e.g., fractures, intra-articular ligament tears). Cases of idiopathic hemarthrosis confined to the antebrachiocarpal and tarsocrural joints have been reported, but this is an infrequent phenomenon. Idiopathic hemarthrosis of the antebriocarpal joint was associated with acute forelimb lameness, whereas hemarthrosis of the tarsocrural joint produced minimal lameness. RBC counts ranged from 4,100,000/μL to 11,100,000/μL, with nucleated cell counts from 7,400/μL to 16,000/μL and protein concentrations from 4.0 g/dL to 5.6 g/dL.[61]

Because platelets (and coagulation factors) are consumed during hemorrhage, hemorrhagic fluid contains no platelets and does not clot, whereas fluid that contains blood from peripheral vessels will contain platelets and will clot. In fluids with high RBC counts, the presence of platelets on cytologic evaluation indicates a component of blood contamination, since platelets are not present in hemorrhagic effusions (Figure 11.16). However, the absence of platelets does not preclude peripheral blood contamination if the sample was collected into a non-anticoagulant tube (e.g., red-top tube) and subsequently clotted *in vitro*. Cytologic findings that support hemarthrosis include the presence of erythrocytes and/or hemosiderin within macrophages (Figure 11.16). Note that if there is a delay in sample processing (>3-4 hours), RBC phagocytosis can occur *in vitro* in the transport tube. Conversely, erythrophagocytosis

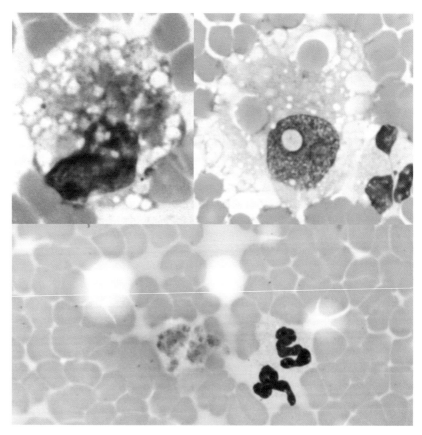

Figure 11.16 Macrophages containing golden-green hemosiderin (upper left) and erythrocytes (upper right) in a hemorrhagic effusion. The presence of platelet clumps (lower center) in another sample indicates peripheral blood contamination.

can be absent in samples from true hemorrhage if there has been insufficient time for RBC phagocytosis within the joint space (i.e., peracute hemorrhage). In general, it takes several hours for erythrophagocytosis to occur; subsequent RBC breakdown into hemosiderin usually takes at least three days.[36] Thus, cytologic interpretations of bloody fluid should be undertaken with knowledge of the type of collection tube used, as well as the amount of time before the sample was processed.

References

1. Brownlow MA, Hutchins DR, Johnston KG. 1981. Reference values for equine peritoneal fluid. *Equine Vet J* 13:127–130.
2. Clark CH, Woodley CH. 1959. The absorption of red blood cells after parenteral injection at various sites. *Am J Vet Res* 20: 1062–1066.
3. Collatos C, Barton MH, Prasse KW, et al. 1995. Intravascular and peritoneal coagulation and fibrinolysis in horses with acute gastrointestinal tract diseases. *J Am Vet Med Assoc* 207:465–470.
4. DeHeer HL, Parry BW, Grindem CB. 2002. Peritoneal fluid. In *Diagnostic Cytology and Hematology of the Horse*, Cowell RL and Tyler RD (eds), 2nd ed. pp 127–162. St. Louis: Mosby.
5. Delesalle C, Dewulf J, Lefebvre RA, et al. 2007. Determination of lactate concentrations in blood plasma and peritoneal fluid in horses with colic by an Accusport analyzer. *J Vet Intern Med* 21:293–301.
6. Delgado MA, Monreal L, Armengou L, et al. 2009. Peritoneal D-Dimer concentration for assessing peritoneal fibrinolytic activity in horses with colic. *J Vet Intern Med* 23:882–889.
7. Delgado MA, Monreal L, Armengou L, et al. 2009. Effects of blood contamination on peritoneal D-dimer concentration in horses with colic. *J Vet Intern Med* 23:1232–1238.
8. Epstein CE, Elidemir O, Colasurdo GN, et al. 2001. Time course of hemosiderin production by alveolar macrophages in a murine model. *Chest* 120: 2013–2020.
9. Estepa JC, Lopez I, Mayer-Valor R, et al. 2006. The influence of anticoagulants on the measurement of total protein concentration in equine peritoneal fluid. *Res Vet Sci* 80:5–10.
10. Freden GO, Provost PJ, Rand WM. 1998. Reliability of using results of abdominal fluid analysis to determine treatment and predict lesion type and outcome for horses with colic: 218 cases (1991-1994). *J Am Vet Med Assoc* 213:1012–1015.
11. Garma-Avina A. 1998. Cytology of 100 samples of abdominal fluid from 100 horses with abdominal disease. *Equine Vet J* 30:435–444.
12. George JW. 2001. The usefulness and limitations of hand-held refractometers in veterinary laboratory medicine: an historical and technical review. *Vet Clin Pathol* 30:201–210.
13. George JW, O'Neill SL. 2001. Comparison of refractometer and biuret methods for total protein measurement in body cavity fluids. *Vet Clin Pathol* 30:16–18.
14. Grindem CB, Fairley NM, Uhlinger CA, Crane SA. 1990. Peritoneal fluid values from healthy foals. *Equine Vet J* 22:359–361.
15. Hunt E, Tennant BC, Whitlock RH. 1985. Interpretation of peritoneal fluid erythrocyte counts in horses with abdominal disease. In: *Proceedings of the 2nd Equine Colic Research Symposium*, University of Georgia, pp. 168–174.

16. La Perle KMD, Piercy RJ, Blomme EAG. 1998. Multisystemic, eosinophilic, epitheliotropic disease with intestinal lymphosarcoma in a horse. *Vet Pathol* 35:144-146.

17. Latson KM, Nieto JE, Beldomenico PM, et al. 2005. Evaluation of peritoneal fluid lactate as a marker of intestinal ischaemia in equine colic. *Equine Vet J* 37:342-346.

18. Malark JA, Peyton LC, Galvin MJ. 1992. Effects of blood contamination on equine peritoneal fluid analysis. *J Am Vet Med Assoc* 201:1545-1548.

19. Matthews A, Dart AJ, Reid SWJ, et al. 2002. Predictive values, sensitivity and specificity of abdominal fluid variables in determining the need for surgery in horses with an acute abdominal crisis. *Aust Vet J* 80:132-136.

20. McSherry BJ, Al-Baker J. 1976. Comparison of total serum protein determined by T/S meter and biuret technique. *Bull Amer Soc Vet Clin Path* 3:4-12.

21. Southwood LL, Kawcak CE, Trotter GW, et al. 2000. Idiopathic focal eosinophilic enteritis associated with small intestinal obstruction in 6 horses. *Vet Surg* 29:415-419.

22. Stockham SL, Scott MA. 2008. Cavitary effusions. In *Fundamentals of Veterinary Clinical*, Stockham SL and Scott MA (eds), 2nd ed. pp 831-868. Ames: Blackwell Publishing.

23. Swansick RA, Wilkinson JS. 1976. A clinical evaluation of abdominal paracentesis in the horse. *Austr Vet J* 52:109-116.

24. Tulleners EP. 1983. Complications of abdominocentesis in the horse. *J Am Vet Med Assoc* 182:232-234.

25. Van Hoogmoed L, Rodger LD, Spier SJ, et al. 1999. Evaluation of peritoneal fluid pH, glucose conentration, and lactate dehydrogenase activity for detection of septic peritonitis in horses. *J Am Vet Med Assoc* 214:1032-1036.

26. Wagner AE, Bennett DG. 1982. Analysis of equine thoracic fluid. *Vet Clin Pathol* 11:13-17.

27. Weimann CD, Thoefner MB, Jensen AL. 2002. Spectrophotometric assessment of peritoneal fluid haemoglobin in colic horses: an aid to selecting medical vs. surgical treatment. *Equine Vet J* 34:523-527.

28. Bain AM. 1963. *Corynebacterium equi* infections in the equine. *Aust Vet J* 39:116-121.

29. Byars TD, Tyler DE, Whitlock RH, et al. 1984. Non-erosive polysynovitis in a horse. *Equine Vet J* 16:141-143.

30. Caron JP. 2005. Intra-articular injections for joint disease in horses. *Vet Clin North Am Equine Pract* 21:559-573.

31. Clayburne G, Baker DG, Schumacher HR Jr. 1992. Estimated synovial fluid leukocyte numbers on wet drop preparations as a potential substitute for actual leukocyte counts. *J Rheumatol* 19:60-62.

32. Climent F, Carmona JU, Cuenca R, et al. 2007. Eosinophilic synovitis of the tarsocrural joint in a horse. *Vet Comp Orthop Traumatol* 20:142-145.

33. Dumoulin M, Pille F, van den Abeele A-M, et al. 2010. Use of blood culture medium enrichment for synovial fluid culture in horses: A comparison of different culture methods. *Equine Vet J* 42:541-546.

34. Dykgraaf S, Dechant JE, Johns JL, et al. 2007. Effect of intrathecal amikacin administration and repeated centesis on digital flexor tendon sheath synovial fluid in horses. *Vet Surg* 36:57-63.

35. Ekmann A, Rigdal M-L, Grondahl G. 2010. Automated counting of nucleated cells in equine synovial fluid without and with hyaluronidase pretreatment. *Vet Clin Pathol* 39:83-89.

36. Epstein CE, Elidemir O, Colasurdo GN, et al. 2001. Time course of hemosiderin production by alveolar macrophages in a murine model. *Chest* 120: 2013-2020.

37. Frees KE, Lillich JD, Gaughan EM, et al. 2002. Tenoscopic-assisted treatment of open digital flexor tendon sheath injuries in horses: 20 cases (1992-2001). *J Am Vet Med Assoc* 220:1823-1827.

38. Fuller CJ, Barr AR, Sharif M, et al. 2001. Cross-sectional comparison of synovial fluid biochemical markers in equine osteoarthritis and the correlation of these markers with articular cartilage damage. *Osteoarthritis Cartilage* 9:49-55.

39. Hunt E, Tennant BC, Whitlock RH. 1985. Interpretation of peritoneal fluid erythrocyte counts in horses with abdominal disease. In: *Proceedings of the 2nd Equine Colic Research Symposium*, University of Georgia, pp. 168-174.

40. Kenney DG, Robbins SC, Prescott JF, et al. 1994. Development of reactive arthritis and resistance to erythromycin and rifampin in a foal during treatment for Rhodococcus equi pneumonia. *Equine Vet J* 26:246-248.

41. Kwan C, Bell R, Koenig T, et al. 2012. Effects of intra-articular sodium pentosan polysulfate and glucosamine on the cytology, total protein concentration, and viscosity of synovial fluid in horses. *Aus Vet J* 90:315-320.

42. LaPointe J, Laverty S, La Voie J. 1992. Septic arthritis in 15 Standardbred race horses after intra-articular injection. *Equine Vet J* 24:430-434.

43. Lloyd KC, Stover SM, Pascoe JR, et al. 1988. Effect of gentamicin sulphate and sodium bicarbonate on the synovium of clinically normal equine antebrachio-carpal joints. *Am J Vet Res* 49:650-657.

44. Lumsden JM. 1990. Suspected immune-mediated polysynovitis and serositis in a horse. *Aust Vet J* 67:470-471.

45. Madison JB, Scarratt WK. 1988. Immune-mediated polysynovitis in four foals. *J Am Vet Med Assoc* 192:1581-1584.

46. Madison J, Sommer M, Spencer P. 1991. Relations among synovial membrane histopathologic findings, synovial fluid cytologic findings, and bacterial culture results in horses with suspected infectious arthritis: 64 cases (1979-1987). *J Am Vet Med Assoc* 198:1655-1661.

47. Madison JB, Ziemer EL. 1993. Eosinophilic synovitis following the intra-articular injection of bacterial antigen in horses. *Res Vet Sci* 54:256-258.

48. Mahaffey EA. Synovial fluid. 2002. In *Diagnostic Cytology and Hematology of the Horse*, Cowell RL and Tyler RD (eds), 2nd ed. pp. 163-170. St. Louis: Mosby.

49. Mills ML, Rush BR, St Jean G, et al. 2000. Determination of synovial fluid and serum concentrations, and morphologic effects of intra-articular ceftiofur sodium in horses. *Vet Surg* 29:398-406.

50. Paradis M. 1997. Cutaneous and musculoskeletal manifestations of Rhodococcus equi infection in foals. *Equine Vet Educ* 9:266-270.

51. Pille F, Martens A, Schouls LM, et al. 2007. Broad range 16S rRNA gene PCR compared to bacterial cluture to confirm presumed synovial infection in horses. *Vet J* 173:73-78.

52. Pusterla N, Pratt SM, Magdesian KG, et al. 2006. Idiopathic immune-mediated polysynovitis in three horses. *Vet Rec* 159:13-15.

53. Schneider R, Bramlage L, Moore R, et al. 1992. A retrospective study of 192 horses affected with septic arthritis/tenosynovitis. *Equine Vet J* 24:436-446.

54. Steel CM. 2008. Equine synovial fluid analysis. *Vet Clin North Am Equine Pract* 24:437-454.

55. Steel CM, Hunt AR, Adams PLE, et al. 1999. Factors associated with prognosis for survival and athletic use in foals with septic arthritis: 93 cases (1987-1994). *J Am Vet Med Assoc* 215:973-977.

56. Stover SM, Pool RR. 1985. Effect of intra-articular gentamicin sulphate on normal equine synovial membrane. *Am J Vet Res* 46:2485-2491.
57. Sweeney CR, Sweeney RW, and Divers TJ. 1987. *Rhodococcus equi* pneumonia in 48 foals: response to antimicrobial therapy. *Vet Microbiol* 14:329-336.
58. Trumble TN, Brown MP, Merritt KA, et al. 2008. Joint dependent concentrations of bone alkaline phosphatase in serum and synovial fluids of horses with osteochondral injury: an analytical and clinical validation. *Osteoarthritis and Cartilage* 16:779-786.
59. Tumalo R, Bramlage L, Gabel A. 1989. Sequential clinical and synovial fluid changes associated with acute infectious arthritis in the horse. *Equine Vet J* 21:325-331.
60. Turner AS, Gustafson SB, Zeidner NS, et al. 1990. Acute eosinophilic synovitis in a horse. *Equine Vet J* 22:215-217.
61. Vallance SA, Lumsden JM, Begg AP, et al. 2012. Idiopathic haemarthrosis in eight horses. *Aus Vet J* 90:214-220.
62. Vrins A, Feldman BF. 1983. Lupus erythematosus like syndrome in a horse. *Equine Pract* 5:18-25.
63. Wagner AE, McIlwraith CW, Martin GS. 1982. Effect of intra-articular injection of orgotein and saline solution on equine synovia. *Am J Vet Res* 43:594-597.
64. White KK, Hodgson DR, Hancock D, et al. 1989. Changes in equine carpal joint synovial fluid in response to the injection of two local anaesthetic agents. *Cornell Vet* 79:25-38.

Chapter 12

Cytology of the Lower Respiratory Tract

Martina Piviani

> **Acronyms and abbreviations that appear in this chapter:**
>
> BAL   bronchoalveolar lavage
> EIPH exercise-induced pulmonary hemorrhage
> IAD   inflammatory airway disease
> PCR   polymerase chain reaction
> RAO   recurrent airway obstruction
> TW   tracheal wash

Indications

Lower airway disease is one of the major causes of poor performance in horses. The clinical diagnosis of equine pulmonary disorders is largely dependent on obtaining an accurate history and performing a thorough clinical examination. Depending on the cause, clinical signs of lower respiratory tract disease may include dyspnea, tachypnea, cough, stridor, nasal discharge, and fever. Auscultation may reveal abnormal sounds. Additional diagnostic steps would include, when possible, radiographic examination and thoracic ultrasound. Other data, such as hemogram and serum biochemistry, would add valuable information about the patient's general health status and may point to a septic inflammatory process if leukocytosis or hyperfibrinogenemia is present. Specific tools for the diagnosis of lower airway disease in horses include bronchoscopy and cytologic analysis of the fluid recovered from the respiratory tract by bronchoalveolar lavage (BAL) and tracheal wash (TW).

Equine Clinical Pathology, First Edition. Edited by Raquel M. Walton.
© 2014 John Wiley & Sons, Inc. Published 2014 by John Wiley & Sons, Inc.

Collection techniques

Bronchoalveolar lavage

Bronchoalveolar lavage (BAL) is a method for the recovery of respiratory secretions that line the lower airways and alveoli. It is usually performed during bronchoscopic evaluation of the lower respiratory tract and requires chemical restraint and the use of topical lidocaine solution during the procedure. The endoscope is passed through the nares, the nasopharynx, and the trachea to be wedged into the most distal small bronchus. Aliquots of 250-300 mL of warm physiologic saline or phosphate-buffered saline are then instilled and immediately re-aspirated with the suction channel of the endoscope.[8,20,32] The fluid is then pooled and submitted for analysis. Variations between different sequential aliquots have been reported in some studies but not in others.[25,28,35,44] In one recent study, there were higher percentages of neutrophils and lower percentages of macrophages in the first aliquot than in the second aliquot, both in healthy horses and horses with recurrent airway obstruction (RAO).[25] Based on these results, the second aliquot is thought to contain less bronchial material, reach broader areas of the lung, and in general be more representative of the bronchoalveolar area in horses.[25] Another study showed that sequential aliquots of saline (100 mL each) did not significantly differ from a pooled sample (300 mL).[35] Pooling all aliquots is still advised by most authors.[20] Studies have shown no difference in most cell types between samples from the left and right lungs, with the exception of mast cells that were more numerous in the left lung in one study and in the right lung in another study.[25,44]

Because the unprotected tube lumen is likely to be contaminated with bacteria found in the upper airways, BAL is used primarily for cytologic examination of nonseptic conditions. It is especially helpful when a diagnosis of diffuse lower airway inflammation such as heaves (RAO), inflammatory airway disease (IAD), or exercise induced pulmonary hemorrhage (EIPH) is sought. The strength of BAL interpretation depends on the assumption that the pulmonary pathology is diffuse in nature rather then localized. In cases of pleuropneumonia, the lesions may be localized to one area of the lungs, thus BAL samples obtained from areas other than the affected bronchus may be not representative of the lung pathology and fail to detect cytologic abnormalities. In addition, the area of the lung lavaged depends greatly on the outer diameter of the bronchoscope. The use of a very small bronchoscope or a catheter passed through the lavage channel results in sampling of a small area of alveoli and bronchioles since wedging occurs in a peripheral bronchiole.

Tracheal wash

Tracheal wash (TW) may be performed during endoscopic evaluation (e.g., prior to BAL) or with a transtracheal approach, which provides a sterile sample that can be used for culture. A sterile catheter is passed through a cannula or large hypodermic needle previously inserted between tracheal rings in the tracheal lumen. Once the catheter reaches the tracheal bifurcation, 10-30 mL of fluid are infused and rapidly re-aspirated.[39] The major indication of TW compared to BAL is a suspected bacterial respiratory process since the sample is collected in a sterile fashion and can be submitted for culture. The association between TW neutrophilic inflammation and cough is acknowledged, but TW is considered less sensitive and specific than BAL to detect inflammation of peripheral airways (i.e., IAD).[2,8,20,25] There is good agreement between BAL cytology and histopathology results, whereas cytology of BAL and TW correlate poorly.[15,23,29] Most established reference intervals for cell differentials refer to BAL samples.

Sample processing

Aspirated fluid can be placed in either glass or EDTA tubes to avoid clotting if there is blood contamination, and should be refrigerated if immediate processing is not possible.[20,37] In general, the use of additives should be avoided but, if refrigeration is not possible, 40% ethanol at a ratio of 1:1 can be added to the sample in case of delayed processing. Formalin can be used but would likely cause a greater alteration of cell morphology. If the sample is to be sent to an external laboratory, sediment or direct smears should be prepared and submitted for evaluation along with the fluid. This may help the clinical pathologist distinguish between *in vivo* and *in vitro* changes (e.g., neutrophil degeneration versus aging; bacterial infection versus contamination and overgrowth). BAL and TW samples are diluted by the saline used during sample collection, thus usually contain low numbers of cells and a low concentration of protein. Cells tend to rupture more easily in low-protein samples. For this reason, some authors recommend adding one or two drops of serum or commercial bovine serum albumin to the pellet obtained by centrifugation in order to obtain higher numbers of viable cells.

BAL and TW sample processing includes macroscopic evaluation, cell count, and the preparation of slides of the cytocentrifuged fluid and/or sediment smears. Normal fluid should appear clear or mildly turbid. BAL samples can contain a layer of foamy surfactant indicating that the alveoli have been sampled. Presence of flocculent material instead of foamy surfactant reflects mucus and cellular debris. The fluid may appear pink-red or yellow-brown in case of recent or chronic hemorrhage, respectively.

Direct smears may be helpful if the fluid contains visible aggregates of mucus that can be smeared directly onto a slide for cytologic evaluation. In our experience, this can increase the possibility of finding larvae, eggs, or aggregates of eosinophils entrapped within mucus. Due to the overall low cellularity of BAL and TW fluids, concentration of the sample is advised and can be performed through centrifugation of the fluid at 300g for 10 minutes and smearing of the pellet obtained after removal of the supernatant. In direct and sedimented smears cells tend to be rounder, smaller, and darker, making their morphologic classification more difficult. Cytocentrifugation is associated with significantly higher percentages of macrophages, mast cells, and eosinophils but lower lymphocyte count compared to direct smear preparation; thus, reference intervals specific for the method used should be adopted.[36] Slides are then rapidly dried before staining to avoid cell crenation, using a fan or by waving the slides in the air manually. Wright-Giemsa and May-Grunwald Giemsa are superior in detecting mast cells compared to quick aqueous Romanowsky stains (e.g., Diff Quik, Baxter Scientific Products). If Diff Quik is used, an additional slide should be stained with toluidine blue for a more sensitive mast cell enumeration.[20]

The cell count can be performed using an automated analyzer or with a hemacytometer. Nucleated cell counts represent an estimate of the true cellularity within airway secretions; the accuracy and precision of the count is limited by the variability of the volume infused and fluid retrieved. The automated count may underestimate the cell count if cell size variation exceeds the window setting of the instrument. Both automated and manual counts are markedly affected by the presence of cell aggregation within the sample. For these reasons the total cell count is not performed in our laboratory, although reference intervals for BAL from healthy horses have been published with reported cell counts lower than 1,000 cells/uL for healthy horses in most studies (Table 12.1).[39]

The American Society of Human Pneumonology and the authors of a recent study in dogs recommend enumerating at least 500 cells to obtain a reliable percentage for all cell types (including mast cells and eosinophils) when performing the differential cell count.[11] No data about the reproducibility of the differential cell count as a function of the number of cells counted have been published for equine BAL samples. However, in most laboratories counting a minimum of 400 nucleated cells is considered acceptable.[20,25,46] Epithelial cells often tend to aggregate unevenly throughout the slide. For this reason in our laboratory the leukocyte count is reported instead of a total nucleated cell count.

Normal findings

Cellular elements

Cells present in respiratory fluid include epithelial cells, macrophages, small lymphocytes, neutrophils, eosinophils, and mast cells. BAL fluid samples from healthy animals are predominantly comprised of macrophages and small lymphocytes admixed with only rare neutrophils. However the first aliquot aspirated, especially if only a small amount of fluid is instilled, may contain higher percentage of neutrophils due to bronchial sampling. Reference intervals for BAL fluid are published (Table 12.1).[39] In general, based on published references, BAL samples from clinically healthy horses should contain 50-70% macrophages, 30-50% small lymphocytes, <5% neutrophils, <2% mast cells, and <1% eosinophils; epithelial cells, usually present in small numbers, may include a few non-ciliated bronchial epithelial and goblet cells but only rare ciliated epithelial cells.[20,41] Predominance of epithelial cells in a BAL fluid with

Table 12.1 Reference Values (mean ± SD) for TW and BAL in Asymptomatic Horses

	Reference	No. of horses	Vol of saline (mL)	TNCC (x10⁶/L)	Differential cell count (%)					
					Neutro	Eos	Lymph	Macro	Mast	EC
BAL	12	10	300	182 ± 578	8.9 ± 3.8	<1.0	43.0 ± 8.5	45.0 ± 8.8	1.2 ± 0.9	3.5 ± 2.2
	16	11	120	ND	7.0 ± 3.3	0.0 ± 0.0	28.0 ± 5.8	65.0 ± 6.2	0.2 ± 0.6	ND
	30	62	65	832 ± 578	8.8 ± 6.4	0.5 ± 3.1	31.3 ± 9.3	59.0 ± 9.7	ND	0.4 ± 0.8
	32	6	300	153 ± 17	3.8 ± 0.7	1.2 ± 2.0	28.3 ± 2.9	64.8 ± 11.2	0.3 ± 0.7	ND
	5	10	200	92.1 ± 142	5.9 ± 4.6	0.5 ± 0.9	36.7 ± 14.8	56.0 ± 13.0	ND	ND
	6	10	250	445 ± 142	3.8 ± 5.5	2.0 ± 1.0	22.9 ± 7.4	68.8 ± 8.8	1.5 ± 0.3	ND
	7	9	250	321 ± 100	6.8 ± 2.7	0.3 ± 0.5	31.4 ± 13.0	57.1 ± 10.3	1.5 ± 0.8	ND
	20 (pasture)	14	300	94 ± 47	3.6 ± 3.5	0.7 ± 1.7	42.6 ± 11.5	41.0 ± 10.8	6.6 ± 5.1	8.1 ± 6.5
	20 (stable)	14	300	89 ± 39	10.3 ± 8.1	1.2 ± 2.2	37.0 ± 9.8	41.4 ± 9.7	4.4 ± 3.9	8.4 ± 9.0
	9	14	120	517 ± 229	15.1 ± 2.8	0.0 ± 0.0	26.2 ± 6.5	50.2 ± 10.4	2.1 ± 1.4	3.4 ± 5.4
	17	26	ND	105 ± 40	9.1 ± 7.9	1.3 ± 5.1	33.9 ± 8.3	47.8 ± 10.3	5.0 ± 2.7	3.8 ± 2.5
	29	15	500	ND	2.5 ± 1.5	0.6 ± 0.7	44.2 ± 12.5	49.4 ± 9.5	1.2 ± 0.5	ND
	39	15	250	255 ± 81	5.1 ± 2.0	0.3 ± 0.5	20.4 ± 9.9	61.9 ± 16.9	0.6 ± 0.5	0.0 ± 0.0
	24	5	500	150 ± 20	8.5 ± 6.7	0.1 ± 0.0	52.3 ± 3.9	37.6 ± 3.9	1.5 ± 0.2	6.1 ± 1.5
TW	27 (endoscopy)	42	30	ND	4.6 ± 4.9	0.7 ± 0.4	2.2 ± 2.4	43.0 ± 10.7	0.1 ± 0.2	49.1 ± 11.5
	27 (transtrach)	15	30	ND	6.4 ± 5.5	1.2 ± 1.4	7.4 ± 3.8	65.0 ± 13.7	0.2 ± 0.4	19.8 ± 6.1
	12	10	20	ND	32.0 ± 28.1	<1.0	8.2 ± 6.0	24.0 ± 12.7	ND	34.0 ± 20.9
	43	66	20	ND	17.8 ± 21.8	0.7 ± 2.2	5.4 ± 4.1	44.1 ± 23.2	0.1 ± 0.2	34.0 ± 24.4
	3	9	20	ND	10 ± 10.8	1.9 ± 1.2	13.0 ± 3.6	74.2 ± 11.1	ND	ND
	39	12	30	ND	9.3 ± 4.9	0.2 ± 0.6	9.3 ± 5.8	79.6 ± 8.2	0.0 ± 0.0	ND

Adapted from Ref 39. *TW*, tracheal wash; *BAL*, bronchoalveolar lavage; *Neutro*, neutrophils; *Eos*, eosinophils; *Lymph*, lymphocytes; *Macro*, macrophages; *Mast*, mast cells; *EC*, epithelial cells; *ND*, not determined.

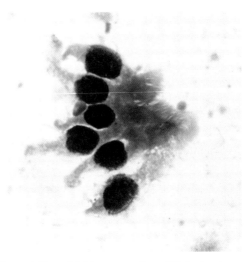

Figure 12.1 Cytocentrifuged BAL preparation. Ciliated columnar epithelial cells. In a BAL, low cellularity and predominance of ciliated epithelial cells may indicate poor technique with inadequate sampling of the alveolar space.

low numbers of leukocytes may indicate poor technique with inadequate sampling of the alveolar space (Figure 12.1). Goblet cells are non-ciliated columnar to pyriform cells with a basally located nucleus, and moderate to abundant cytoplasm with many round magenta mucin granules in the apical region (Figure 12.2). Goblet cells produce mucus and they may be seen in increased numbers with chronic pulmonary irritation.

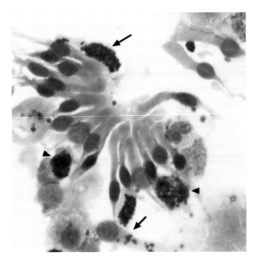

Figure 12.2 Ciliated columnar respiratory epithelial cells with admixed goblet cells (arrows) in a transtracheal wash. The apical portion of goblet cells containing mucin granules may break off and round up, mimicking a mast cell (arrowheads).

There are no accepted published reference intervals for TW differential leukocyte counts, although higher percentages of neutrophils (up to 20%) are normally seen compared to BAL cytology (Table 12.1).[4, 41, 43] Similarly, there are no published reference intervals for the differential cell counts of BAL and TW obtained from foals. Based on old references, TW of foals have a higher number of eosinophils, inflammatory cells, and mast cells than those of adults.[10] In one study, BAL samples in foals of 3 weeks of age had approximately 86% alveolar macrophages. During the first 2 months of life, this proportion decreased to approximately 71%, whereas the relative percentage of lymphocytes increased from 5% to 20%.[48]

Acellular elements

BAL and TW typically contain some amount of mucus, which appears as finely stippled to streaming, pink to lavender material in the background of the slide. Mucus can also form tight spirals, called Curschmann's spirals (Figure 12.3), which are said to represent plugs of inspissated mucus that form within small bronchioles. However, Curschmann's spirals can be present in any sample with abundant mucus, including nasal washes, as a result of persistently increased mucus production or reduced mucus clearance. Occasionally, coarse round magenta granules (typically 1.5 um in diameter) resulting from rupture of Goblet cells may be present free in the background and entrapped within mucus. Occasionally, the apical portion of Goblet cells can detach from the basal portion and nucleus, releasing round cytoplasmic fragments filled with magenta granules that resemble mast cells (Figure 12.2). Occasionally, free cilia or the ciliated apical portion of respiratory epithelial cells may be noted.

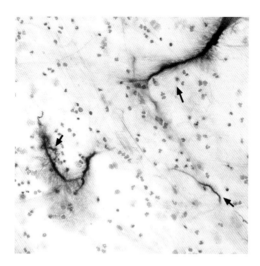

Figure 12.3   Tracheal wash from a horse with IAD. Three Curschmann's spirals (arrows) are present in this field. The background contains numerous variably preserved neutrophils and streaming eosinophilic mucus.

This finding can be artifactual or represent ciliocytophthoria. This term was introduced in 1956 by Papanicolaou to indicate a severe lesion of the columnar epithelial cell characterized by the detachment of the apical portion of the cytoplasm containing cilia from the remainder of the cell. The process was originally associated with viral infections but later was observed with other diseases and lost pathognomonic significance.

Contaminants

Foreign materials can be found in BAL and TW fluids due to contamination during or after the procedure of sample collection (e.g., oropharyngeal contamination, starch granules from gloves), but they may also represent inhalants from the environment. The latter include pollen, elements of saprophytic fungi such as *Alternaria* species, carbonaceous material (e.g., due to pollution or smoke inhalation), and silica crystals.[49] BAL cytology is considered a window on the environment of the horse, and the frequency of mold spores is an indicator of particulate exposure from forage.[20] Inhalants are often noted within the cytoplasm of macrophages and multinucleated cells as a result of phagocytosis (Figure 12.4), while procedural contaminants are usually extracellular, provided that the sample has been processed immediately.

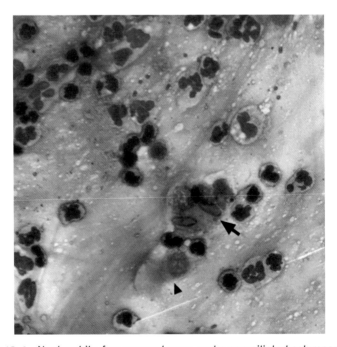

Figure 12.4   Neutrophils, few macrophages, and a non-ciliated columnar epithelial cell (arrowhead) amid a pink background of mucus in a BAL from a horse; note the green fungal elements (likely barn inhalants) phagocytized by a macrophage (arrow).

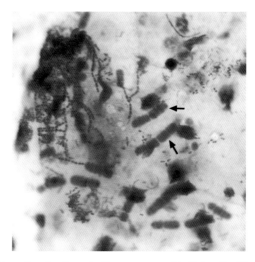

Figure 12.5 Transtracheal wash. Squamous epithelial cell with adherent Simonsiella (arrows) and other mixed bacterial bacilli. This horse coughed during acquisition of the sample, causing the catheter to become displaced into the oropharynx.

Oropharyngeal material that may be seen in BAL and TW include squamous epithelial cells and various types of bacteria, often adherent to the squamous cell surface. *Simonsiella* bacteria are normal inhabitants of the oral cavity that divide lengthwise forming large colonies that appear as a single large cigar-shaped organism with parallel light and dark stripes (Figure 12.5).[49] The presence of oropharyngeal material may just reflect procedural contamination from the mouth, nasal passages, or oropharynx or it may reflect the horse having aspirated oropharyngeal contents into the airway (especially if associated with neutrophilic inflammation).

Interpretation of cytologic patterns

Neutrophilic inflammation

Neutrophils are rare (<5% of total nucleated cells) in BAL samples from healthy horses, and an increased proportion indicates suppurative (neutrophilic) inflammation. Suppurative inflammation is generally considered an acute process but it may also persist for a long time when there is an active stimulus. Neutrophilic inflammation can be seen with septic and nonseptic causes. In septic exudates, neutrophils tend to show degenerative changes such as nuclear swelling and cytoplasmic vacuolation or may appear necrotic. However, evaluation of cell morphology is not considered highly reliable in raising suspicion for a bacterial etiology in BAL and TW fluids because degenerative changes can also occur secondary to collection and handling.

Conversely, a well-preserved neutrophil morphology does not rule out a septic process. Samples characterized by neutrophilic predominance should be cultured to rule out infection. Since any microbes detected usually belong to the normal flora of the upper airway, isolation of bacteria in TW may represent infection, transient lower airway colonization, or contamination of the sample.[39]

Septic etiologies

Septic suppurative inflammation may be due to bacterial, fungal (e.g., *Aspergillus* spp), or, less commonly, viral infection. Often bacteria may be found by microscopic examination of cytologic samples, and the presence of intracellular bacteria within neutrophils (or less commonly macrophages) is strongly supportive of infection as opposed to contamination, provided that the sample has been processed quickly (ideally within 30 minutes, since phagocytosis can also occur *in vitro*). Bacteria found in BAL may include rod-shaped bacilli, round cocci, or microorganisms with a more distinctive morphology, such as *Rhodococcus equi*. *R. equi* organisms are small and pleomorphic, similar to watermelon seeds, rod-shaped to coccoid, with a thin peripheral halo (Figure 12.6). *R. equi*, a Gram-positive facultative intracellular pathogen, is one of the most common causes of pneumonia in foals. This microorganism has the ability to survive and replicate within macrophages by suppression of phagosome-lysosome fusion or phagolysosome acidification.[14,47] This pathogen can be seen cytologically within both neutrophil and macrophage phagosomes.[24] The definitive diagnosis of bronchopneumonia caused by *R. equi* should be based on bacteriologic culture or amplification of the vapA gene using polymerase chain reaction (PCR) from a tracheobronchial sample. Amplification of vapA using PCR may be done in conjunction with (but should

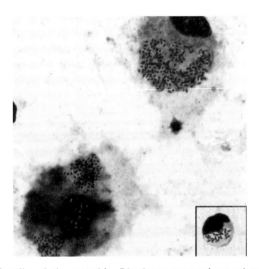

Figure 12.6 Small and pleomorphic, *Rhodococcus equi* coccobacilli are present within lysosomes in macrophages and a moderately degenerate neutrophil (inset).

not replace) bacterial culture because it does not permit identification of other bacterial pathogens or antimicrobial susceptibility testing of *R. equi* isolates. The use of PCR assays based on genes other than vapA is not recommended as these assays would also detect environmental isolates lacking the virulence plasmid, which are not known to cause disease in foals. Both tests may have false positive and false negative results, thus culture or PCR amplification of *R. equi* from tracheobronchial fluid should be interpreted in the context of cytological and clinical findings. In addition, detection of *R. equi* from a foal without clinical signs of respiratory disease, cytological evidence of septic airway inflammation, or ultrasonographic or radiographic evidence of pulmonary lesions may be an incidental finding.[18]

A severe neutrophilic inflammation, often associated with oropharyngeal elements, characterizes BAL fluids obtained from horses with aspiration pneumonia. A secondary bacterial infection, often mixed, is a common sequelum, thus intracellular bacteria may be found and bacterial culture and sensitivity testing are indicated.

Less often, suppurative inflammation can be due to fungal infections, which are usually secondary to immunosuppression or associated with other severe pulmonary and extrapulmonary diseases.[45] Fungal infections may be due to opportunistic fungi, such as *Aspergillus* and *Pneumocystis* spp, or more rarely caused by systemic yeasts, including *Coccidioides immitis*, *Histoplasma capsulatum*, *Blastomyces dermatitidis*, and *Cryptococcus neoformans*. The most common fungal pathogen identified in the lower respiratory tract of horses is *Aspergillus* (Figure 12.7), but other etiologies are possible, including *Penicillium*, *Mucor*, and *Acremonium* spp.[38] Cytology does not permit reliable identification of the specific fungus, thus culture or fungal-specific PCR is required. However, fungal culture results should always be interpreted in light of BAL

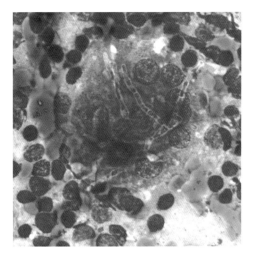

Figure 12.7   A multinucleated giant cell containing septated, branching fungal hyphae surrounded by a mixed neutrophilic and histiocytic inflammation in a TW from a horse with pulmonary aspergillosis (modified Wright-Giemsa stain).

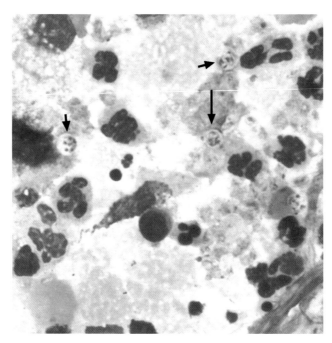

Figure 12.8 Neutrophils and a foamy macrophage amid a background of blue-grey material and chromatin debris in a sedimented smear of BAL fluid from an Arabian foal with *Pneumocystis jirovecii* infection. Several cysts with up to eight internal spores are present extracellularly (arrows).

or TW cytologies because opportunistic fungi can also be cultured in a small percentage of TW samples collected from healthy horses.[42]

Pneumocystis carinii is an opportunistic fungal pulmonary pathogen that can cause pneumonia in immunosuppressed foals or be secondary to bacterial infection. *Pneumocystis* has a complete life cycle within alveoli that includes cyst and trophozoite forms. Cysts are round, measure 5-10 microns, and contain up to eight intracystic bodies (Figure 12.8). Trophozoites are small (2-3 microns in length), pyriform to elongated, light staining, and difficult to distinguish from cellular debris. The associated inflammatory response can be suppurative, predominantly histiocytic, or mixed. *Pneumocystis carinii* was long thought to be a protozoal organism based on the presumption that cystic and trophic forms represented distinctive phases of a protozoan life cycle and on its sensitivity to antiprotozoal drugs. However, mounting evidence, including the identification of genetic sequence homologies with fungi, led to the recategorization of this pathogen as a fungus and its renaming as *Pneumocystis jiroveci*.

Nonseptic etiologies

Nonseptic causes of neutrophilic inflammation include the most common causes of poor performance and airway inflammation: RAO and IAD. RAO is a common condition in stabled mature and old horses, which accounts for more than 50% of all respiratory cases referred and has a reported prevalence of 10-20% in regions with cold or temperate climates.[22,46] RAO or heaves was initially defined as chronic marked breathing difficulty without obvious macroscopic pathologic lung lesions.[1] The disease is characterized by variable recurring airflow obstruction, increased mucus, bronchial hyper-responsiveness, and airway inflammation resulting in increased respiratory efforts at rest, coughing, and exercise intolerance. Clinical signs are triggered in susceptible horses by inhalation of dust particles, aerosolized allergens, and endotoxins that are present in stables, especially those associated with hay feeding. RAO likely results from complex interactions between innate and acquired immune responses, the environment, and genetic susceptibility.[26] RAO is characterized by increased mucus and neutrophilia in respiratory fluids, with the percentage of neutrophils in the BAL usually increasing with the severity of the condition.[27]

IAD is also a nonseptic inflammation of the airways causing poor performance, cough, and variably increased mucus, but, in contrast to RAO, horses of any age may be affected and clinical signs at rest are usually subtle.[8] The pathogenesis of IAD is still poorly defined, but environmental and stable factors may be involved.[8] BAL fluids from horses with IAD are characterized by increased total nucleated cell count with mild neutrophilia, lymphocytosis, and monocytosis. BAL mastocytosis (>2%) and eosinophilia (>1%) are also compatible with a diagnosis of IAD. Based on clinical signs only, it may be difficult to distinguish severe cases of RAO from chronic pneumonia, and early stages of RAO from IAD and other respiratory causes of poor performance. A neutrophilic inflammatory component is common to all these diseases. However, signs of systemic inflammation observed in cases of pneumonia such as fever and leukocytosis are usually lacking in RAO, and BAL neutrophilia is usually less pronounced with IAD (<20%) compared to RAO (>20%).

Mixed neutrophilic and histiocytic inflammation

All the aforementioned diseases can also elicit a histiocytic inflammatory component, which can predominate in chronic phases or with specific etiologic agents (e.g., some fungi). Alveolar macrophages are resident within the alveoli, and they constitute the main cell type in BAL fluids from healthy horses. Thus, increases in macrophages due to proliferation or recruitment from peripheral blood monocytes secondary to inflammation is difficult to recognize, especially if there is a concurrent increase in neutrophils. Assessment of the overall cellularity or phagocytized pathogens may help in these cases.

Eosinophilic and mastocytic inflammation

The differential diagnosis for eosinophilic inflammation includes migrating parasite larvae (e.g., *Dictyocaulus arnfieldi*) and allergic bronchitis. Hypersensitivity seems to be involved in the pathogenesis of both IAD and RAO. Thus,

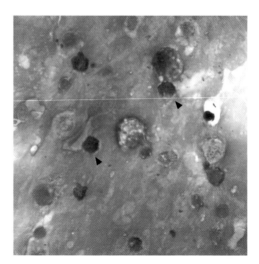

Figure 12.9   Eosinophils (arrowheads) and macrophages admixed with few columnar epithelial cells amid a background of abundant mucus in a sedimented smear preparation of BAL fluid.

an increase in eosinophil and mast cell percentages in BAL fluids may be expected in both conditions, although eosinophilia and mastocytosis seem to be described in IAD more often than RAO and are currently not included in the proposed systems for RAO diagnosis and staging.[8,46]

Eosinophils may be focally distributed and are often entrapped in mucus, thus careful examination of the entire smear may be required to find concentrations of eosinophils (Figure 12.9). It should be noted that in some samples, mast cell granules do not stain with aqueous based Romanovsky stains (e.g., Diff Quik), whereas eosinophil granules stain similarly with either methanol or aqueous-based Romanovsky stains. When evaluating BAL or TW cytologies, care should be taken to avoid confusing fragments of goblet cell cytoplasm with mast cells. As mentioned previously, the apical portion of goblet cells can detach from the basal portion and nucleus, releasing round cytoplasmic fragments filled with magenta granules. Like mast cell granules, goblet cell granules are metachromatic. The two can be distinguished based on the more globular appearance of goblet cell granules and absence of a discernible nucleus.

Hemosiderosis

The presence of hemosiderin-laden macrophages (hemosiderophages) is called hemosiderosis and indicates previous hemorrhage into the airways. The presence of erythrophagocytosis indicates more recent hemorrhage. Staining cytocentrifuged slides with Perl's Prussian blue facilitates the detection of hemosiderophages and is routinely performed in equine TW and BAL samples in our laboratory (Figure 12.10). The major causes of hemosiderosis in BAL

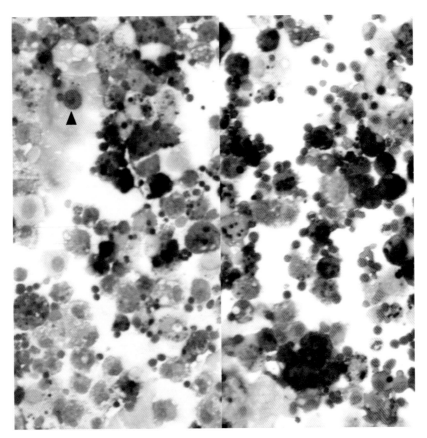

Figure 12.10 Cytocentrifuged preparation of BAL fluid from a horse with EIPH. Left panel (modified Wright-Giemsa stain): macrophages, small lymphocytes, occasional neutrophils, and a mast cell (arrowhead) amid a background of few erythrocytes. Note that most macrophages contain scant to abundant dark-green to black pigment consistent with hemosiderin (hemosiderophages). Right panel (Prussian blue stain): most macrophages contain bright blue to black staining material consistent with hemosiderin.

and TW fluids are exercise-induced pulmonary hemorrhage (EIPH), inhalation of blood due to epistaxis, and bleeding from an ulcerated neoplasm within the respiratory system. The presence of erythrocytes in TW and BAL fluids can also be a consequence of trauma caused by the bronchoscopy or fluid collection procedure.

Exercise-induced pulmonary hemorrhage

EIPH occurs as a consequence of strenuous exercise and is a common cause of poor performance in racehorses.[19] While no clinical or laboratory "gold standard" method has been established, the cytologic diagnosis of EIPH is based on the finding of >50% hemosiderophages in a TW or BAL.[13,34]

Cellular atypia

BAL and TW samples may occasionally contain few clusters of epithelial cells with a cuboidal rather than columnar shape, increased cytoplasmic basophilia, increased nuclear-to-cytoplasmic ratio, and some degree of anisocytosis (Figure 12.11). When associated with the presence of inflammatory cells, these findings are usually interpreted as respiratory epithelial cell hyperplasia and dysplasia secondary to chronic irritation. If marked atypia is present (e.g., pleomorphism, prominent multiple nucleoli, or marked anisocytosis), an epithelial neoplasm may be suspect. However, primary lung tumors are rare in horses and difficult to diagnose on BAL and TW cytology unless the neoplasm has extensively invaded trachea, bronchi, and bronchioli. Other non-epithelial primary and metastatic lung neoplasms include, among others, pulmonary granular-cell tumor, pulmonary chondrosarcoma, bronchial myxoma, malignant melanoma, and fibrosarcoma. Neoplastic cells from these neoplasms do

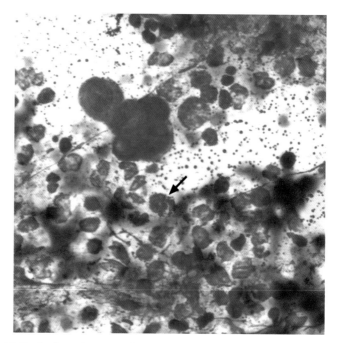

Figure 12.11 Sediment preparation of BAL fluid from a horse with septic suppurative inflammation. A cluster of atypical epithelial cells admixed with degenerate neutrophils and few small lymphocytes amid a background of chromatin debris (pink granular to linear material) and many erythrocytes. Small bacterial cocci in short chains are seen within the cytoplasm of degenerate neutrophils (arrow). Epithelial cells are mildly pleomorphic, with low cuboidal to round shape, increased nuclear to cytoplasmic ratio, immature chromatin, prominent nucleoli, and moderate anisocytosis and anisokaryosis. These features are interpreted as hyperplasia and dysplasia secondary to the inflammatory process.

not tend to exfoliate easily in respiratory fluids and in cases of suspected pulmonary neoplasia percutaneous lung aspirates or biopsy is preferable.

References

1. Bouley H. 1863. In *Nouveau dictionnaire lexicographique et descriptif des sciences médicales et vétérinaires*. Raige-Delorme MM, Daremberg C, Bouley H et al. (eds) pp. 1073-1074. Paris: Asselin.
2. Christley RM, Hodgson DR, Rose RJ, et al. 1996. Coughing in thoroughbred racehorses in training: the relationships between disease and viruses, bacteria and environment. *Vet Rec* 139:308-313.
3. Christley RM, Hodgson DR, Rose RJ, et al. 1999. Comparison of bacteriology and cytology of tracheal fluid samples collected by percutaneous transtracheal aspiration or via an endoscope using a plugged, guarded catheter. *Equine Vet J* 31:197-202.
4. Christley RM, Hodgson DR, Rose RJ, et al. 2001. A case-control study of respiratory disease in Thoroughbred racehorses in Sydney, Australia. *Equine Vet J* 33:256-264.
5. Clark CK, Lester GD, Vetro T, et al. 1995. Bronchoalveolar lavage in horses: effect of exercise and repeated sampling on cytology. *Aust Vet J* 72:249-252.
6. Couëtil LL, Denicola DB. 1999. Blood gas, plasma lactate and bronchoalveolar lavage cytology analyses in racehorses with respiratory disease. *Equine Vet J* 30:77-82.
7. Couëtil LL, Rosenthal FS, DeNicola DB, et al. 2001. Clinical signs, evaluation of bronchoalveolar lavage fluid, and assessment of pulmonary function in horses with inflammatory respiratory disease. *Am J Vet Res* 62:538-546.
8. Couëtil LL, Hoffman AM, Hodgson J, et al. 2007. Inflammatory airway disease of horses. *J Vet Intern Med* 21:356-361.
9. Couroucé-Malblanc A, Pronost S, Fortier G, et al. 2002. Physiological measurements and upper and lower respiratory tract evaluation in French Standardbred Trotters during a standardised exercise test on the treadmill. *Equine Vet J* Suppl 34:402-407.
10. Crane SA, Ziemer EL, Sweeney CR. 1989. Cytologic and bacteriologic evaluation of tracheobronchial aspirates from clinically normal foals. *Am J Vet Res* 50:2042-2048.
11. De Lorenzi D, Masserdotti C, Bertoncello D, et al. 2009. Differential cell counts in canine cytocentrifuged bronchoalveolar lavage fluid: a study on reliable enumeration of each cell type. *Vet Clin Pathol* 38:532-536.
12. Derksen FJ, Brown CM, Sonea I, Darien BJ, et al. 1989. Comparison of transtracheal aspirate and bronchoalveolar lavage cytology in 50 horses with chronic lung disease. *Equine Vet J* 21:23-26.
13. Doucet MY, Viel L. 2002. Alveolar macrophage graded hemosiderin score from bronchoalveolar lavage in horses with exercise-induced pulmonary hemorrhage and controls. *J Vet Intern Med* 16:281-286.
14. Fernandez-Mora E, Polidori M, Luhrmann A, et al. 2005. Maturation of R. equi-containing vacuoles is arrested after completion of the early endosome stage. *Traffic* 6:635-653.
15. Fogarty U. 1990. Evaluation of a bronchoalveolar lavage technique. *Equine Vet J* 22:174-176.
16. Fogarty U, Buckley T. 1991. Bronchoalveolar lavage findings in horses with exercise intolerance. *Equine Vet J* 23:434-437.

17. Gerber V, Robinson NE, Luethi S, et al. 2003. Airway inflammation and mucus in two age groups of asymptomatic well-performing sport horses. *Equine Vet J* 35:491-495.
18. Giguère S, Cohen ND, Keith Chaffin M, et al. 2011. Diagnosis, treatment, control, and prevention of infections caused by Rhodococcus equi in Foals. *J Vet Int Med* 25:1209-1220.
19. Hinchcliff KW, Jackson MA, Morley PS, et al. 2005. Association between exercise-induced pulmonary hemorrhage and performance in Thoroughbred racehorses. *J Am Vet Med Assoc* 227:768-774.
20. Hoffman AM. 2008. Bronchoalveolar lavage: sampling technique and guidelines for cytologic preparation and interpretation. *Vet Clin North Am Equine Pract.* 24:423-435.
21. Holcombe SJ, Jackson C, Gerber V, et al. 2001. Stabling is associated with airway inflammation in young Arabian horses. *Equine Vet J* 33:244-249.
22. Hotchkiss JW, Reid SW, Cristely RM. 2007. A survey of horse owners in Great Britain regarding horses in their care. Part 2: risk factors for recurrent airway obstruction. *Equine Vet J* 39:301-308.
23. Hughes KJ, Malikides N, Hodgson DR, et al. 2003. Comparison of tracheal aspirates and bronchoalveolar lavage in racehorses. 1. Evaluation of cytological stains and the percentage of mast cells and eosinophils. *Aust Vet J* 81:681-684.
24. Hylton PK, Rizzi TE, Allison RW. 2006. Intracellular success: cytologic findings in an ulcerated submandibular mass from a cat. *Vet Clin Pathol* 35:345-347.
25. Jean D, Vrins A, Beauchamp G, et al. 2011. Evaluation of variations in bronchoalveolar lavage fluid in horses with recurrent airway obstruction. *Am J Vet Res* 72:838-842.
26. Leclere M, Lavoie-Lamoureux A, Lavoie JP. 2011. Heaves, an asthma-like disease of horses. *Respirology* 16:1027-1046.
27. Leguillette R. 2003. Recurrent airway obstruction-heaves. *Vet Clin North Am Equine Pract* 19:63-86.
28. Mair TS, Stokes CR, Burne FJ. 1987. Cellular content of secretions obtained by lavage from different levels of the equine respiratory tract. *Equine Vet J* 19:458-462.
29. Malikides N, Hughes KJ, Hodgson DR, et al. 2003. Comparison of tracheal aspirates and bronchoalveolar lavage in racehorses 2. Evaluation of the diagnostic significance of neutrophil percentage. *Aust Vet J* 81:685-687.
30. Mazan MR, Vin R, Hoffman AM. 2005. Radiographic scoring lacks predictive value in inflammatory airway disease. *Equine Vet J* 37:541-545.
31. McKane SA, Canfield PJ, Rose RJ. 1993. Equine bronchoalveolar lavage cytology: survey of Thoroughbred racehorses in training. *Aust Vet J* 70:401-404.
32. Miskovic M, Couëtil LL, Thompson Hoffman CA. 2007. Lung function and airway cytologic profiles in horses with recurrent airway obstruction maintained in low-dust environments. *J Vet Intern Med* 21:1060-1066.
33. Moore BR, Krakowka S, Robertson JT, et al. 1995. Cytologic evaluation of bronchoalveolar lavage fluid obtained from standardbred racehorses with inflammatory airway disease. *Am J Vet Res* 56:562-567.
34. Newton JR, Wood JL. 2002. Evidence of an association between inflammatory airway disease and EIPH in young Thoroughbreds during training. *Equine Vet J* 34:417-424.
35. Pickles K, Pirie RS, Rhind S, et al. 2002. Cytological analysis of equine bronchoalveolar lavage fluid. Part 1: Comparison of sequential and pooled aliquots. *Equine Vet J* 34:288-291.

36. Pickles K, Pirie RS, Rhind S, et al. 2002. Cytological analysis of equine bronchoalveolar lavage fluid. Part 2: Comparison of smear and cytocentrifuged preparations. *Equine Vet J* 34:292-296.
37. Pickles K, Pirie RS, Rhind S, et al. 2002. Cytological analysis of equine bronchoalveolar lavage fluid. Part 3: The effect of time, temperature and fixatives. *Equine Vet J* 34:297-301.
38. Pusterla N, Holmberg TA, Lorenzo-Figueras M, et al. 2005. Acremonium strictum pulmonary infection in a horse. *Vet Clin Pathol* 34:413-416.
39. Richard EA, Fortier GD, Lekeux PM, et al. 2010. Laboratory findings in respiratory fluids of the poorly-performing horse. *Vet J* 185:115-122.
40. Richard EA, Fortier GD, Pitel PH, et al. 2010. Subclinical diseases affecting performance in Standardbred trotters: diagnostic methods and predictive parameters. *Vet J* 184:282-289.
41. Robinson NE. 2003. Inflammatory airway disease: defining the syndrome. Conclusions of the Havemeyer workshop. *Equine Vet Education* 15:61-63.
42. Sweeney CR, Divers TJ, Benson CE. 1985. Anaerobic bacteria in 21 horses with pleuropneumonia. *J Am Vet Med Assoc* 187:721-724.
43. Sweeney CR, Humber KA, Roby KA. 1992. Cytologic findings of tracheobronchial aspirates from 66 thoroughbred racehorses. *Am J Vet Res* 53:1172-1175.
44. Sweeney CR, Rossier Y, Ziemer EL, et al. 1992. Effects of lung site and fluid volume on results of bronchoalveolar lavage fluid analysis in horses. *Am J Vet Res* 53:1376-1379.
45. Sweeney CR, Habecker PL. 1999. Pulmonary aspergillosis in horses: 29 cases (1974-1997). *J Am Vet Med Assoc* 214:808-811.
46. Tilley P, Sales Luis JP, Branco Ferreira M. 2012. Correlation and discriminant analysis of clinical, endoscopic, thoracic X-ray and bronchoalveolar lavage fluid cytology scores, for staging horses with recurrent airway obstruction (RAO). *Res Vet Sci* 93:1006-1014.
47. Toyooka K, Takai S, Kirikae T. 2005. Rhodococcus equi can survive a phagolysosomal environment in macrophages by suppressing acidification of the phagolysosome. *J Med Microbiol* 54:1007-1015.
48. Zink MC, Johnson JA. 1984. Cellular constituents of clinically normal foal bronchoalveolar lavage fluid during postnatal maturation. *Am J Vet Res* 45:893-897.
49. Zinkl JG. 2002. Lower respiratory tract. In *Diagnostic Cytology and Hematology of the Horse*, Cowell RL and Tyler RD (eds), 2nd ed. pp. 73-86. St. Louis: Mosby.

Chapter 13
Cerebrospinal Fluid

Andrea Siegel

Cerebrospinal fluid (CSF) analysis combined with history, physical exam, and other diagnostic tests is an important component of the diagnostic evaluation of patients with central and peripheral neurological disease. CSF should be collected whenever an inflammatory, infectious, traumatic, neoplastic, or degenerative disorder of the brain and the spinal cord is suspected. However, analysis of CSF often only supports the diagnosis of a central nervous system disorder and is rarely definitively diagnostic. Similar to a complete blood count, CSF analysis has good sensitivity for disease detection, but low specificity. CSF analysis is not always abnormal in a horse with central nervous disease if the lesion is extradural, collection occurred early or late in the course of disease, or the CSF collection site is far away from the lesion.

Formation, circulation, absorption, and function

The CSF is a clear, colorless fluid that surrounds and permeates the entire central nervous system (CNS) and therefore protects, supports, and nourishes it. The CSF is produced by ultrafiltration and active transport mechanisms in the choroid plexuses. Fluid formed in the lateral ventricles flows into the third ventricle and then into the fourth ventricle, where the majority of it exits into the subarachnoid space. The CSF also moves caudally, surrounding the spinal cord and leaving the CNS via the dural reflections of the spinal nerve roots. The CSF is absorbed by the arachnoid villi and ultimately directed into the venous system.

The cerebrospinal fluid functions include physical support of the neural structures, excretion of potentially toxic by-products of cerebral metabolism, and intracerebral transport of biologically active substances.[53] New studies have revealed that CSF cells are involved in immunomodulatory mechanisms via production of proinflammatory as well as immunosuppressive cytokines. While IL-6 and TNF-α appear to promote inflammation in the CSF of horses

Equine Clinical Pathology, First Edition. Edited by Raquel M. Walton.
© 2014 John Wiley & Sons, Inc. Published 2014 by John Wiley & Sons, Inc.

with inflammatory or infectious diseases, TGF-β seems to be involved in down-regulation of the inflammatory activity.[45]

Collection

The diagnostic quality of cerebrospinal fluid depends on the site of collection and handling. Cerebrospinal fluid can be collected in horses from the atlanto-occipital or the lumbosacral sites depending on the neurological exam and location of the lesion.[51] An intracranial or cervical lesion is more likely to yield a diagnostic sample if obtained from an atlanto-occipital tap. Lumbosacral aspirates are indicated for lower spinal cord lesions. The atlanto-occipital collection requires general anesthesia, whereas lumbosacral collection usually can be performed in standing horses. In foals, CSF can be collected from either site with the animal in lateral recumbency.[1] Techniques of cerebromedullary cisternal and lumbosacral CSF collection are aptly covered in neuroanatomy and clinical neurology textbooks.

Specific risks of CSF collection include iatrogenic brainstem trauma or spinal cord trauma due to needle puncture, extradural hemorrhage, and herniation of the cerebrum or the cerebellum through the foramen magnum in patients with increased intracranial pressure.[27] An aseptic technique is necessary due to the potential risk of introducing infectious agents into the CNS. A study that compared sequential samples of CSF in horses suggested that in order to minimize blood contamination, a minimum of three 2 ml samples should be collected before submitting the final sample for analysis, even if there is no gross evidence of blood contamination.[50] Artifacts like deteriorated cells and contaminants (including iatrogenic hemodilution) may affect the cytological interpretation.

Laboratory analysis

The routine laboratory analysis of CSF includes gross inspection, cell counts, protein concentration, chemistry assays, and cytological examination. Other tests, such as bacterial and fungal culture, serology, and polymerase chain reaction (PCR), are added depending on the results of the cytological examination, clinical presentation, and neurologic exam.

Due to the low CSF protein and lipid concentrations, cells degenerate and lyse rapidly, causing distortion of cellular morphology and reduction of the total nucleated cell count. For this reason, cell counts and cytological preparations should be performed within 30 minutes of collection.[19] Cells can be preserved by mixing autologous serum with the sample, which will conserve cell morphology for 24 hours when stored at 4°C.[5] The addition of hetastarch at a ratio of 1:1 (vol:vol) or fetal calf serum at a concentration of 20% volume can help stabilize cells in CSF.[19] Samples containing additives to preserve cellular morphology should not be used to measure protein or for antibody titers.

Generally, 1 ml of fluid is sufficient for protein and cellular examination.[8] CSF samples should be collected in sterile plastic or silicon-coated tubes, especially when not processed immediately, because monocytes will adhere to glass and activate.[53] EDTA tubes are not recommended because the additive can falsely elevate the total protein concentration, although submission in an EDTA tube may be required if the sample is for PCR analysis.[14, 46]

Gross appearance

The normal CSF is clear and colorless, has a viscosity similar to water, and does not clot due to the absence of fibrinogen. Turbidity is measured subjectively from 0 or clear to $+4$, which is cloudy enough to preclude reading through the sample. Causes of CSF turbidity include elevated cell count (WBC or RBC or both), presence of microorganisms, markedly increased protein concentration, or aspiration of epidural fat.[29] Nucleated cell counts greater than 400 to 500 cells/µl are necessary to produce a slightly turbid CSF.

Pink or red discoloration suggests the presence of blood, which could result from either iatrogenic blood contamination or pathologic hemorrhage. A clear supernatant after centrifugation indicates iatrogenic hemorrhage or peracute hemorrhage in the subarachnoid space. On the other hand, a red-tinged CSF with a xanthochromic supernatant (yellow-orange coloration) supports prior hemorrhage, likely associated with trauma, neoplasia, vascular disorders, or infectious disease.[37] Xanthochromia is caused by the erythrocyte degradation products oxyhemoglobin and bilirubin. Markedly increased CSF protein ($>$400 mg/dl) and severe icterus are other causes of xanthochromia. Normal neonates may have slightly xanthochromic cerebrospinal fluid.[27] Cytological evidence of pathologic hemorrhage includes the presence of hemosiderin, hematoidin, and/or erythrophagocytes.

Increased fluid viscosity usually results from a very high protein concentration, especially fibrinogen. Cryptococcosis may increase the CSF viscosity due to the polysaccharide capsule of the yeast.[53]

Table 13.1   Reference Values for CSF in Adult Horses

Macroscopic evaluation	Reference values
Color	Colorless
Turbidity	Clear
Total protein	30-80 mg/dl
Microscopic evaluation	
Erythrocytes	0 to small number
Total nucleated cell count	0-8 cells/l
Differential cell count	Small lymphocytes (70%)
	Monocytoid cells (30%)
	Rare erythrocytes

Modified from reference 10.

Protein concentration

Reference intervals for CSF total protein concentration can vary with the laboratory and testing method used. Therefore, laboratory-established reference ranges should be used. Normal CSF has very low protein concentration compared to plasma and other body cavity fluids, and most of the protein in normal CSF is albumin. Refractometric methods are not accurate for the measurement of CSF protein content. Refractive index of CSF can be artifactually increased by suspended particles (cells, bacteria), hemoglobin, or radiographic contrast media.[6,37] Urine protein dipsticks have been used to estimate CSF protein concentration; however, they are highly specific for albumin detection and less specific for globulins.[32] The Pandy and Nonne-Apelt tests are qualitative methods that screen for the presence of globulins. These tests have been replaced by quantitative methods that measure immunoglobulins.

Quantitative methods that measure both albumin and globulin in CSF include turbidimetric procedures (trichloroacetic acid) and dye-binding assays (Coomassie brilliant blue, Ponceau S acid red, and pyrogallol red). Dye-binding protein methods are simple, rapid, and more accurate for the measurement of CSF protein concentration.[37,53] The pyrogallol red assay gives a more uniform response to albumin and globulin and therefore is the preferred method.[38] Reported equine CSF protein values range from 10 mg/dl to 120 mg/dl (generally 20-80 mg/dl), which are much higher than those reported in other domestic animals. CSF protein concentration in foals less than 1 week old ranges from 90 mg/dl to 180 mg/dl, decreasing gradually to adult horse levels by 2 weeks of age.[1] Enhanced transport of albumin into CSF from blood or increased permeability of the blood-brain barrier (BBB) may be the reason for the difference between adult and neonatal CSF concentration.[1,3]

Nonpathologic elevation of protein in CSF occurs with blood contamination during collection. Pathologic causes of elevated CSF protein include damage to the BBB, intrathecal hemorrhage, increased local synthesis of immunoglobulins, degeneration of neural tissue, and obstruction of the CSF circulation (e.g., cervical vertebral malformations, abscess, or tumor).

Because albumin is not synthesized intrathecally, increased CSF albumin indicates damage to the BBB, iatrogenic blood contamination, or intrathecal hemorrhage. If hemorrhage or blood contamination is not present, the ratio between CSF albumin and serum albumin (albumin quotient) can be used to assess the functionality of the BBB:

$$\textbf{AQ} \text{ (albumin quotient)} = \frac{\text{CSF albumin}}{\text{Serum albumin}} \times 100 \qquad (13.1)$$

BBB damage in horses is suggested by CSF albumin concentration greater than 2.45 with an albumin quotient greater than 2.35. However, due to the normal variability of CSF albumin in horses, the use of this index is limited.[3]

Electrophoretic techniques define the gamma-globulins as a heterogeneous group of proteins with similar migration rates; this fraction contains the immunoglobulins. High-resolution agarose gel electrophoresis (HRE) produces sharper bands and definition of CSF protein fractions.[21] Electrophoresis should be performed on CSF and serum simultaneously to compare the distribution of proteins. Three major immunoglobulins are found in CSF: IgG, IgM, and IgA. IgG is the major cerebrospinal fluid immunoglobulin present in normal CSF. Since CSF IgG originates from plasma, elevated concentrations of IgG in CSF may indicate an abnormal BBB or increased intrathecal synthesis by inflammatory cells. An IgG index is used to determine whether the IgG present is due to local synthesis or originates from the plasma (alteration in the blood-brain CSF barrier, intrathecal hemorrhage, or iatrogenic blood contamination):

$$\textbf{IgG index} = \frac{\text{CSF IgG/Serum IgG}}{\text{CSF albumin/serum albumin}} \qquad (13.2)$$

An IgG index greater than 0.3 with a normal albumin quotient suggests intrathecal IgG production, which is generally caused by infectious inflammatory diseases.[20] The IgG index may be useful in differentiating inflammatory lesions from noninflammatory diseases.

Recent studies have described other techniques, the antibody index and C-value, that use antigen-specific antibody titers rather than total IgG that are believed to be more accurate than the IgG index.[22] The antibody index relates a specific IgG titer to the total IgG concentration, allowing a the detection of a fraction of specific antibody made in the CNS. Movement of a specific antibody into the CSF due to leakage across a porous barrier or blood contamination during sample collection would not be expected to affect the antibody index.[30,36] The C-value theory is that the ratio of antigen-specific antibody to total IgG in CSF is equal to the ratio in the serum. Values >1.7 are suggestive of intrathecal antibody production.[20]

The presence of IgM is an abnormal finding in the CSF and is considered more specific than IgG or total immunoglobulin levels for detection of active or recent infectious disease.[6] Serum IgM capture ELISA (MAC-ELISA) is the preferred method for the diagnosis of West Nile virus infection in vaccinated and unvaccinated horses due to high sensitivity and specificity. Because there is 100% agreement between serum and CSF results, there is no clear advantage in testing CSF rather than serum. However, future introduction of live attenuated vaccines that may elicit a serologic IgM response suggest that CSF testing may become the gold standard for diagnosing West Nile disease in vaccinated horses.[43]

Elevated CSF protein concentration may be found in cases of encephalitis, neoplasms, meningitis, and trauma. Typically, neoplasms or trauma produce an increase of albumin because of disruption of the BBB. In contrast, in inflammatory diseases such as encephalitis and meningitis, globulins are the primary protein increased, due to intrathecal production.[43] The CSF nucleated cell count and CSF protein concentration tend to increase proportionately. However, in some disorders the cell count remains normal, whereas the total protein concentration may be increased. This condition is called albuminocy-tological dissociation, which has been described in viral non-suppurative en-cephalomyelitis such as equine herpes virus meningoencephalitis (EHV-1), neoplastic disease, traumatic, vascular, degenerative, and compressive spinal cord lesions.[6,14]

Antibody titers

A variety of antibody and antigen tests are available for viruses, fungi, rick-ettsia, protozoa, and parasites.[17] In order to evaluate antibody titers, two samples taken two weeks apart should be analyzed. Antibodies detected in CSF may be derived from vaccination, antigen exposure, or actual disease. Interpretation of CSF antibody titers should be done in light of the vaccination history, serum titers, BBB integrity, intrathecal immunoglobulin production (IgG index), and CSF IgM levels.

Antibody titers for equine herpesvirus 1 (EHV-1), togavirus, West Nile virus, and equine protozoal myelitis (*Sarcocystis neurona*) can be measured in CSF.[2,27,39] Titers can be measured using Western blot, a semi-quantitative antibody-based test, or indirect immunofluorescence (IFAT), which is a quan-titative antibody test. Because there is evidence of passive movement of antibodies across the blood-CSF barrier, CSF antibody titers can be influ-enced by serum antibody titers and yield a false positive result.[42] Moreover, even minimal iatrogenic blood contamination during collection (8 RBC/μl of CSF) has been shown to be the source of positive CSF Western blot for anti-bodies against *S. neurona* in equine serum and cerebrospinal fluid.[40] As dis-cussed previously, the intrathecal production of an antigen-specific antibody can be evaluated using the antibody index, which reflects the ratio between the CSF/serum-specific Ig and CSF/serum total Ig. An index >1 suggests the intrathecal origin of the specific antibody.[47]

The Western blot test for *S. neurona* antibodies has low specificity but high sensitivity. While a positive result does not necessarily indicate active equine protozoal myelitis (EPM), a horse with a negative CSF Western blot is prob-ably not infected with *S. neurona*, ruling out the disease.[11] Clinically normal neonatal foals born to seropositive mares may be positive for CSF Western blot antibodies against *S. neurona*, likely secondary to increased transport of passively transferred serum immunoglobulins across the blood-CSF bar-rier.[9] The indirect fluorescent antibody test (IFAT) for *S. neurona* antibodies is more specific and accurate than the Western blot test for diagnosis of EPM.[16] Higher serum and CSF IFAT titers are more frequent in horses with EPM than in uninfected horses, thus helping differentiate exposure/vaccination from active infection.

Cell counts

Because the cellular concentration of normal and sometimes abnormal CSF is too low to be detected by standard hematological analysis, red and white blood

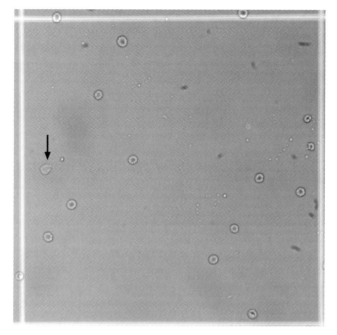

Figure 13.1 Microscopic identification of WBCs and RBCs in the hemocytometer chamber. The light tan, round, crenated cells are RBCs. There is one WBC (arrow) that has irregular borders and a granular opaque cytoplasm (magnification ×400).

cell counts are performed using a hemocytometer. Undiluted CSF is added to the counting chamber. After 10-15 minutes the cells settle and are visible in the same plane of focus. Then, RBCs and WBCs are counted in both chambers (18 squares) and the average total count of each cell type is multiplied by 1.1 to obtain the number of cells per μl. Erythrocytes are recognized as small, refractile, light tan, and generally crenated (Figure 13.1). White blood cells have irregular cell borders with a granular texture. Small lymphocytes may be difficult to differentiate from erythrocytes.

Normal CSF does not contain erythrocytes, but they may present due to subarachnoid hemorrhage or, more commonly, with iatrogenic blood contamination. Blood contamination may affect the leukocyte and differential counts. A formula using the RBC count in blood and CSF along with the peripheral blood WBC count to correct the measured white blood cell count in the cerebrospinal fluid has been used.[50] However, the use of this formula is controversial, and studies have shown that white blood cells are often overcorrected in blood-contaminated CSF, obscuring an underlying inflammatory process.[50,55]

The total white cell count in CSF of normal horses ranges from 0 to 8 depending on the reference. A normal hemocytometer count does not necessarily reflect normal CSF; abnormalities in cell types or cell proportions may be present.[7] "Pleocytosis" is the term used to indicate increased cellularity in cerebrospinal fluid. The severity of pleocytosis is determined by the etiology and location of the lesion with respect to the subarachnoid space or ventricular system. Therefore, although often severe, deep parenchymal lesions that do not communicate with the subarachnoid space generally have CSF nucleated cell counts within reference limits.

Glucose

CSF glucose concentration varies proportionally with blood glucose values. Normal glucose cerebrospinal concentration in horses ranges from 30 mg/dl to 70 mg/dl (30-75% of plasma glucose concentrations).[27,37] Therefore, CSF results must be interpreted in light of the serum glucose values. However, since CSF equilibration with plasma glucose requires 1 to 2 hours, CSF glucose concentration reflects serum glucose values 1 hour prior to CSF collection.[53] The main differential diagnoses for decreased CSF glucose are increased glucose utilization (associated with bacterial meningitis or marked neutrophilic pleocytosis) and hypoglycemia. Due to the lack of specificity of glucose measurement, more specific tests such as cytologic evaluation and bacterial culture are recommended to assess for evidence of sepsis in the cerebrospinal fluid.

Enzymes

Enzymes in the CSF may originate from the blood, neural tissue, or cerebrospinal fluid cellular components. Therefore, interpretation of enzyme results should consider the integrity of the blood-brain CSF barrier, blood contamination, and the cytologic examination. Creatine kinase (CK) concentration is very low in normal CSF. Because CK is a large macromolecule and does not cross the BBB, the most likely source of increased activity of this enzyme in the CSF is nervous tissue damage. One study suggests that CK is often increased with protozoal myelitis, helping differentiate this condition from compressive neurological disease.[24] However, other studies in horses have failed to demonstrate a correlation between nucleated cell counts, serum CK, or CSF protein concentration and a specific disease. Moreover, contamination of CSF with epidural fat or dura during CSF collection may falsely increase CSF CK activity.[33]

Lactic acid

Lactic acid is produced during anaerobic glycolysis by the enzymatic conversion of pyruvic acid. Because lactic acid diffuses very slowly through the intact blood-brain CSF barrier, increased CSF lactate levels indicate anaerobic glycolysis in the brain. In a study of horses with confirmed neurologic disease, CSF lactate concentrations were significantly elevated in several diseases. Thus, although sensitive for neurological disease, this assay lacks specificity.[53]

Polymerase chain reaction

Polymerase chain reaction (PCR) is a very sensitive molecular genetic test that amplifies short sequences of DNA (or RNA). In horses, PCRs for bacteria, protozoa, and viruses are available in many diagnostic laboratories.[42,53] PCR testing for *S.neurona* in the CSF is highly specific for the diagnosis of equine protozoal myeloencephalitis (EPM); however, many false negative results have been reported, probably because intact merozoites rarely enter the CSF and free-parasite DNA is destroyed rapidly by enzymatic action.[22] In contrast, PCR testing of neural tissue has been shown to be useful as a post-mortem test for EPM. The diagnostic sensitivity of West Nile virus PCR in the CSF is very low probably because viremia is often very short-lived. Collecting the sample early during the disease process may increase the sensitivity of this test.[44] EHV-1 real-time PCR testing of whole blood is able to differentiate neuropathogenic strains from non-neuropathogenic strains.[34]

Phenotyping

Immunophenotypic markers can be used to characterize the lymphocyte sub-populations in CSF and their association with disease. However, individual variation and the large volume of sample necessary makes this test clinically impractical.[23] In horses, T cells comprise about 80% of the lymphocyte population in CSF, which is similar to that found in humans.

Cytological examination

Cytological assessment of the CSF provides information regarding cellularity, types of cells, and presence or absence of infectious agents or inclusions. Due to the low cellularity of normal CSF, concentration of cells by cytocentrifugation, sedimentation, simple centrifugation, or membrane filtration is necessary for morphological evaluation.[13] The diagnostic quality and cell recovery of slides made by simple centrifugation is generally poor, thus this technique is not recommended. Membrane filtration methods produce the best cellular recovery (90-100%), and addition of 40% ethanol after collection eliminates the need for immediate processing.[18] Membrane filtration methods are not recommended, however, because they produce poor cellular morphology and are technically difficult. Sedimentation is the recommended technique when there is limited access to a laboratory or when a cytocentrifuge is not available. With this technique the cellular yield is adequate and cellular morphology is well preserved. An inexpensive chamber has been described for in-house use.[25] Cytocentrifugation is the ideal method in human and veterinary medicine because it preserves cellular morphology, thereby facilitating cellular identification; however, it requires special equipment and the cellular yield is relatively low.[7]

Slides containing sample are stained with Romanowsky stains (Wright's, Wright-Giemsa, and Diff-Quik®). The use of special stains like Gram's, India ink, and luxol fast blue may be helpful in identifying bacteria, Cryptococcus, and myelin, respectively. Cytological examination of the cerebrospinal fluid is recommended even if the cell count is not increased, because abnormalities in cell proportions or cell type may still be present.

Normal findings

Most of the cells in normal CSF are mononuclear (80-90%), comprised predominantly of small lymphocytes with fewer monocytoid cells (Figure 13.2). Lymphocytes (small mononuclear cells) are 9-15 um in diameter and have a scant amount of pale-blue cytoplasm and a dark, dense, round to slightly oval or indented nucleus. Monocytoid cells (large mononuclear cells) are large (12-15 um), with oval, sometimes kidney-shaped, nuclei. They have moderate to abundant light-blue cytoplasm that may be foamy or finely vacuolated.

Eosinophils are not found in normal CSF, whereas the presence of few neutrophils is controversial. While some authors suggest that rare neutrophils may be normally present, others suggest that finding neutrophils is indicative

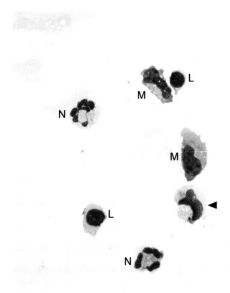

Figure 13.2 **Mixed inflammatory cell response from a CSF from a foal with head trauma. Two neutrophils (N), two lymphocytes (L), two monocytoid cells (M), and one ruptured cell (arrowhead) are present (magnification ×1000). Courtesy of Dr. Theresa E. Rizzi, Oklahoma State University.**

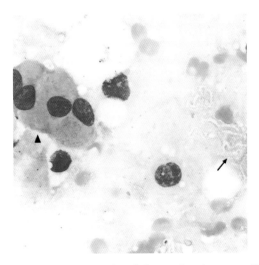

Figure 13.3 Meningeal cells (arrowhead) from a touch preparation of tissue in the cerebellomedullary cistern. These, along with extracellular eosinophilic myelin (arrow), can be present in normal CSF as procedural contaminants.

of an abnormality.[4,7,29,37] Occasionally, ependymal cells, choroid plexus cells, and meningeal lining cells are seen (Figure 13.3).

Abnormal findings

A marked pleocytosis with predominance of neutrophils is suggestive of bacterial meningitis (Figure 13.4). Cytological identification of the bacteria or a positive culture result is confirmatory of septic meningitis. However, neutrophilic pleocytosis in the absence of degeneration and bacteria does not rule out sepsis, even if the Gram stain and culture are negative.[1,52] Neutrophils may also be found in noninfectious processes such as necrosis, early stages of eastern equine viral meningoencephalitis, central nervous system hemorrhage, and post myelography with iodinated contrast agents.[29]

In pathological conditions, monocytes are transformed into macrophages that contain varying amounts of phagocytized material such as lipid droplets, erythrocytes, microorganisms, or cellular debris in various stages of digestion. Activated monocytoid cells and macrophages may appear in clusters mimicking epithelial cells. Phagocytic cells might be expected where there is extensive damage to nervous tissue.

Lymphocyte counts may be elevated in cases of spinal cord compression, axonal degeneration, infections, and immune-mediated disorders such as polyneuritis.[2,29] Plasma cells are not a normal finding and may be observed with reactive lymphocytes in viral encephalitis, chronic protozoal or rickettsial infections, and immune-mediated diseases when there is a humoral response to inflammation. When a mixed pleocytosis with eosinophils is present, fungal

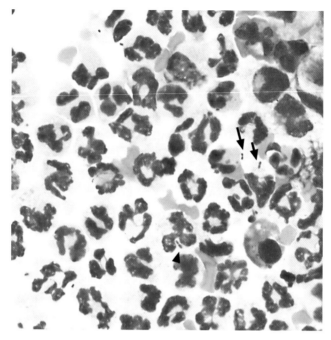

Figure 13.4 CSF from a foal with septic meningitis. The field shows numerous degenerative neutrophils, one of which contains a phagocytized bacillus (arrowhead). Extracellular bacterial bacilli are also present (arrows). Courtesy of Dr. Robin W. Allison, Oklahoma State University.

or protozoal infection or parasite migration should be included in the differential diagnosis.

Cerebrovascular accidents can be suspected with a xanthochromic sample, increased protein concentration, presence of erythrocytes, and erythrophagocytosis (Figure 13.5). Hemorrhage can occur secondary to trauma, infection, parasite migration, coagulopathy, or neoplasia. In horses, CNS neoplasia is uncommon, with the exception of pituitary adenoma. Therefore, finding neoplastic cells in the CSF is rare. Melanin pigment and lymphoblasts are occasionally seen with CNS melanomas and lymphomas, respectively.[41]

CSF in specific diseases

Viral infections

Many viral diseases of the central nervous system are associated with mononuclear pleocytosis, high protein concentration, or both. However, the CSF of acute eastern and Venezuelan equine encephalomyelitis is typically neutrophilic but becomes predominantly monocytic within 2-3 days.[49] CSF changes in equine herpesvirus encephalomyelopathy are consistent with

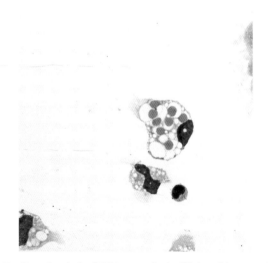

Figure 13.5 Erythrophagia in CSF from a foal with head trauma. Two monocytoid cells and one small lymphocyte are also present (magnification ×1000). Courtesy of Dr. Theresa E. Rizzi, Oklahoma State University.

a vasculopathy and are characterized by marked xanthochromia and al-buminocytological dissociation.[34,53] CSF findings in horses with West Nile meningoencephalitis are more likely to be abnormal when collected from the lumbosacral site, and consist of a predominantly lymphocytic, mononuclear pleocytosis with mildly increased protein concentration.[54]

Bacterial infections

Bacterial meningoencephalitis occurs most frequently in foals, secondary to neonatal septicemia. The CSF analysis is characterized by moderate to marked elevations of the nucleated cell counts, with a predominance of degenerative or nondegenerative neutrophils. Protein concentration is generally elevated. Although bacteria are occasionally seen on cytological preparations, bacterial culture is often negative.[48] PCR assays may be used to detect bacterial DNA.

Fungal infections

Rarely, mycotic encephalitis may occur secondary to guttural pouch mycosis via hematogenous spread. In one report a focal area of encephalitis caused by *Aspergillus* spp. was attributed to direct transfer from the frontal sinuses rather than to hematogenous spread from the guttural pouch.[31] In two horses with cryptococcal meningoencephalitis, the CSF findings were characterized by markedly increased protein concentration and profound neutrophilic pleo-cytosis.[28,52] Increased CSF viscosity has been reported with cryptococcosis due to the polysaccharide capsule of the yeast.[53]

Parasitic infections

CSF changes in horses with equine protozoal encephalomyelitis are not consistent. There may be a mild to moderate mononuclear pleocytosis with increased total protein or the fluid may be normal. CSF analysis is more useful in differentiating other neurologic diseases from EPM.[35] The CSF of horses with parasitic migration through the central nervous system, such as cerebrospinal nematodiasis (*Halicephalobus gingivalis* previously *Micronema deletrix*), may be xanthochromic with a mixed pleocytosis and a normal to increased protein level.[12]

Other diseases

The CSF of horses with equine motor neuron disease may be normal or show albuminocytological dissociation, which may reflect necrosis of motor neurons and degeneration in the spinal roots.[10,15] The CSF appearance in horses with cauda equina neuritis (polyneuritis equi) may be xanthochromic or cloudy with a moderately mixed (predominantly lymphocytic) pleocytosis and moderately increased protein concentration.[2] CSF analysis was normal in a report of four horses with cervical vertebral spinal hematomas.[26]

Although CSF findings may help formulate a differential diagnosis, abnormalities are often not specific and can also occur with other disease processes. Therefore, other diagnostic tests such as imaging, serology, and PCR are often necessary to identify the etiologic agent or disease present.

References

1. Adams R, Mayhew IG. 1985. Neurological diseases. *Vet Clin North Am Equine Pract* 1:209-234.
2. Aleman M, Katzman SA, Vaughan B, et al. 2009. Antemortem diagnosis of polyneuritis equi. *J Vet Intern Med* 23:665-668.
3. Andrews FM, Geiser DR, Sommardahl CS, et al. 1994. Albumin quotient, IgG concentration, and IgG index determinations in cerebrospinal fluid of neonatal foals. *Am J Vet Res* 55:741-745.
4. Beech J. 1983. Cytology of equine cerebrospinal fluid. *Vet Pathol* 20:553-562.
5. Bienzle D, McDonnell JJ, Stanton JB. 2000. Analysis of cerebrospinal fluid from dogs and cats after 24 and 48 hours of storage. *J Am Vet Med Assoc* 216:1761-1764.
6. Chrisman CL. 1992. Cerebrospinal fluid analysis. *Vet Clin North Am Small Anim Pract* 22:781-810.
7. Christopher MM, Perman V, Hardy RM. 1988. Reassessment of cytologic values in canine cerebrospinal fluid by use of cytocentrifugation. *J Am Vet Med Assoc* 192:1726-1729.
8. Cook JR, DeNicola DB. 1988. Cerebrospinal fluid. *Vet Clin North Am Small Anim Pract* 18:475-499.
9. Cook AG, Maxwell VB, Donaldson LL, et al. 2002. Detection of antibodies against *Sarcocystis neurona* in cerebrospinal fluid from clinically normal neonatal foals. *J Am Vet Med Assoc* 220:208-211.

10. Cummings JF, de Lahunta A, George C, et al. 1990. Equine motor neuron disease; a preliminary report. *Cornell Vet* 80:357-379.

11. Daft BM, Barr BC, Gardner IA, et al. 2002. Sensitivity and specificity of western blot testing of cerebrospinal fluid and serum for diagnosis of equine protozoal myeloencephalitis in horses with and without neurologic abnormalities. *J Am Vet Med Assoc* 221:1007-1013.

12. Darien BJ, Belknap J, Nietfeld J. 1988. Cerebrospinal fluid changes in two horses with central nervous system nematodiasis (*Micronema deletrix*). *J Vet Intern Med* 2:201-205.

13. Deisenhammer F, Bartos A, Egg R, et al. 2006. Guidelines on routine cerebrospinal fluid analysis. Report from an EFNS task force. *Eur J Neurol* 13:913-922.

14. Di Terlizzi R, Platt SR. 2009. The function, composition and analysis of cerebrospinal fluid in companion animals: Part II—Analysis. *Vet J* 180:15-32.

15. Divers TJ, Mohammed HO, Cummings JF, et al. 1992. Equine motor neuron disease: a new cause of weakness, trembling, and weight loss. *Comp Contin Educ Vet* 14:1222-1226.

16. Duarte PC, Daft BM, Conrad PA, et al. 2003. Comparison of a serum indirect fluorescent antibody test with two Western blot tests for the diagnosis of equine protozoal myeloencephalitis. *J Vet Diagn Invest* 15:8-13.

17. Duarte PC, Ebel ED, Traub-Dargatz J, et al. 2006. Indirect fluorescent antibody testing of cerebrospinal fluid for diagnosis of equine protozoal myeloencephalitis. *Am J Vet Res* 67:870-876.

18. Freeman KP, Brewer B, Slusher SH. 1989. Membrane filter preparations of cerebrospinal fluid from normal horses and horses with selected neurologic diseases. *Comp Contin Educ Vet* 11:1100-1109.

19. Fry MM, Vernau W, Kass PH, et al. 2006. Effects of time, initial composition, and stabilizing agents on the results of canine cerebrospinal fluid analysis. *Vet Clin Pathol* 35:72-77.

20. Furr M. 2007. Humoral immune responses in the horse after intrathecal challenge with ovalbumin. *J Vet Intern Med* 21:806-811.

21. Furr M, Chickering WR, Robertson J. 1997. High resolution protein electrophoresis of equine cerebrospinal fluid. *Am J Vet Res* 58:939-941.

22. Furr M, Mackay R, Granstrom D, et al. 2002. Clinical diagnosis of equine protozoal meningoencephalitis (EPM). *J Vet Intern Med* 16:618-621.

23. Furr M, Pontzer C, Gasper P. 2001. Lymphocyte phenotype subsets in the cerebrospinal fluid of normal horses and horses with equine protozoal myeloencephalitis. *Vet Ther* 2:317-324.

24. Furr M, Tyler RD. 1990. Cerebrospinal fluid creatine kinase activity in horses with central nervous system disease—69 cases (1984-1989). *J Am Vet Med Assoc* 197:245-248.

25. Garma-Avina A. 2004. An inexpensive sedimentation chamber for the preparation of cytologic specimens of cerebrospinal fluid. *J Vet Diagn Invest* 16:585-587.

26. Gold JR, Divers TJ, Miller AJ, et al. 2008. Cervical vertebral spinal hematomas in 4 horses. *J Vet Intern Med* 22:481-485.

27. Green EM, Constantinescu GM, Kroll RA. 1993. Equine cerebrospinal fluid: analysis. *Comp Contin Educ Vet* 15:288-301.

28. Hart KA, Flaminio MJBF, Williams CO, et al. 2008. Successful resolution of cryptococcal meningitis and optic neuritis in an adult horse with oral fluconazole. *Vet J Intern Med* 22:1436-1440.

29. Hayes TE. 1987. Examination of the cerebrospinal fluid in the horse. *Vet Clin North Am Equine Pract* I3:283-291.

30. Heskett KA, MacKay J. 2008. Antibody index and specific antibody quotient in horses after intragastric administration of *Sarcocystis neurona* sporocysts. *Am J Vet Res* 69:403-409.

31. Hunter B, Nation PN. 2011. Mycotic encephalitis, sinus osteomyelitis, and guttural pouch mycosis in a 3-year-old Arabian colt. *Can Vet J* 52:1339-1341.

32. Jacobs RM, Lumsden JH, Cochrane SM, et al. 1990. Relationship of cerebrospinal fluid protein concentration determined by dye-binding and urinary dipstick methodologies. *Can Vet J* 31:587-588.

33. Jackson C, de Lahunta A, Divers T, et al. 1996. The diagnostic utility of cerebrospinal fluid creatine kinase activity in the horse. *J Vet Intern Med* 10:246-251.

34. Johnson AL. 2011. Update on infectious diseases affecting the equine nervous system. *Vet Clin North Am Equine Pract* 27:573-587.

35. MacKay RJ, Granstrom DE, Saville WJ, et al. 2000. Equine protozoal myeloencephalitis. *Vet Clin North Am Equine Pract* 16:405-425.

36. MacKay RJ, Tanhauser ST, Gillis KD. 2008. Effect of intermittent oral administration of ponazuril on experimental *Sarcocystis neurona* infection of horses. *Am J Vet Res* 69:396-401.

37. MacWilliams PS. 2002. Cerebrospinal fluid. In *Diagnostic Cytology and Hematology of the Horse*, Cowell R, Tyler R (eds.) pp. 171-179. St. Louis: Mosby.

38. Marshall T, Williams KM. 2000. Protein determination in cerebrospinal fluid by protein dye-binding assay. *Brit J Biomed Sci* 57:281-286.

39. Miller MM, Sweeney CR, Russell GE, et al. 1999. Effects of blood contamination of cerebrospinal fluid on Western blot analysis for detection of antibodies against *Sarcocystis neurona* and on albumin quotient and immunoglobulin G index in horses. *J Am Vet Med Assoc* 215:67-71.

40. Murphy JE, Marsh AE, Reed SM, et al. 2006. Development and evaluation of a *Sarcocystis neurona*-specific IgM capture enzyme-linked immunosorbent assay. *J Vet Intern Med* 20:322-328.

41. Paradis MR. 1998. Tumors of the central nervous system. *Vet Clin North Am Equine Pract* 14:543-561.

42. Pellegrini-Masini A, Livesey LC. 2006. Meningitis and encephalomyelitis in horses. *Vet Clin North Am Equine Pract* 22:553-589.

43. Porter MB, Long M, Gosche DG, et al. 2004. Immunoglobulin M-capture enzyme-linked immunosorbent assay testing of cerebrospinal fluid and serum from horses exposed to west Nile virus by vaccination or natural infection. *J Vet Intern Med* 18:866-870.

44. Pusterla N, Madigan JE, Leutenegger CM. 2006. Real-time polymerase chain reaction: a novel molecular diagnostic tool for equine infectious diseases. *J Vet Intern Med* 20:3-12.

45. Pusterla N, Wilson W, David C, et al. 2006. Comparative analysis of cytokine gene expression in cerebrospinal fluid of horses without neurologic signs or with selected neurologic disorders. *Am J Vet Res* 67:1433-1437.

46. Rand JS, Parent J, Percy D, et al. Clinical, cerebrospinal fluid, and histological data from thirty-four cats with primary noninflammatory disease of the central nervous system. *Can Vet J* 35:174-181.

47. Reiber H, Lange P. 1991. Quantification of virus-specific antibodies in cerebrospinal fluid and serum: sensitive and specific detection of antibody synthesis in the brain. *Clin Chem* 37:1153-1160.

48. Smith JJ, Provost PJ, Paradis MR. 2004. Bacterial meningitis and brain abscesses secondary to infectious disease processes involving the head in horses: seven cases (1980-2001). *J Am Vet Med Assoc* 224:739-742.

49. Smith JM, DeBowes RM, Cox JH. 1987. Central nervous system disease in adult horses. III. Differential diagnosis and comparison of common disorders. *Comp Contin Educ Vet* 9:1042-1054.

50. Sweeney CR, Russell GE. 2000. Differences in total protein concentration, nucleated cell count, and red blood cell count among sequential samples of cerebrospinal fluid from horses. *J Am Vet Med Assoc* 217:54-57.

51. Thomson CE, Kornegay JN, Stevens JB. 1990. Analysis of cerebrospinal fluid from cerebromedullary and lumbar cisterns of dogs with focal neurological disease: 145 cases (1985-1987). *J Am Vet Med Assoc* 196:1841-1844.

52. Toth B, Aleman M, Nogradi N. 2012. Meningitis and meningoencephalomyelitis in horses: 28 cases (1985-2010). *J Am Vet Med Assoc* 240:580-587.

53. Vernau W, Vernau KA, Bailey CS. 2008. Cerebrospinal fluid. In *Clinical Biochemistry of Domestic Animals*, Kaneko JJ, Harvey JW, and Bruss ML (eds), 6th ed., pp. 769-819. Burlington: Academic Press.

54. Wamsley HL, Alleman AR, Porter MB, et al. 2001. Findings in cerebrospinal fluids of horses infected with west Nile virus: 30 cases (2001). *J Am Vet Med Assoc* 221:1303-1305.

55. Wilson JW, Stevens JB. 1977. Effects of blood contamination on cerebrospinal fluid analysis. *J Am Vet Med Assoc* 171:256-258.

Index

Equine Clinical Pathology, First Edition. Edited by Raquel M. Walton.
© 2014 John Wiley & Sons, Inc. Published 2014 by John Wiley & Sons, Inc.

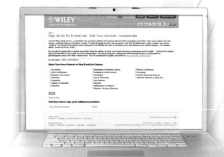